THE PHYSIOLOGY OF
HUMAN PREGNANCY

The Physiology of
Human Pregnancy

FRANK E. HYTTEN

M.D.(Sydney)   Ph.D.(Aberdeen)

Research Physiologist
Obstetric Medicine Research Unit (M.R.C.)
Aberdeen Maternity Hospital

AND

ISABELLA LEITCH

O.B.E.   M.A.   D.Sc.(Aberdeen)

Commonwealth Bureau of Animal Nutrition
Bucksburn, Aberdeen

WITH A FOREWORD BY

SIR DUGALD BAIRD

B.Sc.   M.D.   LL.D.(Hon.) Glas.
D.Sc.(Hon.) Manchester   D.P.H.   F.R.C.O.G.

Regius Professor of Midwifery
University of Aberdeen

BLACKWELL
SCIENTIFIC PUBLICATIONS
OXFORD

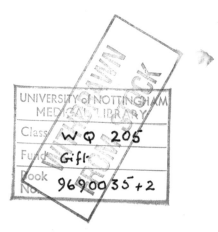

Printed in Great Britain by
WILLMER BROTHERS AND HARAM LTD, BIRKENHEAD
and bound by
THE KEMP HALL BINDERY, OXFORD

Contents

Foreword

Until about thirty years ago, the most urgent problem facing the obstetrician was the high rate of maternal mortality, mainly from infection, haemorrhage and obstructed labour. The antibiotics have brought infection under control; haemorrhage is much less dangerous, thanks to blood transfusion; and difficult labour can be safely avoided or overcome by caesarean section. The reduction of maternal mortality to a small fraction of what it used to be has been accompanied by a less dramatic yet substantial fall of perinatal mortality, brought about mostly by a reduction of deaths from birth trauma. The main causes of foetal wastage are now abortion, premature birth, defective foetal growth, congenital malformations and such serious complications as antepartum haemorrhage and hypertension. It seems possible that many of these pathological states encountered in clinical obstetrics result from failure of the mother to achieve the adaptive changes needed. We therefore need to know much more about the changes in body composition and function which occur in human pregnancy.

In animal studies the physiologist would probably use a carefully chosen inbred strain of animal with a high reproductive performance and maintain it in uniform and healthy conditions. In the human it is clearly impossible to have such well controlled conditions and this imposes severe limitations on the scope of work in the human field. It is impossible at present to allow for genetic factors nor can environment be controlled accurately. Epidemiological research has shown, however, that some groups of women are more vulnerable in pregnancy than others. For example, the risks of difficult labour and of stillbirth from all causes, are much higher in a first than a second or third pregnancy and in 'elderly' primigravidae. At any age and parity risks are greater in women from the lowest socio-economic groups. The social gradient is associated with gradients in physique and in general health, women from the more affluent classes being, on the average, taller and healthier than those from the poorer classes.

In studies which deal with the 'normal' or physiological changes in the mother during pregnancy, great care must be taken to select as the subjects for investigation women who are most likely to show the highest level of reproductive efficiency. For example, primigravidae should be between the ages of about twenty and thirty, tall and in good health and, if possible, from the upper socio-economic groups. This, in practical terms, is as near as we can get in the human to the more stringent procedures used in similar studies in animals.

Our epidemiological studies have shown, however, that even in such carefully selected women obvious differences in response to pregnancy occur. For example, there is considerable variation in the amount of weight gained during pregnancy and this is associated with differences in perinatal mortality and prematurity rates. It is therefore of great importance when drawing conclusions from an intensive physiological study of a few patients to have an accurate epidemiological study of the total population from which the patients are drawn. Again it is most important for the physiologist to work in an obstetrical atmosphere, since not only may the normal physiological response to pregnancy give insight into the aetiology of the pathological but the pathological response may help us to understand the normal.

How is this work to be organised? Suitable patients, when chosen, must be persuaded to undergo procedures which call for their active co-operation. Even the sampling of blood from a superficial vein at regular intervals is not quite painless, and usually requires that the patient must attend a clinic under specified conditions. She must be told that measurements are being made for research purposes, and are unlikely to benefit her directly. Nevertheless, she expects some 'reward', if only unconsciously, and it is necessary to stage research in circumstances where the highest standards of clinical care can be offered, not only in terms of obstetric techniques, but also in terms of personal attention. Either the research physiologist must himself be a competent obstetrician, or he must work in close co-operation with his obstetric colleagues.

Beds should be set aside in hospital so that when the needs of research require it, patients who otherwise do not have to be in hospital, can be admitted. In this way the best timing of observations is made possible by ensuring that a bed is available when it is required. In the Aberdeen Maternity Hospital eight beds have been set aside for research purposes alone. Care is taken to give patients in these beds an exceptionally high standard of comfort and personal attention, for the severely practical reason that research plans often make it necessary to persuade women to stay in hospital for longer periods than is clinically essential. The special 'research beds' are serviced by a group of nurses who are trained in unusual procedures, and who recognise the need for meticulous accuracy. In addition to beds, a research unit devoted to the physiology of pregnancy needs out-patient facilities and it is convenient to have the laboratories adjacent to the clinical accommodation.

The assembly of the proper team essential to research into both the physiological changes in pregnancy and the significance of deviation from the 'normal' presents the difficulties common to all clinical research in depth in any field. The solution to the problem must depend on circumstances. Few practising obstetricians have the time or the special experience that is necessary for many forms of physiological investigation. On the other hand, it is not easy to persuade professional physiologists to leave their classrooms and laboratories to face the difficulties of working with human subjects. If they are attached to the obstetric staff when at a relatively junior stage, they may come to feel that they are isolated from their own profession. Yet the study of human physiology requires prolonged devotion to it. In Aberdeen, we have been fortunate in obtaining the support of the Medical Research Council which by establishing a research unit in a maternity hospital is able to offer career posts to staff who are not obstetricians. The possibility of isolation is reduced by a system of joint appointments between the research unit and the appropriate University departments.

It is becoming more and more difficult to study 'normal' pregnancy since the intensification of medical care in an attempt to reduce mortality and morbidity to a minimum may lead to forms of treatment which modify 'natural' response to pregnancy. A few examples are prophylactic use of iron or folic acid, the giving of other vitamin preparations, calcium or diuretics, or the restriction of weight increase by dietary control.

The needs of therapy and research call for close co-operation between physiologists and obstetricians so that on the one hand the patient, on whom difficult and elaborate measurements have been made, is not given advice or treatment which may change the whole situation; on the other there must be no delay in instituting treatment which the clinician thinks is necessary. Changes in treatment will give rise to fresh physiological problems. For example, if a patient is made to lose weight by eating less, is she losing fat or water or both? Does dietary restriction affect the growth of the foetus and if not why not? If it is beneficial in clinical terms, why is this so? In this connection a great deal of work needs to be done in the evaluation of conventional methods of treatment during the antenatal period so that the research outlook should permeate the whole hospital. Records of all cases must be carefully planned and systematically compiled with a view to subsequent analysis.

Perhaps the most interesting material in this book is its account of the adaptations that take place during the course of pregnancy. Many of them occur so early that they cannot be responses to an immediate need, but must represent fundamental changes that are necessary to secure the safe development of the foetus at a later stage of gestation. To unravel their nature and to determine their meaning will be a prolonged but fascinating task. Meanwhile the authors have made a notable contribution to these fundamental problems not only by their valuable critical review of the literature but also by much original work.

Further progress in obstetrics must be founded on an understanding of the true nature of the physiological processes involved in pregnancy so that discoveries in other fields of medicine, chemistry or pharmacology may be applied rationally.

I therefore hope that this book will be read and carefully studied by practising obstetricians and all others interested in human reproductive physiology.

DUGALD BAIRD

Preface

In his foreword, Professor Sir Dugald Baird has outlined the background against which this book has been thought out and written. It remains for us only to say a little about the book itself.

This is not a review textbook. Certainly it is a synthesis of research and clinical observation, but the literature cited and the research results used to explain a finding or support a point of view are not usually all that might be quoted. We believe we cannot be accused of unfair selection, but the selection has been *ad hoc*. We have been critical and we hope provocative. A distressingly high proportion of published studies are worthless simply because the techniques used have been either intrinsically poor, or unsuitable for pregnancy. For this reason we have placed great emphasis on technical method. We do not wish to encourage an interest in method for its own sake, but in pregnancy perhaps more than in some other situations it is important to consider results in the light of how they were derived.

We have deliberately restricted our field to the physiology of the mother in pregnancy, excluding labour which deserves a book to itself, and the still poorly studied winding-down processes which follow delivery. And except where reference to the foetus was needed to clarify the maternal situation we have made no attempt to include foetal physiology.

It will be plain to those who are kind enough and patient enough to read the book that there are two main themes: first, measurements, and second, requirements and their satisfaction. The first twelve chapters are devoted primarily to measurements of the pregnant woman and of the changes that take place in her physiological processes and metabolism; the last two to the specific requirements that may be derived from these changes and the environmental circumstances in which those needs are to be met.

We have written the book primarily for the interested obstetrician, particularly registrars engaged on research problems; but we hope too that it may appeal to others, from the more interested medical student to the professional physiologist.

The growth of ideas is always slow and uncertain compared to the prodigiously rapid growth of facts. Ideas and concepts we have developed here have evolved not only from years of personal research and the assimilation of published research results but also from talking and arguing with many people. To all of them we owe some debt of gratitude. Here we can only give our thanks to those who have helped us directly by criticizing the manuscript and giving advice during the writing of the book or by giving us their data. Dr Angus Thomson has been of inestimable help in detailed criticism of the whole book; others have helped with specific sections: Dr S.G.Anderson, Dr S.Aboul-Khair, Dr J.B.Brown, Dr P.S.Brown, Mr W.Z.Billewicz, Dr J.M.Crawford, Dr H.F.Helweg-Larsen, Dr A.I.Klopper, Dr B.F.Matthews, Dr D.R.Mishell, Dr D.B.Paintin, Dr R.V.Short, Dr J.M.Stowers and Dr W.A.W. Walters.

Above all, our gratitude is due to Professor Sir Dugald Baird for creating the environment that made the book possible.

Finally we are grateful to Miss Margaret Porter who has devoted so much of her spare time to typing and retyping the manuscript.

Aberdeen Maternity Hospital   F.E.H.
October 1963   I.L.

CHAPTER 1

The Volume and Composition
of the Blood

BLOOD VOLUME

In a paper describing one of the earliest attempts to measure the increase of blood volume in human pregnancy, Miller, Keith and Rowntree (1915) stated that the 'plethora' of pregnancy had been recognised early in the nineteenth century and quoted German work as far back as 1854 which showed a rise of blood volume in pregnant laboratory animals. But until the early 20th century the evidence for plethora in women rested primarily on the demonstration of a reduced concentration of solids and cells in the blood.

The measurement of blood volume

Both the major components of blood, the red cells and the plasma, may be measured by methods based on the dilution principle, but they have seldom been measured together. Usually one is measured and the other is estimated from packed cell volume. The volume of white cells is usually ignored.

PLASMA AND SERUM

A great deal has been written about techniques of measuring the volume of plasma or serum and Gregersen and Rawson (1959) have recently made a detailed review. We will attempt no more than a description of the main principles. In theory any substance that spreads evenly in the plasma and does not leak out of the blood vessels during the time required for mixing is suitable for use and many such substances have been tried. Only two or three have come into common use. Evans blue dye (T1824) has been, and probably still is, the most popular. It fulfils the theoretical requirements of a tracer by attaching itself firmly and selectively to plasma albumin, and the amount that leaves the circulation during the mixing phase is negligible. About 70 per cent has disappeared in 48 hr (Wyers and van Munster, 1961) so that plasma

I

volume may be measured again after such an interval. Equilibration in the plasma is complete in less than 10 minutes after injection of the dye (Strumia, Colwell and Dugan, 1958) and the final concentration can be estimated on a single sample, taken at 10 minutes, or by extrapolating to zero time the results for a number of samples taken between, say 10 and 30 minutes. In theory, the extrapolation method, which takes account of dye lost from the circulation during the mixing phase, is the more accurate and is preferred by many of the most experienced workers in the field (for example, Reeve, 1947–48; Gregersen and Rawson, 1959); but a careful comparative study by Senn and Karlson (1958) suggests that the method with one ten-minute sample, which is much more convenient in clinical practice, has an error which is no greater than that of the extrapolation method. Caton et al. (1951) suggested that 10 minutes was insufficient for complete mixing of the dye in pregnancy and they allowed 15 minutes. Other studies, for example that of Roscoe and Donaldson (1946) and an unpublished Aberdeen study, have shown complete mixing in 10 minutes and that time is now almost universally accepted as sufficient.

Most workers use anticoagulant in the blood samples and are therefore estimating plasma volume. Direct reading of the concentration of dye in plasma or serum is subject to errors due to the presence of fat, to haemolysis and to changes in plasma colour. For this reason many workers have abandoned direct reading in favour of one of the many methods (for example that of Allen, 1951) by which the blue dye is extracted from the plasma on cellulose columns and eluted in an aqueous solution. Recovery of the dye is not complete nor of constant proportion, but tends to be about 97 per cent.

The use of serum instead of plasma reduces to a minimum the errors due to lipaemia (Murray and Shillingford, 1958) and, in our experience, if the subject is fasting and if blood samples are taken with care, direct reading of the dye in serum, taken 10 minutes after injection and compared with standards made up in blank serum from the same subject, gives results of a consistency which compares favourably with that of any of the more sophisticated techniques. Repeated estimates of the serum volume in any one subject should not show a range of more than 5 per cent from the mean.

Another tracer which is widely used to estimate plasma volume is albumin labelled with ^{131}I, that is radioactive, iodinated serum albumin (RISA). This method has its own difficulties (see Gregersen and Rawson's review) but has the advantage that the state of the plasma does not affect the count of radioactivity as it may affect the reading of a dye concentration. A number of workers have compared RISA with Evans blue dye, for example Senn and Karlson (1958) and Overall and Williams (1959). The two methods they say give much the same answer, but Senn and Karlson claim that there is a greater error in the Evans blue method because of variations in the optical density of plasma. Nor is that the only trouble.

From an analysis of results published by Zipf, Webber and Grove (1955) and Inkley, Brooks and Krieger (1955) Overall and Williams concluded that 'techniques of estimating plasma volume are significantly influenced by the technicians employing them. Evans blue dye and RISA are not two standard techniques but instead represent two families of techniques, members of which must be identified according to the investigators using them'. This is an important conclusion which might explain in part the wide range of mean values for plasma volume found at different stages of normal pregnancy by different workers. In any case it is clearly unwise to compare directly estimates made in one laboratory with estimates made in another by a technique broadly similar but differing in many details. Fortunately for our purposes in this book, the absolute values for plasma volume are of less interest than the extent of the change during pregnancy.

There are other methods of measuring plasma volume but less is known of their characteristics. Many different tracers have been used; for example Geigy Blau 536 is popular in continental European countries, and recently dextran and iron-dextran as described by Semple, Thomsen and Ball (1958) and Mackenzie and Tindle (1959).

None of the tracers used in the measurement of plasma volume crosses the placenta, at least during the time needed for equilibration in the maternal blood. Measurements in pregnancy are therefore of maternal plasma only.

RED CELL VOLUME

In the earliest method of measuring red cell volume haemoglobin was labelled with carbon monoxide (CO). It has seldom been used in pregnancy and has two characteristics which make it difficult to compare its results with those of other methods. First, carbon monoxide has been shown by Nomof *et al.* (1954) to overestimate red cell volume by 12 to 16 per cent when compared with direct labelling of cells (see below), because it attaches itself to myoglobin and other body pigments; second, it crosses the placenta and the measurement therefore includes foetal haemoglobin and myoglobin. Since radioactive labels suitable for red cells became available in the 1940s, the use of CO as a label has almost disappeared. The current application of the dilution principle to the measurement of red cell volume requires labelled red cells which can be injected into a subject in known quantity and may be easily identified in a sample of blood after mixing has taken place.

Radioactive isotopes of iron, ^{55}Fe and ^{59}Fe, have the advantage of being built into the haemoglobin molecule; they cannot be eluted and lost from the circulation during equilibration. But they have two great disadvantages: (1) donor cells are needed and there is therefore a risk, however careful the cross-typing may be, of the clumping or lysis of the injected cells and (2) there are the hazards of a long-lived source of radiation (^{55}Fe has a half-life of nearly 3 years, ^{59}Fe of 45 days) which cannot be excreted. The latter risk is greater when these isotopes are used in pregnancy because some is transferred to the foetus. They are now seldom used to label cells.

The two most popular techniques at present are the *in vitro* labelling of a sample of the subject's own red cells with ^{51}Cr or ^{32}P. Considerable experience with these isotopes has been amassed and their characteristics are now well understood. Chromium is the better tracer and is lost from the cells at the rate of only 1 per cent per day compared to a rate of about 6 per cent per hour for phosphorus. The chromium labelling technique has been described in detail by Nomof *et al.* (1954).

TOTAL BLOOD VOLUME

Without doubt the best estimate of total blood volume is obtained when plasma volume and red cell volume are measured simultaneously, say with Evans blue dye and red cells labelled with ^{51}Cr. But the two measurements are rarely made together and the majority of published reports of blood volume in pregnancy are based on estimates of either plasma volume or red cell volume. The fraction not directly estimated is calculated from an estimate of the proportion of red cells in the blood, which proportion is often termed the 'body haematocrit'. That term is now in the literature although the expression 'over-all cell percentage' used by Gregersen and Rawson (1959) is more specific and to be preferred. The over-all cell percentage in blood is derived from the cell percentage (packed cell volume or haematocrit) of a sample of peripheral venous blood. Two corrections must be made. The first is purely technical: plasma is trapped between the red cells in the packed cell column of the centrifuged blood and may cause an over-estimate of the cell percentage by up to 5 per cent. The value depends on the centrifugal force and time of centrifugation; with some modern high speed equipment there may be no appreciable trapping of plasma.

The second correction is necessary since the cell percentage in venous blood and all large vessels is higher than the over-all cell percentage because of the relatively high proportion of plasma in the smaller blood vessels and capillaries. The physics of blood flow is such that plasma tends to line the vessel wall while red cells congregate and flow in the centre of the vessel. The sorting out is negligible in large vessels but becomes important in small vessels and capillaries where there is a relatively wide zone of plasma surrounding a concentrated core of more rapidly moving red cells, which results in a permanently increased proportion of plasma in small vessels. The effect is accentuated when red cells tend to clump as they do in pregnancy (see below). Chaplin, Mollison and Vetter (1953) found that the over-all cell percentage in non-pregnant adults was 91 per cent of the venous cell percentage (i.e. the 'haematocrit ratio' was 0.91) when the red cell volume was estimated with cells labelled with ^{32}P and the plasma volume with Evans blue dye by a technique that involved correction for the dye leaving the circulation during equilibration. Where plasma volume and total red cell volume have been measured simultaneously in pregnancy by Caton et al. (1951) and by Verel, Bury and Hope (1956) the ratio between the over-all and the venous cell percentages varied widely; the range found by Verel et al. for 13 subjects was from 87 per cent to 103 per cent, and Caton et al. found a range of from 71 per cent to 124 per cent. More recently, Paintin (1963) has shown that, if the total red cell volume is estimated with cells labelled with ^{51}Cr and if the serum volume is

B

estimated without making a correction for dye leaving the circulation during the equilibration period, the ratio varies no more in pregnant than in non-pregnant subjects. His value of 88 per cent differs from that of Chaplin *et al.* only because of differences in detail of technique. Failure to use these corrections can lead to substantial errors; yet they have seldom been applied in published studies.

So far we have been discussing only laboratory techniques. These are now highly developed and errors are, for biological measurements, small. But differences due to physiological changes may be large. It is essential that physiological conditions be standardized if measurements from different subjects and from time to time in the same subject are to be comparable. Here, briefly, are some of the circumstances which must be taken into account.

Plasma volume is temporarily reduced by exercise. Kaltreider and Meneely (1940) found reductions of up to almost a litre within a few minutes after the start of vigorous exercise. Bed rest also reduces plasma volume; Taylor, Erickson, Henschel and Keys (1945) found a mean fall of over 500 ml in 6 healthy young men strictly rested in bed for 3 weeks, with a gradual return to previous values after a week or more of normal activity. Athletic training raises the plasma volume (Sjöstrand, 1953). The effect of posture is such that plasma volume falls when a subject stands quietly by loss of plasma into the extravascular space in the lower limbs and rises when the subject lies down (Waterfield, 1931). There are seasonal variations; plasma volume rises in warm weather and falls in cold weather (Yoshimura, 1958). Red cell volume falls with prolonged bed rest and is raised by physical training and by acclimatization at high altitudes.

The packed cell volume can be raised locally to high levels by venous stasis due, for example, to application of a tourniquet for more than one minute when blood samples are being taken.

It may not be possible to standardize all these variables, but they should not be ignored. In pregnancy, good reproducibility is obtained when the subject is brought fasting to the laboratory at, say 9 a.m. after a normal night's rest and the measurements are made after she has rested in a warm bed for 15 or 30 minutes.

It is, unfortunately, necessary to add that reported values may include numerical errors. For example, we have found several apparent errors of addition or transcription in the frequently-quoted data of Caton *et al.* (1951).

The measurement of haemoglobin

The techniques of blood sampling and of haemoglobin estimation are not usually described in detail in published papers and yet results from different investigations cannot properly be compared without full knowledge of the procedures used. The technical pitfalls of haemoglobinometry have often been discussed. Readings are most likely to be affected by errors of calibration and observer errors can also be large. The errors of estimating haemoglobin concentration were measured and discussed in detail by MacFarlane (1943). As he points out errors in routine practice may be large 'when a relatively inexperienced technician, after forcing a drop of blood from a reluctant patient, and using an unstandardized pipette hurriedly matches the resultant (possibly undergassed) solution in an uncalibrated diluting tube with a colour standard of uncertain value'. And, even if one may assume that the technique of estimating haemoglobin has been reliable, there are seasonal and diurnal variations in venous haemoglobin concentration. Walsh *et al.* (1953) found the mean haemoglobin level in Sydney women in summer to be about 0.5 g per 100 ml below the winter mean; in 34 women the mean haemoglobin concentration at 9 a.m. was 0.34 g per 100 ml higher than the mean at 3 p.m., and the difference between morning and afternoon readings in some women was as high as 1 g per 100 ml. Kerr and Davidson (1958) found the mean haemoglobin in winter to be from 0.7 to 1.0 g per 100 ml higher than the summer mean in a large series of Edinburgh women at different stages of pregnancy and the occurrence of diurnal changes has been confirmed by Stengle and Schade (1957). Physical exercise can cause transitory haemoconcentration and lying down a fall of haemoglobin level in peripheral blood. A tourniquet round the arm causes a progressive rise in the haemoglobin concentration of blood distal to it, obvious after half a minute of constriction. Capillary blood from the finger tip has a lower haemoglobin concentration than venous blood in pregnant women; Lund (1951) found an average difference of about 0.5 g per 100 ml.

It can be appreciated from this summary of the known pitfalls that substantial differences in haemoglobin values between groups of women can be introduced by differences of technique. For example, blood samples obtained by finger prick at an afternoon antenatal clinic are bound to show much lower readings than

TABLE 1

Author	Method	Pregnant Subjects	Control Subjects (non-pregnant)
Thomson *et al.* (1938)	Evans blue	14 clinically normal subjects. Serial studies.	3 of the same subje 30 days or more post-partum
Roscoe and Donaldson (1946)	Evans blue	20 normal subjects 17 primigravidae No clinical detail Serial studies	20 'normal' non-pregnant women
Freis and Kenny (1948)	Evans blue	7 women in last trimester. 4 had widespread oedema, 2 weighed 91 and 105 kg.	6 nurses and labora tory technicians
Werkö *et al.* (1948)	Evans blue	4 women in 'normal' late pregnancy. No detail.	9 healthy non-pregnant women
Lowenstein *et al.* (1950)	Evans blue	35 'unselected' subjects measured 'shortly before delivery' and again post-partum. Ages range from 17–42. Parity from 0 to 7.	Same subjects 8 day post-partum
McLennan and Corey (1950)	Evans blue	33 normal subjects at 35–36 weeks. 56 normal subjects at 39–40 weeks. (Including 23 of the 33 at 35–36 weeks.)	10 'normal non-pregnant women'
Tysoe and Lowenstein (1950)	Evans blue	14 'normal' subjects. Ages 20–38. 2 primigravidae. No other details. Serial studies.	Same subjects 2 months post-partum
White (1950)	Evans blue	56 women at various stages of 'normal' pregnancy. Cross-sectional data.	10 'normal non-pregnant women'

lasma Volume in Pregnancy

Mean Control lasma olume al	Maximum mean plasma volume reported		Mean Plasma volume at term (37 weeks +)	Remarks
	ml	Time in pregnancy		
,600	3913	31–60 days before delivery.	3620	
500	3450	Mean duration 35.6 weeks.	Not stated	
587	4286	'Last trimester'	Not stated	
:500	3800	'8–10 months'	Not stated	Values calculated from total blood volume and haematocrit
.690	No data		3377	
?385	3372	35–36 weeks.	3316	Probably includes subjects in earlier paper by McLennan and Thouin, 1948
?772	4000	8th calendar month	3900	Pregnancy figures not given; read from a graph
?362	3194	'3rd trimester'	No data	From graph, probably only 27 measurements in 3rd trimester

TABLE 1.

Author	Method	Pregnant Subjects	Control Subjects (non-pregnant)
Bucht (1951)	Evans blue	13 'normal' subjects. Cross-sectional data	23 non-pregnant women, nurses or patients in medical wards with minor conditions
Caton et al. (1951)	Evans blue	12 'normal' subjects. Serial studies	5 of the same subject 40–80 days post-partum
Berlin et al. (1953)	^{32}P-labelled red cells and venous haematocrit	157 women at all stages of pregnancy —no clinical information. Cross-sectional data	1. 16 healthy non-pregnant women 2. 17 women at 6 weeks post-partum
Adams (1954)	Evans blue	31 normal subjects with no history or sign of cardiac disease. No other data. Cross-sectional data	8 non-pregnant gynaecological patients
Verel et al. (1956)	Evans blue	7 normal subjects between 36 and 40 weeks	7 normal non-pregnant women age 18–28
Cope (1958)	Evans blue	38 normal subjects. Serial studies	None
Pritchard et al. (1960)	^{51}Cr-labelled cells and haematocrit	24 women at term no clinical detail	None
Hytten and Paintin (1963)	Evans blue	39 healthy young primigravidae with no clinical abnormality. Serial studies	Same subjects 6–8 weeks post-partum

ntinued)

ean ontrol asma lume ‖	Maximum mean plasma volume reported		Mean Plasma volume at term (37 weeks +)	Remarks
	ml	Time in pregnancy		
‖90	4260	9th and 10th months	No data	No explanation for high values. Done in conjunction with cardiac output and renal clearance studies
‖50	4120	40–79 days before delivery.	3950	
2140	3305	'9th month'	3118	
2249				
‖93	3396	34 weeks	3260	Value at 40 weeks read from a graph
‖06	No data		3401	Case numbers 6, 7, 8, 9, 10, 12 and 13 from the paper
o data.	3500	70 days before delivery	3180	Values read from graph
o data.	No data		2631	This study was designed to measure blood loss at delivery and not to define normal values. No correction applied to haematocrit
‖00	4000	33–36 weeks	3800	Figures for plasma volume rounded

venous samples taken in the morning from the same women, possibly of the order of a gram per 100 ml or more.

Plasma or serum volume in pregnancy

The first systematic serial study was made by Dieckmann and Wegner (1934) using Congo Red dye as the tracer, but the modern era of measurement of plasma volume in pregnancy began with the introduction of Evans blue dye, and since the first published study by Thomson *et al.* (1938), many further investigations have been made. Data from sixteen of those which published absolute values are shown in Table 1.1. Few studies have improved either technically or in the selection of subjects on the original one by Thomson and his colleagues. Their 14 subjects appear to have been young women of average weight and height who were clinically normal and who had good sized babies. They were unfortunately of mixed parity but the only important criticism to be made is that the time in pregnancy at which measurements were made was calculated backwards from the date of delivery on the assumption that delivery took place at 40 weeks and the timing is therefore not comparable with that in most other studies where the last menstrual period has been used as the fixed point. There was a good deal of individual variation but the averages suggest that plasma volume reached a maximum of about 3900 ml between 31 and 60 days before delivery and then declined to about 3600 ml in the last month. Taking the mean plasma volume of these subjects a month or more after delivery, 2600 ml, as the non-pregnant value, the pregnancy increase at its maximum was 1300 ml.

Other studies where apparently normal women have had serial measurements made of plasma volume in pregnancy, have shown a similar increase. Tysoe and Lowenstein (1950) found a mean maximum increase of 1228 ml; Caton *et al.* (1951), 1270 ml; Hytten and Paintin (1963), 1230 ml. These increases are measured in relation to 'control' values which may be from a sample of non-pregnant women or from the pregnant subjects after delivery. It seems likely that on the average the plasma volume has returned to about the non-pregnant level by 6 to 8 weeks after delivery (Hytten and Paintin, 1963). More information is needed on blood volume changes in early pregnancy. A valid picture can be established only by serial measurements starting before the subjects become pregnant, but the data of Hytten and Paintin suggest that there is little or no change before 10 weeks, although an increase is apparent by 12 weeks.

Some cross-sectional data are in agreement with the serial studies: Werkö et al. (1948) show a mean rise of 1300 ml and Berlin et al. (1953) of 1165 ml. The agreement between these six studies is the more remarkable because, in most of them, measurements were made at intervals of several weeks and the peak value, which may occur at any time in the last third of pregnancy, must often have been missed. There is more agreement about the size of the increase in plasma volume than about the actual size of the plasma volume itself. For example the mean control values given in Table 1.1 show a wide range; much of the variation is probably due to differences of technique, although differences of body size may play a part. The very low values of Berlin et al. (1953) were derived from direct measurement of the red cell volume apparently without applying a correction for the ratio of body haematocrit to venous haematocrit; the correction would raise these values by more than half a litre. Pritchard, Wiggins and Dickey (1960) who used the same procedure found a plasma volume at term of only 2631 ml; they did not give a value for non-pregnant subjects. At the other end of the scale, Bucht (1951) found a non-pregnant mean of 3390 ml. We cannot explain such a value but Bucht's measurements of plasma volume were incidental to a study of cardiac output and renal clearances and he admits 'a certain amount of unpleasantness' in the procedures. Certainly his figures for cardiac output (see below) were strikingly high, and his subjects were in a state obviously far from 'basal'. Minor differences of technique probably account for the differences in mean values found in most of the other studies. All that can be said at present is that the increase in plasma volume of 1100 to 1500 ml is from mean non-pregnant volume of between 2500 and 2700 ml.

The data of Hytten and Paintin (1963), for healthy primigravidae, were examined statistically to determine the pattern of change in plasma volume. Since plasma volume is related to body size the individual values were adjusted, by regression, to the mean height and weight of the group (162.4 cm; 58.2 kg) and the adjusted data are plotted in Figure 1.1. The fitted curve is expressed by the formula: Plasma volume (ml) $= 2819 - 69.17 \, w + 6.814 \, w^2 - 0.1151 \, w^3$ where $w =$ weeks of gestation between 12 and 38.

The curve is similar in shape to most published curves and shows a peak at about 34 weeks, as did the data of Adams (1954). It is also in agreement with Thomson *et al.* (1938) and Berlin *et al.* (1953) who describe the peak as occurring between 32 and 36 weeks, with Tysoe and Lowenstein (1950) who say it occurs in the '8th calendar month' and with Caton *et al.* (1951) whose peak occurred in the subdivision of 40–79 days before term (29–34 weeks). There is a considerable decline from the peak value to term, averaging about

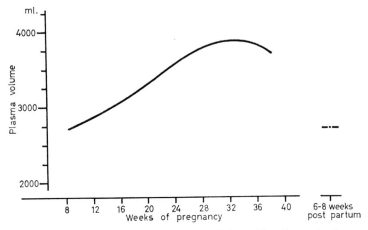

FIGURE 1.1. Plasma volume in normal primigravidae. From the data of Hytten and Paintin (1963)

200 ml [Thomson *et al.* (1938), 300 ml; Tysoe and Lowenstein (1950), 100 ml; Caton *et al.* (1951), 170 ml; Berlin *et al.* (1953), 187 ml; Adams (1954), 136 ml; Cope (1958), 320 ml and Hytten and Paintin (1963), 220 ml].

Although the fitted curve described above probably gives a valid picture of the general pattern of change, it underestimates the extent of the increase in plasma volume. The mean value for the measured maximum increase for individual subjects was 1230 ml, and the distribution is shown in Figure 1.2; the range was 630 ml to 1940 ml. Hytten and Paintin pointed out that since the plasma volume of their subjects was not measured frequently in the last trimester, the maximum volume achieved must often have been missed; this may explain the asymmetry of the distribution. They suggest that the true maximum increase for normal healthy primigravidae is probably about 1350 ml.

For multigravidae the increase is almost certainly more than this.

A parity difference seems never to have been specifically investigated, or even remarked upon when found, yet in every study where it is possible to make comparisons multigravidae show a bigger average change. Dieckmann and Wegner (1934) found a mean increase in plasma volume of 17.4 per cent for their primigravidae and 31.6 per cent for multigravidae. Thomson *et al.* (1938) claimed no parity difference, but when their results are graphed, 4 of the 5

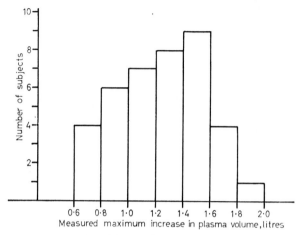

FIGURE 1.2. Distribution of the maximum measured increase of plasma volume in normal primigravidae. From the data of Hytten and Paintin (1963)

multigravidae have values that lie above the average curve. McLennan and Thouin (1948) found increases of 23.5 per cent and 33 per cent and Lowenstein, Pick and Philpott (1950) increases of 20.5 per cent and 29 per cent for primigravidae and multigravidae. Adams (1954) and Kjellberg *et al.* (1950) who measured whole blood volume, found the same pattern. Cope (1958) also describes a parity difference but attributes it to age; he does not present the data. Some of the primigravidae who were the subjects of Hytten and Paintin's series are having their plasma volumes measured in subsequent pregnancies; preliminary unpublished results confirm that, in general, there is a greater response.

It has been usual, in the past, to describe changes in plasma volume in terms of percentage change from the non-pregnant level. Hytten and Paintin found that this practice is misleading, because there is no correlation between the non-pregnant plasma volume and the amount by which it increases during pregnancy. Therefore, the smaller the non-pregnant plasma volume, the greater the increase expressed as a percentage tends to be. We refer to percentage changes in the discussion which follows only because absolute figures are not always published.

It will be evident from what has been said earlier in this chapter and in the Foreword that careful standardization of the type of subject and of the conditions under which she is examined is as important as accurate laboratory technique, and for pregnancy this means the selection of young healthy women of good physique, having a clinically normal pregnancy. Lack of discrimination in the choice of subjects has probably caused much of the confusion about what should be regarded as 'normal'. Several authors describe a huge range of response. For example, Dieckmann and Wegner (1934) found the change in plasma volume to range from -1 per cent to $+106$ per cent of the non-pregnant level, Lowenstein, Pick and Philpott (1950) -4 per cent to $+77$ per cent and Lund (1951) $+14$ per cent to $+121$ per cent. This sort of range makes little physiological sense; both extremes cannot be equally appropriate to the needs of pregnancy. If the average increase of 40 to 50 per cent is physiologically desirable, then an absence of increase represents physiological failure and an increase of as much as 121 per cent suggests gross abnormality, possibly to maintain blood volume in the presence of a red cell deficiency as happens in a gross anaemia. Dieckmann and Wegner's 23 subjects were a motley assortment which included thin and obese women, white and negro, primigravidae and multigravidae. Of Lund's subjects 90 per cent were negro and 'exclusively from the low income groups'. There is little information given for the subjects studied by Lowenstein, Pick and Philpott but they ranged from first to eighth pregnancies, from 17 to 42 years of age and were described as 'unselected'. The use of 'unselected' subjects is often taken to indicate statistical integrity and lack of bias. In a physiological study one must be consciously biased and there must be rigorous selection.

The healthy young subjects of Thomson *et al.* (1938) were within a much smaller range than those just quoted, and in Hytten and Paintin's series the range, in terms of percentage increase, was from 25 per cent to 80 per cent; more than half of the subjects fell in the range of increase 41 to 60 per cent.

There is little doubt that the amount of increase in plasma volume is correlated with clinical performance. Hytten and Paintin (1963) showed, for example, that the increase was quite closely related to the birth weight of the baby, and some women with a history of stillbirth or abortion, or who give birth to underweight babies, have a generally much smaller increase in plasma volume than normal pregnant women (Hytten, unpublished).

To sum up: Healthy women in a normal first pregnancy increase their plasma volume from a non-pregnant level of about 2600 ml by an average of at least 1250 ml; in subsequent pregnancies the increase is greater and may average nearly 1500 ml. The maximum is reached at about 34 weeks with considerable individual variation; after the maximum there is a decline towards term averaging about 200 ml.

Red Cell Volume in Pregnancy

Data from the literature are presented in Table 1.2 and it is obvious that there is no agreed picture for red cell volume. Values are higher where the estimate has been derived from measurement of plasma volume and venous haematocrit than when a direct estimate has been made with labelled red cells, presumably because of failure to correct for the haematocrit ratio (see p. 5). But even where techniques are apparently similar, the range is still extraordinarily wide. For example, averages of estimates made more than a month after delivery vary from 1268 ml (Paintin, 1962) to 1745 ml (Tysoe and Lowenstein, 1950). Much of this range may be due to differences of body size and physique of the groups or to the results of iron medication.

The average maximum increase above non-pregnant control values ranges from 110 ml (Roscoe and Donaldson, 1946) to 560 ml (Werkö et al. 1948) with some concentration of values round 400 ml: Thomson et al. (1938), 353 ml, Lowenstein et al. (1950), 385 ml; Caton et al. (1951), 445 ml; Berlin et al. (1953), 412 ml; Verel et al. (1956), 394 ml, and Pritchard and Adams (1960), 345 ml.

A round figure of 400 ml would seem to be a good representative value, but the concord is misleading because the increase in pregnancy varies according to what is taken as the baseline. For example, for the three studies by Thomson et al., Caton et al. and Roscoe and Donaldson the mean increases of red cell volume from the first measurement in early pregnancy to the maximum in late

TABLE I

Author	Method	Pregnant subjects	Control subjects (non-pregnant)
Thomson *et al.* (1938)	Evans blue and haematocrit	14 clinically normal subjects. Serial studies	3 of the same subje 30 days or more post-partum
Roscoe and Donaldson (1946)	Evans blue and haematocrit	20 'normal' subjects, 17 primigravidae. No clinical detail Serial studies	20 'normal' non-pregnant women
McLennan and Thouin (1948)	Evans blue and haematocrit	20 'normal' subjects, 38–40 weeks. Para 0–15, Body weight 110–203 lb. Ages 17–40	10 non-pregnant women from gynaecological war
Werkö *et al.* (1948)	Evans blue and haematocrit	4 women in 'normal' late pregnancy. No clinical detail	9 healthy non-pregnant women
Lowenstein *et al.* (1950)	Evans blue and haematocrit	35 'unselected' subjects measured shortly before delivery and again post-partum	Same subjects 8 day post-partum
Tysoe and Lowenstein (1950)	Evans blue and haematocrit	14 'normal' subjects. Ages 20–38. 2 primigravidae. Serial studies	Same subjects 2 months post-partum
White (1950)	Evans blue and haematocrit	56 women at various stages of 'normal' pregnancy. Cross-sectional data	10 'normal' non-pregnant women
Caton *et al.* (1951)	Cells labelled with ^{55}Fe	12 'normal' subjects. Serial studies	5 of the same subje 40–80 days post-partum

d Cell Volume in Pregnancy

·an ·trol ume	Maximum mean red cell volume found		Mean red cell volume at term	Remarks
	Volume	Time in pregnancy		
	ml			
52	1805	31–60 days post-partum	1681	Minimum average value found at '151 + days' before delivery: 1314 ml
·0	1950	Mean duration 35.6 weeks.	Not stated	Minimum average value found in first trimester (av. 12.4 weeks): 1650 ml
·9	No data		1978	Measured just before, or early in labour
·0	2160	'8–10 months'	Not stated	
·0	No data		1965	
·5	2023	9th lunar month	1982	
·0	1941	'3rd trimester'	No data.	From graph, probably only 27 measurements in 3rd trimester
·5	1780	0–39 days before delivery	No data.	Minimum average value found 200–240 days before delivery: 1285 ml

TABLE I

Author	Method	Pregnant subjects	Control subjects (non-pregnant)
Berlin et al. (1953)	Cells labelled with ^{32}p.	157 women at all stages of pregnancy Cross-sectional studies	1. 16 healthy non-pregnant women 2. 17 subjects 6 weeks post-partu
Verel et al. (1956)	Cells labelled with ^{32}p.	7 normal subjects between 36 and 40 weeks	7 normal non-pregnant women
Pritchard et al. (1960)	Cells labelled with ^{51}Cr.	32 women at the end of pregnancy—no clinical details	4 non-pregnant women
Paintin (1962)	Cells labelled with ^{51}Cr.	20 healthy primigravidae	Same women 8 weeks post-partum

pregnancy were 491, 495 and 330 ml compared to 445, 353 and 110 ml when the increase is measured from the post-partum value. That is, the post-partum value, was in each case considerably above the early pregnancy value. Berlin et al. have argued that there is a real fall in early pregnancy, 'a true anaemia', although all their subjects were 'routinely placed on oral iron at the time of the first visit'. There is no convincing evidence for a fall of red cell volume in early pregnancy. The study by Berlin et al. was cross-sectional and the small drop from 1422 ± 122 ml for 6 women in the first month to 1352 ± 49 ml for 12 women in the second month is far from statistical significance. The studies by Thomson et al. and Caton et al. were nominally serial studies but the red cell volume was not measured over the same period of pregnancy in all subjects. Of the 14 women studied by Thomson et al. only 3 had measurements made more than 30 days post-partum and not one of these had an estimate made before mid-pregnancy. Similarly only 5 of the *tinued)*

:an trol ume	Maximum mean red cell volume found		Mean red cell volume at term	Remarks
	Volume	Time in pregnancy		
	ml			
562	1833	'9th month'	1657	All subjects on oral iron medication throughout pregnancy
421				
;o	No data		1844	Case numbers 6, 7, 8, 9, 10, 12 and 13 from the paper
ʻ9	No data		1600	This study was designed to measure blood loss at delivery and not to define normal values
ʻ2	1521	37 weeks	No data.	No iron treatment in pregnancy. At least two of these women probably anaemic

12 subjects studied by Caton *et al.* had a measurement made more than 40 days post-partum and in 3 of them that measurement was less than the first made in early pregnancy. The non-pregnant control subjects of Roscoe and Donaldson had a bigger red cell volume than the pregnant subjects in the first trimester but details are not given of either group and it is not possible to judge to what extent they were comparable.

Individual variation, as recorded, is large. McLennan and Thouin describe a range of increase in their 20 women of from − 190 to + 1265 ml, Caton *et al.* a range of from − 125 to + 1600 ml in 12 women, and Lowenstein *et al.* a range in their 35 subjects of − 160 to + 752. In the serial study of individual women by Caton *et al.* where red cell volume was measured directly with labelled cells, the pattern of change for many subjects was so bizarre (a drop of 700 ml in 7 days and a rise of 1200 ml in 25 days are recorded without comment) that averages must be accepted with extreme

c

caution. How much of the variation is due to real differences between subjects and how much to vagaries of technique is hard to say. Paintin (1962) studied 20 apparently healthy primigravidae by a chromium-labelling technique which gave consistent levels in consecutive measurements. Fourteen increased their red cell volume by an average of 241 ml between early and late pregnancy. The other six showed a mean loss of 135 ml in red cell volume, and Paintin gives evidence suggesting that at least two of these had an iron deficiency anaemia.

Interpretation of this material is further bedevilled by the fact that the red cell volume can be increased by iron treatment, a common routine in obstetric practice. Lund (1951) for example, showed that while total haemoglobin increased by 15 per cent in pregnancy when iron was not taken, it increased by 23 per cent in women who took iron. There is no way of knowing how much the figures in Table 1.2 are influenced by iron treatment. Only Berlin et al. state that they gave iron; in other papers nothing is said about it. There are many advocates of iron treatment in both America and Britain; its application is probably more widespread in America, which may explain why the smallest average increases (Roscoe and Donaldson, 1946, White, 1950 and Paintin, 1962) were in British studies. Paintin (unpublished data) suggests that the mean rise in red cell volume for women not having iron medication is about 250 ml; when iron treatment is given the mean rise is probably from 400 to 450 ml. If we accept from those studies where direct estimates were made, a figure of about 1400 ml for the quantity of red cells in the average woman before pregnancy, then the rise for women not given iron is about 18 per cent; for those treated with iron, about 30 per cent. For the moment, we are inclined to regard the increase of 250 ml, which occurs without artificial stimulation, as the physiological.

It is not possible from the available data to determine the shape of the curve of increase, but it is probably linear from about the end of the first trimester to term. Tentatively, we would suggest as average figures a rise of 50 ml by 20 weeks, 150 ml by 30 weeks and 250 ml at term.

Nothing is known about the effects of such variables as age, parity and other maternal characteristics on the increase of red cell volume. It need hardly be said that there is large scope for careful research in this field.

Pritchard and Adams (1960) have given evidence of more rapid red cell production in late pregnancy. Labelled iron, given by injection, was incorporated into cells more rapidly than in the non-pregnant and more of the red cells near term appeared to be young; there were more reticulocytes and a higher mean glycolytic and cholinesterase activity. The rate of red cell destruction was not different from that in non-pregnant women.

Total Haemoglobin in Pregnancy

The concentration of haemoglobin in the red cell (the mean cell haemoglobin concentration) is little, if at all, affected by pregnancy (see below). It is therefore to be expected that the rise of total circulating haemoglobin is parallel to the rise of red cell volume. It has been calculated by several authors, without correction of the venous haematocrit, which applies as much to haemoglobin concentration as to the packed cell volume when peripheral blood is used. If we assume a mean cell haemoglobin concentration of 34 per cent, each 100 ml of red cells will contain 34 g of haemoglobin and the total gain of circulating haemoglobin, for the mother, who is not treated with iron, will be about 85 g by the end of pregnancy. Lund (1951) in his 'poor class' women found a rise of only 69 g in those not given iron compared to 152 g in the iron-treated group. Roscoe and Donaldson (1946) found a rise of 95 g between the 1st and 3rd trimesters, and Tysoe and Lowenstein (1950) a maximum rise of 172 g between the 2nd and 7th months.

Kjellberg et al. (1950) who measured red cell volume with carbon monoxide found the difference between the non-pregnant controls and women in the last 8 weeks of pregnancy to be 153 g, but carbon monoxide crosses the placenta and foetal haemoglobin must be included in that estimate. Assuming a blood volume for the foetus of 400 ml (Smith, 1959) and a haemoglobin concentration of 16.5 g per 100 ml (Walker and Turnbull, 1953) foetal haemoglobin will amount to about 66 g. That would make Kjellberg's estimate of the increase of maternal haemoglobin about 90 g, which may be artificially low because Kjellberg measured his haemoglobin concentration in capillary blood.

The same criticism can be made of the study by Gemzell, Robbe and Sjöstrand (1954). These workers also used carbon monoxide and capillary blood in a serial study of 17 women in pregnancy. The mean total haemoglobin rose from about 497 g at 8 weeks to a maximum of 552 g at 20 weeks and then fell to 509 g at 36 weeks. This picture seems physiologically unlikely and the violent fluctuations from month to month in individuals suggest that the technique may have been faulty. The same workers, in a later paper (Gemzell, Robbe and Ström, 1957) criticize their earlier method as systematically overestimating haemoglobin by about 12 per cent and in the second study showed a rise from 421 g to 627 g in a group of women given iron in pregnancy.

The published evidence for the rise in total haemoglobin is so unsatisfactory, that until better figures are available we will adhere to our own mean estimate of 85 g.

Blood Volume in Pregnancy: Summary

We have arrived at the best estimates we can make for the increase in plasma and red cell volume, and these need only be added to give the best estimate of blood volume. To prepare Table 1.3 we

TABLE 1.3. Plasma Volume, Red Cell Volume, Total Blood Volume and Haematocrit in Pregnancy

	Non-pregnant	Weeks of pregnancy			
		20	30	34	40
Plasma volume ml	2600	3150	3750	3830	3600
Red cell volume ml	1400	1450	1550	1600	1650
Total blood volume ml	4000	4600	5200	5430	5250
'Body haematocrit' per cent	35.0	31.5	29.8	29.5	31.5
Venous haematocrit* per cent	39.8	35.8	34.0	33.5	35.8

* Assuming a haematocrit ratio of 0.88.

have used Hytten and Paintin's figures for plasma in primigravidae, and the table shows, in addition, the change in 'body haematocrit' or overall cell percentage. Assuming a haematocrit ratio of 0.88 (p. 6) we have derived an estimate for the haematocrit of venous blood, which agrees well with actual measurements of venous haematocrit. These are discussed below.

THE COMPOSITION OF THE BLOOD
Changes in Peripheral Blood

The measurement of plasma and red cell volume is technically too difficult for clinical use and the changes in plasma and red cell volume we have described are of little more than academic interest to the clinician who must almost always rely on what can be learnt from a sample of peripheral blood. And since it is a simple matter to withdraw some blood and take it to a laboratory, many studies have been made of changes in the composition of venous blood in pregnancy.

RED CELLS AND HAEMOGLOBIN

Because the increase in the total red cell volume during pregnancy is proportionately less than the increase in plasma volume, the concentration of red cells in the blood falls. The size and haemoglobin content of the cells show little if any change (see below) so that the haemoglobin concentration and haematocrit fall in parallel with the red cell count.

These changes are shown in Tables 1.4, 1.5 and 1.6 compiled from a representative selection of recent publications. Most studies have been made of what is, at least in terms of laboratory time, the easiest measurement: haemoglobin concentration.

HAEMOGLOBIN CONCENTRATION

In healthy non-pregnant women the haemoglobin concentration, measured by standard techniques, is on the average about 13.7 to 14.0 g per 100 ml (Table 1.4: Whitby and Britton, 1957; Verloop, Blokhuis and Bos, 1959a). The lowest average levels recorded during pregnancy are between 11 and 12 g per 100 ml in most series, and where the data have been treated statistically the standard deviation of the mean is about 1 g. Exceptions to this generalization occur in the series published by Rath et al. (1950) from Boston, where the mean haemoglobin concentration did not fall below 12.7 g, and two Australian series, those of Walsh et al. (1953) from New South Wales and Morgan (1962) from Western Australia, who found average minima of 12.1 and 12.4 g per 100 ml. It is possible that these differences may be due to iron medication, the effects of which will be discussed later, but differences of calibration cannot by excluded.

TABLE 1.4. Haemoglobin Concentrat[ion]
(Number of wom[en])

Authority and Place	Non-pregnant		
Medical Research Council (1945) (United Kingdom)	13.9 ± 1.4 (770)	*Month 1* 13.4 (13)	*2* 13.2 (92)
Hamilton (1950) (Edinburgh)	13.3 (23)		*Weeks 6–9* 12.3 (32)
Rath et al. (1950) (Boston, U.S.A.)			*Month 2* 13.5 (12)
Lund (1951) (New Orleans, U.S.A.)			
Ventura and Klopper (1951a) (London)	14.34 ± 1.48 (25)		*Weeks 0–10* 13.93 ± 1.4 (15)
Benstead and Theobald (1952) (Bradford)			
Darby et al. (1953) (Nashville, U.S.A.)	13.09 ± 1.26 [7 weeks post-partum] (1279)		*Weeks 5–9* 13.13 ± 1.37 (131)
Walsh et al. (1953) (New South Wales)	13.93 ± 1.11 (595)		
Edgar and Rice (1956) (Nottingham)			
Sturgeon (1959) (Los Angeles, U.S.A.)	13.3 ± 0.60		
Morgan (1961) (Western Australia)			*Weeks 5–8* 13.5 (7)

Von-Pregnant Women
orackets)

Haemoglobin: g per 100 ml

Pregnant

	4	5	6	7	8	9	
.2	12.6	12.8	12.0	12.1	12.1	12.2	
)	(58)	(71)	(103)	(88)	(140)	(75)	

	4–17	18–21	22–25	26–29	30–33	34–37	38–40
–13	14–17						
.0	12.9	12.3	12.1	11.5	12.9	12.1	12.1
)	(43)	(47)	(41)	(39)	(43)	(41)	(31)

	4	5	6	7	8	9
–4	12.7	12.7	12.7	12.9	12.7	12.8
3)	(9)	(16)	(15)	(18)	(17)	(9)

	16	20	24	28	32	36	40
eek 12	13	12	12	12	11	11	11.5
	(8)	(9)	(6)	(6)	(7)	(7)	(8)

	11–20	21–30	31–40
	13.50 ± 1.29	12.67 ± 1.07	11.62 ± 1.12
	(25)	(25)	(40)

	Week 16	20	24	28	32	36	40
	13.2	13.0	12.4	11.6	11.4	11.3	12.0
	(36)	(36)	(36)	(36)	(36)	(36)	(36)

	14–19	20–26	27–32	33+
–13	12.01	11.94	11.43	11.55
.95	± 1.06	± 1.07	± 1.30	± 1.43
1.15	(674)	(691)	(1395)	(562)
06)				

	13–16	17–20	21–24	25–28	29–32	33–36	37–40
eeks 8–12	12.71	12.62	12.34	12.26	12.10	12.19	12.23
.26	± 0.88	± 1.01	± 0.94	± 0.81	± 1.05	± 1.02	± 1.13
1.00	(116)	(108)	(118)	(124)	(155)	(171)	(107)
44)							

	Week 16	20	24	28	32	36	40
	12.5	12.2	11.6	11.2	10.8	10.8	11.1
	(25)	(25)	(25)	(25)	(25)	(25)	(25)

					8		
onths 3					11.4		
.2							

	13–16	17–20	21–24	25–28	29–32	33–36	37–40
–12	13.1	13.0	12.9	12.8	12.4	12.9	12.7
.7	(26)	(33)	(29)	(25)	(40)	(36)	(27)
9)							

TABLE 1.5. Packed Cell Volume
(Number of wom⬛

Authority and Place	Non-pregnant		
Hamilton (1950) (Edinburgh)	41.5 (23)	*Weeks 6–9* 42.8 (32)	*10–13* 42.0 (45)
Lundström (1950) (Uppsala, Sweden)	39.0 ± 0.22 (98)	*Weeks up to 8* 38.3 ± 0.59 (17)	
Rath *et al.* (1950) (Boston, U.S.A.)		*Month 2* 39.5 (12)	*3* 38.8 (13)
Lund (1951) (New Orleans, U.S.A.)			*Week 12* 40 (3)
Benstead and Theobald (1952) (Bradford)			
Darby *et al.* (1953) (Nashville, U.S.A.)	40.5 ± 2.9 [7 weeks post-partum] (1279)		*Weeks 5–⬛* 39.2 ± 3.4 (131)
Edgar and Rice (1956) (Nottingham)			
Paintin (1962) (Aberdeen)	37.2 ± 3.2 [7–8 weeks post-partum]		*Week 11.⬛* 36.7 (20)

on-Pregnant and Pregnant Women
brackets)

Packed cell volume: per cent

Pregnant

4-17	*18-21*	*22-25*	*26-29*	*30-33*	*34-37*	*38-40*
o.9	39.8	39.8	38.3	39.3	38.8	40.0
43)	(47)	(41)	(39)	(43)	(41)	(31)
6		*24*		*32*		*40*
7.2 ± 0.23		35.2 ± 0.26		33.7 ± 0.26		33.7 ± 0.28
98)		(115)		(119)		(123)
	5	*6*	*7*	*8*	*9*	
7.2	37.0	36.7	37.2	37.0	37.9	
9)	(16)	(15)	(18)	(17)	(9)	
6	*20*	*24*	*28*	*32*	*36*	*40*
9	37	35.5	35.2	34.2	34.4	35.7
8)	(9)	(6)	(6)	(7)	(7)	(8)
Week 16	*20*	*24*	*28*	*32*	*36*	*40*
9.8	38.3	37.1	35.5	34.6	35.5	36.8
36)	(36)	(36)	(36)	(36)	(36)	(36)
0-13	*14-19*	*20-26*	*27-32*	*33 +*		
8.5 ± 3.1	35.8 ± 3.0	35.5 ± 2.8	34.8 ± 3.4	35.1 ± 3.5		
206)	(674)	(691)	(1395)	(562)		
Week 16	*20*	*24*	*28*	*32*	*36*	*40*
7.8	36.2	34.4	34.2	33.0	33.0	36.3
25)	(25)	(25)	(25)	(25)	(25)	(25)
	20.5		*28.9*		*36.8*	
	34.6		32.9		32.6	
	(20)		(20)		(20)	

TABLE 1.6. Red Cell Count
(Number of wome

Authority and Place	Non-pregnant		
Lundström (1950) (Uppsala, Sweden)	4.20 ± 0.03 (98)	*Weeks up to 8* 4.16 ± 0.10 (17)	
Rath *et al.* (1950) (Boston, U.S.A.)		*Month 2* 4.46 (12)	*3* 4.43 (13)
Darby *et al.* (1953) (Nashville, U.S.A.)	4.55 ± 0.45 (216)	*Weeks 5–9* 4.38 ± 0.45 (131)	
Edgar and Rice (1956) (Nottingham)			
Sturgeon (1959) (Los Angeles, U.S.A.)	4.8 ± 0.34	*Months 3* 4.19	

The fall of haemoglobin concentration is usually apparent in the first three months of pregnancy and is of the order of 0.5 g per 100 ml. The minimum concentration is reached at about 30 to 32 weeks, a little later in some studies, and there is a rise in the last few weeks of up to 0.5 g. This pattern could be predicted from the relative changes in the plasma and red cell volumes; the red cell concentration decreases until the maximum plasma volume is reached at about 34 weeks, and then increases as plasma volume falls towards term, while the red cell volume continues to increase.

HAEMATOCRIT, PACKED CELL VOLUME

The haematocrit falls in parallel with the haemoglobin concentration to reach an average of about 34 per cent from a generally accepted non-pregnant norm of 40 to 42 per cent (Table 1.5). The average lowest values found by Rath *et al.* (1950), 36.7 per cent and by Hamilton (1950), 38.3 per cent, were exceptional and may have been due to failure to correct for trapped plasma. Like haemoglobin-

on-Pregnant and Pregnant Women
brackets)

Red cell count: millions per mm³

		Pregnant				
6		*24*		*32*		*40*
.05 ± 0.03		3.79 ± 0.03		3.69 ± 0.02		3.82 ± 0.03
98)		(115)		(119)		(123)
	5	*6*	*7*	*8*	*9*	
.24	4.17	4.17	4.20	4.17	4.30	
9)	(16)	(15)	(18)	(17)	(9)	
'0–13	*14–19*	*20–26*	*27–32*	*33 +*		
.29 ± 0.45	4.04 ± 0.44	3.98 ± 0.45	3.88 ± 0.41	4.08 ± 0.49		
206)	(103)	(184)	(220)	(72)		
Week 16	*20*	*24*	*28*	*32*	*36*	*40*
.39	4.15	4.02	3.85	3.70	3.80	3.80
25)	(25)	(25)	(25)	(25)	(25)	(25)
				8		
				4.07		

concentration the haematocrit rises slightly towards term. These values are in reasonable agreement with what would be expected from the changes in plasma and red cell volumes (Table 1.3).

RED CELL COUNT

The counting of red cells is tedious and has a relatively large error. It is therefore not surprising that there is little information about red cell count. More studies will probably be made now that automatic counting is possible. The evidence available suggests that the number of red cells per unit volume of blood like the packed cell volume runs parallel to haemoglobin concentration (Table 1.6).

MEAN CELL HAEMOGLOBIN CONCENTRATION (MCHC)

The MCHC appears to vary little during pregnancy from an average of about 32 to 33 per cent. Lundström (1950), Rath et al. (1950), Tysoe and Lowenstein (1950), Lund (1951), Darby et al. (1953) and Morgan (1961) found no appreciable change.

Benstead and Theobald (1952) and Davis and Jennison (1954) reported a fall of about 0.5 per cent during the last trimester in two small series of women, and Edgar and Rice (1956) in 25 women a mean fall from 32.6 per cent at 16 weeks to 30.2 per cent at term. Sturgeon (1959) found a fall from 31.7 in early pregnancy to 30.9 in late pregnancy in women who received no iron; an iron-treated group showed no such fall. Roscoe and Donaldson (1946) on the other hand, found a small rise during pregnancy in a series of 20 women. Any change reported for small numbers of subjects should be regarded with caution. The MCHC is extremely sensitive to small errors in the estimation of haemoglobin and haematocrit. An error of ±5 per cent in the haemoglobin estimate with a ±2 per cent error in the haematocrit can cause variations of ±8 per cent in the MCHC. With this in mind it can be said that there is no certain evidence of a change in MCHC in pregnancy.

MEAN CELL HAEMOGLOBIN (MCH)

The mean cell haemoglobin similarly remains almost constant, although Rath *et al.* (1950), Lundström (1950) and Darby *et al.* (1953) reported a small decrease towards the end of pregnancy.

MEAN CELL VOLUME

There is general agreement that the mean cell volume does not change (Roscoe and Donaldson, 1946; Wills *et al.* 1947; Rath *et al.* 1950; Merivale and Richardson, 1950; Darby *et al.* 1953); but Tysoe and Lowenstein (1950) found that the size of cells 'increased throughout pregnancy, although the values remained within normal limits'; Edgar and Rice (1956) found a similar small rise and Lundström (1950) and Sturgeon (1959) recorded a decrease. The mean cell diameter as measured by Merivale and Richardson (1950) was slightly below the mean for non-pregnant women, which means that the cells were more spherical; Elliott (1944) found no deviation from the non-pregnant.

To summarize, the red cell is apparently little, if at all, changed by pregnancy and probably contains the same amount of haemoglobin. The concentration in the blood of red cells, and therefore of haemoglobin, falls because the increase of plasma volume is relatively greater than the increase of red cell volume. The lowest concentration is reached within ten weeks of term, probably at about 34 weeks, when plasma volume is greatest. There is a slight rise from the lowest point to term, corresponding to the decline in plasma volume at this time.

'Physiological anaemia'

The reduced concentration of red cells and haemoglobin is often called the 'physiological anaemia of pregnancy', a meaningless term which, while it strives to avoid offence to those who believe the phenomenon to be normal, yet implies a pathological state. A large body of opinion considers the fall to indicate iron-deficiency and we must examine the evidence for that view. The keystone of the evidence is that the changes in blood which we have described above can be considerably modified when extra iron is given to the pregnant woman.

THE EFFECT OF IRON

Haemoglobin concentration. Lundström (1950), Benstead and Theobald (1952), Davis and Jennison (1954), Fisher and Biggs (1955), Edgar and Rice (1956), Verloop, Blokhuis and Bos (1959b) and Morgan (1961) have all reported that the mean haemoglobin concentration in women given therapeutic doses of iron by mouth rose during pregnancy, sometimes to non-pregnant levels; and Wills *et al.* (1947), Lund (1951), Magee and Milligan (1951) and Sturgeon (1959) were able to arrest or modify the usual fall. Gerritsen and Walker (1954) say that Bantu women, with an exceptionally high intake of iron in the diet, have no fall in mean haemoglobin concentration during pregnancy. The very small fall in haemoglobin concentration found for a group of Boston women by Rath *et al.* (1950) and in the two Australian series is remarkably close to that in other series in which medicinal iron was given, and suggests that those women may have been taking iron supplements of their own accord.

Other values. The usual falls in packed cell volume and red cell count can be similarly modified by iron (Lundström, 1950; Lund, 1951; Benstead and Theobald, 1952; Wills *et al.* 1947; Davis and Jennison, 1954; Edgar and Rice, 1956; Verloop, Blokhuis and Bos 1959b). The mean cell haemoglobin concentration and mean cell volume may be raised slightly by iron; Lundström and Edgar and Rice found higher values in their patients given iron, and Benstead and Theobald were able to raise the average mean cell haemoglobin concentration to the high value of 34 to 36 per cent by the end of pregnancy.

OTHER EVIDENCES OF IRON DEFICIENCY

The finding that the haemoglobin concentration of the blood can be increased by giving iron raises the question whether the usual fall in pregnancy is truly normal or should be regarded as a sign of iron deficiency. It suggests cure by replacement, the classical test of deficiency, and other evidence is believed to support that suggestion.

Free Protoporphyrin. For example, the mean concentration of free protoporphyrin in the red cell was found to be raised during pregnancy (Fay *et al.* 1949; Lund, 1951; Ventura and Klopper 1951a; Sturgeon, 1959) and is known to be increased in hypochromic anaemia (Cartwright *et al.* 1948), but the rise in pregnancy, which varies widely in magnitude, is not necessarily analogous. Ventura and Klopper stated that free protoporphyrin values 'are increased whenever the linkage between iron and protoporphyrin is disturbed. Anaemia is not the only condition which may disturb this linkage; it is just as reasonable to assume that pregnancy may itself be the disturbing factor.'

Serum Iron. The average serum iron concentration is reduced at term to about 35 per cent below the mean in non-pregnant women (Fay *et al.* 1949; Lundström, 1950; Ventura and Klopper, 1951b; Mukherjee and Mukherjee, 1953; Verloop, Blokhuis and Bos, 1959b; Sturgeon, 1959 and Morgan, 1961), and the iron-binding capacity is raised, so that the percentage saturation of iron-binding protein is low. Similar changes are found in iron-deficiency anaemias (Laurell, 1947; Smith, 1952). Taken together with the fact that the serum iron can be raised by iron in pregnancy, as in iron-deficiency anaemia (Lundström, 1950; Davis and Jennison, 1954; Mukherjee and Mukherjee, 1953; Verloop, Blokhuis and Bos, 1959b), and does not fall at all in women on diets rich in iron (Gerritsen and Walker, 1954), these findings are assumed by many to be strong evidence that the usual changes in the blood in pregnancy are due to deficiency of iron, but the analogy must be drawn with great caution. In health, serum iron shows immense individual variability, even from hour to hour (Jacot, 1951; Fowler and Barer, 1952; Howard, 1953; Rechenberger and Hevelke, 1955), and the processes which determine the changes are not understood. Serum iron is low during the first week of the menstrual cycle (Powell, 1944; Dahl, 1948; Smith, 1952) and during acute infections. It falls whenever production of red cells rises (Wasserman *et al.* 1952; Finch and Finch, 1955), and may be low even when large stores of iron can be demonstrated histologically in the marrow (Davidson and Jennison, 1952). Goldeck *et al.* (1954) have shown that the concentrations of haemoglobin and serum iron are not correlated in pregnancy. In any event, the total amount of iron circulating in the plasma is probably raised, because of the increased plasma volume of pregnancy.

Iron-binding capacity. The iron-binding capacity of the blood is even less well understood. It is now known to depend on the β_1-globulin transferrin, which is thought to act specifically as an iron transporter. Ventura and Klopper (1951a) attributed the raised iron-binding capacity to 'the vastly increased turnover of iron in late pregnancy', but it may simply be associated with the rise in the concentration of plasma globulin. Gerritsen and Walker (1954) found the iron-binding capacity raised in the blood of Bantu pregnant women who showed no reduction of either haemoglobin or serum iron.

The concept of saturation of iron-binding capacity is not helpful, since saturation occurs only when large quantities of iron are released into the bloodstream, either by haemolysis or after intravenous injection of iron. Laurell (1947) believed that the low saturation during deficiency of iron and in pregnancy presents a condition favourable for absorption of iron from the gut, but the saturation in non-pregnant women of 30 or 40 per cent should leave an adequate margin for any further transport of iron which is required. A more plausible explanation might be that additional facilities for carriage of iron and 'enhanced power and speed in coping with an influx of iron' (Ventura and Klopper, 1951b) are needed to deal with the relatively large amount of iron returned to stores at the end of pregnancy, when the excess of red cells is destroyed and the blood volume returns to normal.

Serum copper. The copper content of serum in pregnancy is above that of non-pregnant women (Fay *et al.* 1949; Röttger, 1950; Ventura and Klopper, 1951a; Lahey *et al.* 1953; Sturgeon, 1959), as it is in iron-deficiency anaemia (Cartwright *et al.* 1948). But the copper content of plasma is raised in many other conditions also (Lahey *et al.* 1953) and is not related to serum iron. Its role is not well understood.

What, then, are the grounds for regarding the fall in haemoglobin concentration during pregnancy, which occurs in healthy normal women, as an indication of deficiency of iron? The low serum iron, the increased iron-binding capacity, the high serum copper and the high free protoporphyrin in red cells have been discussed. None of these specifically indicates deficiency of iron, nor does the peripheral blood picture. The cells are of normal size and the mean cell haemoglobin concentration, regarded by Whitby and Britton (1957) as 'the true indicator of iron deficiency', is normal. There remains the belief that because the haemoglobin concentration in the blood can be raised by giving iron, there must be deficiency of iron. Widdowson and McCance (1936), Fowler and Barer (1941), Garry *et al.* (1954); and Verloop, Blokhuis and Bos (1959a), have shown that iron can raise haemoglobin concentration even in normal persons, and in one of Fowler and Barer's series the haemoglobin fell again to its initial level even while iron was still being given. Iron in sufficient amounts appears to provide a specific, though temporary, stimulus to erythropoiesis. Wills *et al.* (1947), commenting on the rise of haemoglobin level which followed administration of iron in their series of pregnant women, say that '. . . judging from the nature of the changes in the haematological picture, [the iron] cannot have acted by correcting a latent hypochromic anaemia'. Lund (1951) too saw that the total mass of haemoglobin could be increased in pregnancy by giving iron even when there was no evidence of deficiency.

The fact that the fall of haemoglobin concentration in normal multigravidae has been found to be greater than in primigravidae (Goodall and Gottlieb, 1936; Wills *et al.* 1947; Magee and Milligan, 1951) has been interpreted as indirect evidence of depletion of iron, accentuated by repeated pregnancy. But the blood pictures of primigravidae and multigravidae are not directly comparable; we have shown (p. 15) that multigravidae have a greater rise of plasma volume than primigravidae and a correspondingly lower haemoglobin concentration is to be expected.

All these findings emphasize the important principle that 'normality' in pregnancy cannot be judged by reference to non-pregnant standards. Physiologically the only meaningful criterion of red cell sufficiency is that oxygen carrying capacity should be adequate in the circumstances; arbitrary levels of haemoglobin or of red cell concentration have no physiological significance in themselves although the practice of giving to an arbitrary reading on a particular scale, the value 'roo per cent' may give that impression. Within wide limits there is no reason for any fixed relation between plasma and red cells. The two components of the blood perform quite different functions and are controlled by different mechanisms. Curiously enough only 'haemodilution' seems to cause anxiety; a relative increase in red cell volume such as occurs at high altitudes never seems to cause concern for a plasma deficiency. Moreover a 'satisfactory' level of haemoglobin concentration may indicate no more than an unsatisfactory increase of plasma volume.

In the next chapter we will show that the average changes in red cell volume and plasma volume are entirely appropriate to the changed circumstances of pregnancy and in fact the margin of safety for oxygen carriage is probably raised. As one might expect from this, the woman with so-called 'physiological anaemia of pregnancy' does not feel any benefit from having her haemoglobin raised by administration of iron, as is freely admitted, even where medication with iron in pregnancy is recommended as a routine. Fisher and Biggs (1955) say that the women in their series, who did not respond to iron and whose haemoglobin fell throughout pregnancy, were nevertheless 'clinically well at all stages', and Magee and Milligan (1951) commented that in their large series 'the great bulk of women, whether taking iron or not, were perfectly healthy and had no complaints, which raises the question whether a haemoglobin level raised by iron therapy is in itself an advantage.'

It has been claimed for a high level of haemoglobin in pregnancy that the woman is in a stronger position to withstand haemorrhage and even that she has less tendency to haemorrhage post-partum. But here also evidence is confused and inconclusive. Wills *et al.* (1947) reported a greater incidence of haemorrhage in women who took no additional iron, but Lund (1951) found no significant difference in the incidence of haemorrhage between treated and untreated women, and Benstead and Theobald (1952) say that 'the only disadvantage of maintaining the haemoglobin level at its normal value throughout pregnancy would appear to be a slightly increased risk of post-partum haemorrhage'.

In general, there is no convincing published evidence that the normal pregnant woman is at an advantage if she takes extra iron. Perhaps the real benefit is not to the woman at all, but lies in that

D

'... the confidence of both doctor and midwife, particularly in domiciliary practice, is greatly increased by the knowledge that the haemoglobin level is high at term' (Fisher and Biggs, 1955), a benefit which should not be despised, since iron-deficiency anaemia in pregnancy does occur and in some places is a major problem. The diagnosis of true anaemia presents considerable difficulty and is discussed by Hytten and Duncan (1956).

Blood viscosity. The change in the concentration of red cells affects the viscosity of the blood. Hamilton (1950) has shown that the relative blood viscosity (relative to distilled water) fell from 4.61 in non-pregnant women to 4.20 in early pregnancy and then to 3.84 at 22 to 28 weeks when the mean haemoglobin concentration in her series was lowest. Plasma viscosity changed little and the viscosity of whole blood appeared to depend almost entirely on the concentration of red cells. It should be remembered that viscosity of blood measured in a glass viscometer tube may give an exaggerated impression of its viscosity in small blood vessels (MacFarlane, 1961) and the change in red cell concentration occurring in pregnancy may have little or no real effect on viscosity. If there is any reduction of viscosity it must diminish considerably the work of the heart and should help to keep arterial blood pressure normal as the cardiac output rises. Artificial raising of the haemoglobin concentration by iron medication will reduce this advantage.

Changes in leucocyte concentrations

Andrews and Bonsnes (1951) quote Nasse as having shown as early as 1835 that pregnancy was associated with leucocytosis. Since then there have been numerous confirmations. Andrews and Bonsnes found a rise from a mean of 7,100 per mm^3 in non-pregnant women to 10,500 in late pregnancy. The rise was mostly due to an increased number of neutrophil polymorphonuclear cells; these rose in number from a mean of 4,500 per mm^3 in non-pregnant women to 7,700 in late pregnancy. Lymphocytes rose only from 2,000 to 2,300 per mm^3, a change which was not statistically significant. No significant change occurred in the numbers of monocytes or of eosinophilic polymorphonuclear leucocytes. Thonnard-Neumann (1961) concluded that the number of basophilic polymorphonuclear leucocytes was reduced in pregnancy.

Apart from the gross changes associated with infections, little is known about variations in leucocyte populations and it is not possible to offer any interpretation of the changing picture in pregnancy.

Changes in composition of plasma and serum

As plasma volume increases, there are changes also in its composition. The term 'haemodilution' is freely used in discussions of the blood in pregnancy, and by usage, has the meaning of 'dilution' of the red cell mass by the relatively greater increase of plasma. There is also a true dilution of the plasma with water. Paaby (1959) in a careful serial study showed that both serum and plasma water rose from about 91.5 per cent in early pregnancy to over 92 per cent at the maximum, which was reached for different women at various points between the middle and end of pregnancy. The water content always fell sharply before delivery, usually to below 91 per cent but it is not clear whether this is a particularly low value or a return to the non-pregnant level. Dilution is by no means a simple excess of water but the result of a number of complex changes in the composition of the plasma. We are not able to give a comprehensive account

TABLE 1.7. Changes in Plasma Electrolytes During Pregnancy
(from Newman, 1957)

Electrolyte mEq/l	Non-pregnant	First trimester	Second trimester	Third trimester
Na$^+$	143.3	138.9	139.1	139.5
K$^+$	4.25	4.07	4.00	3.97
Ca^{++}	4.86	4.94	4.81	4.69
Mg^{++}	1.67	1.57	1.53	1.47
HCO$_3^-$	25.9	24.6	23.9	23.2
Cl$^-$	104.7	102.7	104.2	104.2
HPO$_4^=$	1.96	1.95	1.78	1.82
Protein$^-$	16.5	16.4	15.4	15.1
Total cations	154.08		149.34	
Total anions	149.06		144.85	

of these changes because while some components like protein have been the object of numerous studies there are few figures available for changes in electrolyte patterns; levels of some nutrients such as vitamins and amino-acids not particularly relevant to a discussion of gross composition will be considered later (Chapter 13).

ELECTROLYTES

Newman (1957) made an extensive analysis of the blood of 27 women throughout pregnancy and compared the results with analyses of blood from non-pregnant women. His results for electrolytes, except sulphate which he did not measure, are shown in Table 1.7. In general there is a fall in the concentration of electrolytes in pregnancy; some appear to fall earlier than others and some more steeply than others. The overall change is small, a fall of about 5 mEq for cations and the same for anions. Now that flame photometry and other methods for the measurement of electrolytes have been developed to a state of great efficiency there should be a welcome increase in our knowledge of electrolyte chemistry in pregnancy. At present so little is known that we cannot discuss the significance of most of the recorded changes. Bicarbonate is presumably reduced to compensate for the low blood CO_2 which will be discussed in more detail in Chapter 3. Protein will be considered below.

CONCENTRATION OF PLASMA AND SERUM PROTEIN

It has long been known that the concentration of protein in the serum and plasma is reduced in pregnancy, and since the introduction of paper electrophoresis there have been many studies of protein fractions, most of them in serum.

TOTAL PROTEIN IN PLASMA AND SERUM

Although there is complete agreement that serum protein concentration falls in pregnancy there are extraordinary differences of opinion about the extent and pattern of the fall. Figure 1.3 shows the average results in three recent studies in three countries: MacGillivray and Tovey (1957) in Britain; Paaby (1960) in Denmark; and de Alvarez, Afonso, and Sherrard (1961) in the United States. None of these studies was entirely satisfactory; all were, at least in part, serial measurements in 'normal' pregnancy but the numbers were too few to give confidence in the averages. It is most unlikely that the differences between them are biological; presumably the variation is due to technique, although it is difficult to see what sort of differences in a relatively simple technique could give disagreement of such an order. The extent of the confusion can be further gauged from a review article by Macy (1958) where two sets of results, both presumably from her laboratories in Detroit, are

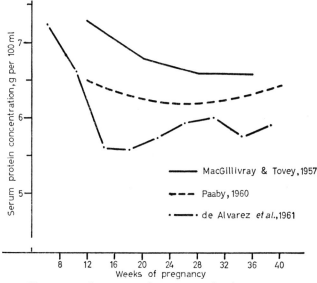

FIGURE 1.3. Serum protein concentration in pregnancy

used as illustrations. One, a figure, shows a fall from a non-pregnant mean of about 7.0 g per 100 ml to about 6.3 g per 100 ml at 3 months and a continuing fall to below 6 g per 100 ml at term. The second, a table, quotes average figures (for plasma, the amount of fibrinogen being subtracted) of 7.01, 6.99 and 6.85 g per 100 ml for the three trimesters of pregnancy. Clearly, more research, including an enquiry into fundamentals of method, is required. Personal experience of many estimations in normal pregnancy (Hytten unpublished) supports the findings of de Alvarez et al. that there is a rapid fall in early pregnancy from a non-pregnant level of over 7 g per 100 ml to less than 6 g per 100 ml.

PROTEIN FRACTIONS

A number of studies have been made, with simple electrophoretic methods, of the main protein fractions, albumin, α_1, α_2, β and γ globulins. More refined techniques have revealed many sub-divisions inside these main groups but they have not yet been applied to sera from pregnant women.

Serum albumin. Figure 1.4 shows the results for albumin of the same

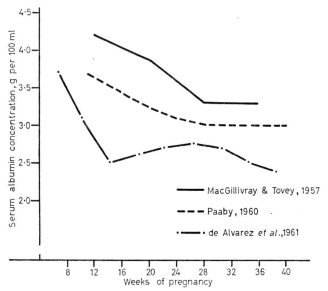

FIGURE 1.4. Serum albumin concentration in pregnancy

three studies presented in Figure 1.3. There is agreement that the albumin falls in concentration and the pattern is similar to that for total protein. The same systematic differences between the studies in absolute values occur, as they would be expected to, because albumin was not estimated chemically but as a proportion of total protein, judged from electrophoretic patterns.

The fall in albumin concentration is proportionately greater than that of total protein; for example de Alvarez *et al.* found the proportion of albumin in total serum protein to fall from about 50 per cent in early pregnancy and non-pregnant controls to about 40 per cent at the end of pregnancy.

α_1-*globulin*. There is general agreement that the proportion of α_1 globulin in total protein rises slightly but its concentration in serum is not significantly affected by pregnancy. Only Paaby claims an absolute rise from about 0.4 g per 100 ml in early pregnancy to 0.5 g per 100 ml at the end of pregnancy.

α_2-*globulin*. There is a slight rise in the proportion of α_2-globulin and its concentration in serum also may rise slightly during pregnancy.

β-*globulin*. The β-globulin fraction rises conspicuously during pregnancy both as a proportion of total protein and in absolute concentration. de Alvarez *et al*. found a rise from about 1 g per 100 ml in early pregnancy to more than 1.3 g per 100 ml in late pregnancy and both Paaby, and MacGillivray and Tovey describe rises of a similar order. The results of these three studies are shown in Figure 1.5.

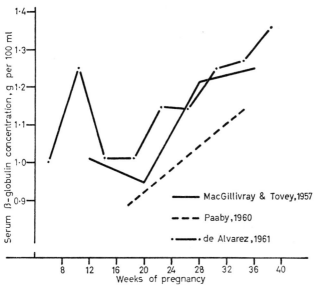

FIGURE 1.5. Serum β-globulin concentration in pregnancy

γ-*globulin*. γ-globulin may be reduced in pregnancy but the difference is probably small. Only MacGillivray and Tovey showed a consistent fall. In Paaby's study there was no real change and, if the first point in the study by de Alvarez *et al*. which is based on only 2 observations be excluded, no convincing change can be claimed, although their level throughout pregnancy lay considerably below their non-pregnant average.

Fibrinogen. de Alvarez *et al*. found a continuous rise during pregnancy from about 0.26 g per 100 ml to about 0.38 g per 100 ml; Gillman, Naidoo and Hathorn (1959) found a rise from 0.35 g in non-pregnant women to 0.56 g in late pregnancy, and Phillips and Skrodelis (1958) a rise from 0.30 g in the first trimester to 0.40 g at term.

In summary, the total concentration of plasma protein measured in serum falls steeply in pregnancy, probably with the major part of the fall occurring at the beginning. Most of that fall is due to a relatively large decline of serum albumin. The globulin fractions behave quite differently. There are slight rises in the alpha fractions and a definite rise in beta globulin; gamma globulin probably changes little but may fall. Fibrinogen concentration rises throughout pregnancy.

The significance of the changes in blood protein

There is not sufficient information available for us to offer an interpretation of these changes and indeed little is known of the precise physiological functions of the several blood proteins. Tovey (1959) suggests, without evidence, that the fall in albumin may be due to increased renal catabolism. It is perhaps surprising that such a dramatic change in the one protein fraction which is thought to have an important effect on plasma oncotic pressure, should not be attended by a more obvious change in water balance. Bennhold, Peters and Roth (1954) describe a patient with congenital absence of serum albumin who had no apparent disturbance of water balance and Haurowitz (1961) suggests that compensating mechanisms may exist or that the importance of serum albumin in the regulation of water balance may have been overestimated.

Circulating globulin increases in amount throughout pregnancy. Even if there were no increase in the concentration of the alpha fractions their absolute quantity would be raised in proportion to the expansion of serum volume. Beta globulin may rise in concentration by about 40 per cent so that the total amount circulating may be doubled.

Proteins are known to act as carriers in the blood. For example, metals, lipids, carbohydrates and hormones are all carried in association with proteins, mostly globulins, and it would be easy to say that the increase in carrier capacity is demanded by the increased turnover of substances to be carried. But we cannot offer any evidence to support such a view and a great deal of further research is necessary before interpretation of changes is possible. One thing is certain: the fall of plasma protein is not due to 'dilution' as the plasma volume expands. Albumin is the only fraction which is significantly 'diluted' and its concentration appears to fall abruptly at a time in pregnancy when plasma volume is just beginning to rise (see also Chapter 13).

ERYTHROCYTE SEDIMENTATION RATE

It seems appropriate at this point to mention the erythrocyte sedimentation rate (ESR), which has long been known to be raised in pregnancy. For example, Furuhjelm (1956), in a study of 185 women in late pregnancy found the ESR for whole blood to vary from 44 to 114 mm in the first hour with a mean of 78 mm. For citrated blood the range was 30 to 98 mm, the mean 56 mm. For normal non-pregnant women the ESR does not exceed 20 mm for whole blood or 10 mm for citrated blood (Whitby and Britton, 1957).

It is not at all clear what determines the ESR except that a high sedimentation rate implies clumping of red cells, the clumps falling faster than individual cells. According to MacFarlane (1961) clumping can be caused by increase of plasma fibrinogen and also by increase of globulin, which may explain the raised ESR of pregnancy. In pregnancy, therefore, ESR is of little or no value as diagnostic of disease.

BLOOD CLOTTING

The present information about clotting mechanisms is confusing and difficult to interpret. MacFarlane (1961) in an excellent summary, points out that many 'factors' postulated as necessary for blood clotting, and there is a large and increasing number of them, are no more than hypothetical. Few have been identified chemically and a number have been inferred when only an activity has been observed. There is little detailed information about these mechanisms in pregnancy but we have already shown that the pregnant woman has a considerable increase in circulating fibrinogen. If we accept as an example the rise described by Gillman, Naidoo and Hathorn of from 350 mg per 100 ml before pregnancy to say 550 mg per 100 ml in late pregnancy with an average expansion of the plasma, this would mean a rise in circulating fibrinogen from under 10 g to more than 20 g.

As far as it has been investigated fibrinolytic activity is considerably reduced in pregnancy (Biezenski and Moore, 1958; Gillman Naidoo and Hathorn, 1959). Biezenski and Moore found less than 10 per cent of women in late pregnancy to have lytic activity and both investigations showed a rapid return to normal fibrinolytic activity in the puerperium. Biezenski (1960) found no increase in antifibrinolytic activity in pregnancy and concludes that there must be 'an actual reduction in the circulating lytic enzyme'. Phillips and Skrodelis (1958) found an increase in circulating profibrinolysin, a precursor of fibrinolysin, but the increase was matched by a similar increase of profibrinolysin inhibitor.

The increased fibrinogen in pregnancy may therefore be a direct result of a reduced rate of destruction. It has often been suggested that some fibrin is formed continuously in the normal person and is removed by continuous fibrinolysis. As MacFarlane (1961) says: 'If this is so, then the relative rates of fibrin formation and removal become important in the maintenance of vascular patency and integrity, and fibrinolysis becomes an important anti-thrombotic activity, any decrease of which might be disastrous.'

Acceptance of this idea would suggest that the pregnant woman

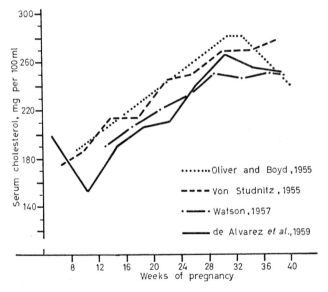

FIGURE 1.6. Serum cholesterol concentration in pregnancy

lives continually in danger of widespread thrombosis, and yet there is no clinical indication of it and a more comforting view for the obstetrician would be that she has increased protection against blood loss. His confidence in this is supported by the fact that there is an increased number of platelets in pregnancy. Mor *et al.* (1960) found the platelet count to rise from a non-pregnant mean of 187,000/mm^3 to 210,000 in the first trimester, 276,000 in the second trimester and 316,000 in the third trimester.

There is, as usual, considerable room for research.

BLOOD LIPIDS

Total lipid. It seems to have been recognised for many years that the fat content of blood is raised in pregnancy. Total lipid, which is no more than the material in blood which is soluble in solvents such as petroleum ether is, as Peters and Van Slyke (1946) have said 'such a heterogeneous conglomeration of loosely related compounds that it has little chemical or functional significance'. de Alvarez *et al.* (1959) found total lipid concentration to rise from a mean of between 650 and 700 mg per 100 ml serum up to 16 weeks to a little over 1000 mg per 100 ml at the end of pregnancy, and von Studnitz (1955) describes a similar rise in his cross-sectional study.

Cholesterol. There is general agreement that the concentration of cholesterol in serum rises considerably during pregnancy. The results of four recent studies are shown in Figure 1.6 (Oliver and Boyd, 1955; von Studnitz, 1955; Watson, 1957; de Alvarez *et al.* 1959). Oliver and Boyd obtained their blood samples at mid-day after their subjects had fasted for 3 hours; Watson had blood taken at a routine afternoon antenatal clinic; de Alvarez *et al.* took blood from their subjects before breakfast and after they had fasted for at least 12 hours; there is no information as to how and when von Studnitz obtained his samples. Yet the similarity of the findings is impressive. The increase in cholesterol concentration probably begins in early pregnancy. The fall shown by de Alvarez *et al.* before 12 weeks is based on only four observations, but Peters, Heinemann and Man (1951) also claimed that there was a tendency for the level to fall in early pregnancy before rising some time after the 12th week. More information is needed to confirm the early fall. There seems to be no doubt that the level of cholesterol declines somewhat or at least stops rising between the 30th week and term.

It is interesting to note that the cholesterol level at 6 to 8 weeks post-partum is still considerably above the level in early pregnancy and the generally accepted non-pregnant level. Even 20 weeks after delivery the mean level in Oliver and Boyd's subjects was still a little above the mean in early pregnancy.

Peters and Van Slyke (1946) have pointed out that there is a close association between the amount of free cholesterol and the amount of cholesterol ester. The relation apparently holds for pregnancy: de Alvarez *et al.* found free cholesterol to vary only between about 22 and 25 per cent of the total cholesterol and Oliver and Boyd similarly found free cholesterol to increase approximately in proportion to total cholesterol.

Phospholipid. Phospholipid, which is usually measured and often expressed as lipid phosphorus, rises in much the same way as cholesterol. de Alvarez *et al.* (1959) showed a small and statistically non-significant rise for lipid phosphorus from about 10 mg per 100 ml serum before 8 weeks to about 11 mg at 20 weeks, after which the level rose more rapidly to about 14 mg per 100 ml at the end of pregnancy. This is equivalent to an overall rise in phospholipid from about 250 mg in early pregnancy to about 350 mg per 100 ml at term and is similar to von Studnitz's (1955) finding that phospholipids rose from 245 mg in early pregnancy to 398 mg at term. Oliver and Boyd (1955) found the phospholipid to rise by 'about 25 per cent' from about 250 mg per 100 ml of plasma at 9 weeks, to its peak level at 33 weeks, a much smaller rise than that found by either de Alvarez *et al.* or von Studnitz.

Just as free and total cholesterol are closely related in health, so are cholesterol and phospholipid. The relation has been ascribed to a mutual antagonism between these two substances in their action on membranes which necessitates the maintenance of a constant balance. 'A proper balance between the lipids appears to be more sedulously protected and is, therefore, presumably more important than the absolute concentration of any one or all of the lipid components' (Peters and Van Slyke, 1946). It is not possible from the available evidence to say how well this balance is preserved in pregnancy. Oliver and Boyd found the ratio of cholesterol to phospholipid to rise from 0.74 at 9 weeks to 0.92 at 31 weeks, and to fall again to 0.79 at term, and Peters, Heinemann and Man found the mean ratio of lipid phosphorus to free cholesterol to be both higher and more variable in pregnancy than in the healthy non-pregnant subject. In the studies by de Alvarez *et al.* and von

Studnitz on the other hand, the ratio of lipid phosphorus to cholesterol seemed to be constant.

Neutral fat. There seems to have been no recent study of neutral fat in the blood in pregnancy. Peters, Heinemann and Man (1951) found that neutral fat showed the biggest proportionate rise of all the lipid fractions, 'unmistakable and consistent in all subjects'.

Distribution of fractions. Lipid is carried in blood attached to protein. There are two primary types of lipoprotein, α-lipoprotein which migrates electrophoretically with α-globulin and β-lipoprotein which migrates with β-globulin. The relative proportion of β-lipoprotein increases during pregnancy so that there is an increase in the $\beta:\alpha$-lipoprotein ratio (Russ, Eder and Barr, 1954; Oliver and Boyd, 1955; von Studnitz, 1955; Watson, 1957). Possibly there is a shift in the distribution of lipid in favour of β-lipoprotein as suggested by Russ, Eder and Barr. Oliver and Boyd found the distribution of cholesterol between α and β-lipoprotein to rise from 1:2 in the non-pregnant to 1:5 at the 32nd week of pregnancy.

The significance of the changes in blood lipid in pregnancy is quite unknown although there is no shortage of speculation invoking most of the hormones. We do not wish to add further to the spate of theory but it is of interest that cholesterol is probably the major precursor of the steroid hormones whose turnover in pregnancy is tremendously increased.

CHAPTER 2

Cardiovascular Dynamics

In this chapter we deal with changes of blood flow in pregnancy: cardiac output, regional changes in blood vessels and blood flow and changes in intravascular pressure during pregnancy.

CARDIAC OUTPUT

TECHNIQUES OF STUDY

All methods for the measurement of cardiac output require considerable expertise if they are to give reliable results; none is simple. What we have said about the standardization of conditions of study in Chapter 1 deserves even greater emphasis here because large changes in blood flow can occur quickly in response to many different stimuli and not all of them are easy to control. For example, cardiac output may be quickly increased in response to even slight emotional excitement or muscular activity and, if measurements in different subjects, or in the same subject at different times, are to be comparable, they must be made as far as possible under 'basal' conditions, i.e. when the subject is resting, completely relaxed and preferably fasting. In pregnancy these conditions are more than usually difficult to meet. The pregnant woman is emotionally more labile than usual and more easily excited and her enhanced appetite, particularly in early pregnancy, may make fasting hard to tolerate. In late pregnancy, she finds it difficult to lie comfortably in one position for more than a short time and position may have some effect on cardiac output: for example a few women suffer an acute fall of blood pressure when lying on their backs, the 'supine hypotensive syndrome' which we will discuss later, and recently Vorys, Ullery and Hanusek (1961) showed that cardiac output was considerably reduced when subjects in late pregnancy lay on their backs or in the lithotomy or Trendelenburg positions, in comparison with output when they lay on their sides. Palmer and Walker (1949) presented convincing evidence that in late pregnancy painless uterine contractions can have a large and sudden effect on the oxygen content of venous blood returning to the heart which would affect the estimation of cardiac output. Contractions in labour greatly increase cardiac output (Hendricks, 1958).

An excellent review of methods of measuring cardiac output was made in a symposium published in 1945 (Cournand, 1945) and only modifications of detail have been added since. The indirect application of the Fick principle,* with acetylene, was developed in Denmark by Krogh and Lindhard and was the most popular and respected means of measuring cardiac output until the end of the 1930s, at least in America where most of the early studies in pregnancy were made. It is now recognized that this method gives estimates which are too low and it has been abandoned. With the development of the technique of passing a catheter into the heart it became possible to measure cardiac output by direct application of the Fick principle. If, for example, arterial blood leaving the heart contains 19 ml of oxygen per 100 ml and mixed venous blood returning to the heart contains 14 ml of oxygen, then the arterio-venous difference is 5 ml per 100 ml or 50 ml per litre. If in these circumstances the body is consuming 250 ml of oxygen per minute, then the volume of blood which must pass through the lungs to carry this oxygen is 250/50 or 5 litres per minute. Assuming dynamic equilibrium, the left heart output is equal to the right heart output and the systemic circulation will also be at the rate of 5 litres per minute. It is possible to measure oxygen consumption with reasonable accuracy and arterial oxygen content can be measured in a sample from any large artery, but mixed venous blood can be obtained only from the heart. The oxygen content of the inferior vena cava is frequently different from that of the superior vena cava

---

* The Fick principle, briefly, is this: the quantity of a substance X, taken up by the body (or by an organ) in a given time equals the amount carried to it in the arterial blood, minus the amount carried away in the venous blood. The quantity of X retained therefore equals blood flow multiplied by the mean arterio-venous difference in concentration of X, and

$$\text{Blood flow} = \frac{\text{Quantity of X retained}}{\text{Arterio-venous difference in X}}$$

For cardiac output, oxygen is used as the test substance and it therefore equals,

$$\frac{\text{Quantity of oxygen taken up by the body, or oxygen consumption}}{\text{Mean arterio-venous oxygen difference}}$$

and there is no doubt that adequate mixing of the two streams does not occur in the right atrium. The venous sample must be obtained from the right ventricle, or preferably the pulmonary artery and unless the end of the catheter is known from X-ray examination to be beyond the atrium considerable inaccuracies may be introduced.

Although cardiac catheterization is now accepted as a generally safe procedure which causes little or no discomfort, it is not entirely without risk and is sufficient of a surgical undertaking to deter physiologists from using it repeatedly in the same subjects during pregnancy and no longitudinal study is available with this method.

Another, simpler, method with a dye indicator has been used in pregnancy; this will probably displace cardiac catheterization. A small volume of dye is injected quickly into a vein and the time of its appearance, and its concentration in arterial blood is estimated either by frequent sampling or more recently by continuous monitoring of the optical density of the blood with a photocell. Flow rate can be calculated if the amount of dye injected is known and the concentration as a function of time is accurately determined. The method is more difficult than this simplified description suggests and requires meticulous attention to detail, but it cannot be criticized on theoretical grounds and its results have been shown to correlate well with those of the direct Fick method both in pregnant and non-pregnant subjects (Hamilton *et al.* 1948; Werkö *et al.* 1949). Now that dye on the output side of the heart can be measured by an external monitor, a modified ear oximeter, the subject need suffer no more trauma than a venipuncture and it should be more easily possible in future to make longitudinal studies of normal pregnant women.

Other methods of measuring cardiac output have not been applied to pregnant subjects. Brehm and Kindling (1955) estimated cardiac output from a modification of the pulse pressure method in which calculations are based on pulse amplitude and frequency. The method involves so many assumptions which are of doubtful validity that we do not propose to consider the results here.

Where the technique of estimation of blood flow in specific organs or regions of the body is important to the understanding of the results they have been dealt with in the chapters dealing specifically with these organs. Renal blood flow is discussed in Chapter 4.

CARDIAC OUTPUT IN PREGNANCY

It can be said at once that the data available are not satisfactory and it is not possible to give a confident estimate of changes in cardiac output during normal pregnancy.

The picture which has been firmly established in current teaching, for example that described by Burwell and Metcalfe (1958), is due largely to Burwell who, during the 1930s, made intensive studies of a few women with the acetylene method. Individual changes during pregnancy in these women were haphazard but the average trend suggested a steady rise in cardiac output to a peak about the 30th week, after which there was a decline towards non-pregnant values at the end of pregnancy. It is characteristic of this method that the absolute estimates are lower than those from direct application of the Fick principle and Burwell has selected from recent studies that by Hamilton (1949) to support his thesis. Hamilton's figures, while considerably above the Burwell estimates, follow a somewhat similar pattern, but the pattern is not confirmed by other studies.

Table 2.1 shows estimates of cardiac output in pregnancy from four studies where sufficient data were published to allow adequate analysis. A study by Adams (1954) who used the dye dilution technique has not been included because his results were not published; only a graph was shown which presents a most erratic pattern, but suggests a trend similar to that of Burwell. The study by Bucht (1951) will not be considered further; his high figures can almost certainly be attributed to the fact that his subjects were not 'basal'. Renal clearances were measured concurrently with the cardiac output and Bucht admits that the procedures, which included numerous injections and catheterization of the bladder, caused 'a certain amount of unpleasantness'.

The three remaining studies all used the direct Fick principle with cardiac catheterization. Those by Hamilton (1949) and Palmer and Walker (1949) could be criticized in that in both venous blood was sampled from the right atrium and not the pulmonary artery, and in both the oxygen saturation of the arterial blood was assumed to be 95 per cent. As far as can be determined from the description both these studies followed an identical procedure— both workers were trained by Professor John McMichael in the Postgraduate Medical School, London. The subjects in both

E

TABLE 2.1. Average Cardiac Output in Pregnancy
Number of subjects in each group in brackets

Author	Not pregnant	Weeks of pregnancy — Cardiac output, litres per minute									Remarks
		−8	9–12	13–16	17–20	21–24	25–28	29–32	33–36	37–40	
(1) Palmer and Walker (1949)	4.6 (8)		6.2 (8)	6.1 (6)	5.5 (8)	6.4 (9)	4.7 (7)	5.8 (5)	5.7 (8)	5.7 (8)	Direct Fick. Catheter in right atrium Arterial oxygen saturation assumed to be 95 per cent
(2) Hamilton (1949)	4.51 (24)	4.29 (4)	5.14 (5)	5.45 (8)	5.65 (8)	5.71 (5)	5.73 (6)	5.54 (11)	5.5 (8)$_0$	4.6 (13)$_0$	Number of subjects in each group taken from graph and may not be exact. Direct Fick Catheter in right atrium Arterial oxygen saturation assumed to be 95 per cent
(3) Bader, Bader, Rose and Braunwald (1955)				5.05 (1)	6.97 (3)	6.57 (4)	6.82 (11)	6.38 (12)	5.20 (6)	5.72 (9)	Direct Fick. Catheter in pulmonary artery Arterial oxygenation measured
(4) Bucht (1951)	7.4 (20)	6.7 (1)	8.2 (10)	8.6 (3)	— (0)	7.2 (1)	6.3 (1)	7.5 (2)	8.9 (4)	8.9 (9)	Dye injections. Subjects almost certainly not basal—see text
Means of 3 studies with direct Fick (1), (2), (3) above	4.53 (32)	4.29 (4)	5.79 (13)	5.67 (15)	5.80 (19)	6.25 (18)	5.93 (24)	5.95 (28)	5.49 (22)	5.23 (30)	

studies appear to have been normal healthy women and considerable efforts were made to achieve ideal 'basal' conditions; the numbers of subjects were similar. In these circumstances it is not easy to see why the two sets of results should be so different. Hamilton's followed a smooth trend; that of Palmer and Walker was much more erratic and generally at a higher level. Palmer and Walker attribute the unexpectedly low average during the seventh month to the 'effect of posture'. It is difficult to understand why this should have happened only at that point. The type of subject in the two studies may have been different but evidence is lacking. Most of the women studied by Palmer and Walker were apparently primigravidae but details of age or parity, or of body size, are not given for either study. There is a big individual variation in the cardiac output figures in both studies and the differences may be due to no more than small numbers of subjects in the groups.

The study by Bader, Bader, Rose and Braunwald (1955) was technically superior in that the mixed venous blood sampled from the pulmonary artery and oxygen saturation of arterial blood was estimated directly. Unfortunately, no estimate was made in early pregnancy; only one subject had her cardiac output measured before 18 weeks: a 38-year-old woman studied at 14 weeks. Also, it seems likely from the relatively high heart rates that these women were not in a basal state and this may be inevitable with the more elaborate technique which involved for example, X-ray location of the catheter and sampling of arterial blood.

It is not easy to summarize these data. Cardiac output almost certainly declines during the last two or three months of pregnancy although the change is variable; the suggestion (Hamilton, 1949; Adams, 1954; Brehm and Kindling, 1955) that it declines to non-pregnant levels is not proven. Nor is there good evidence of the traditionally accepted peak of cardiac output at 28–32 weeks. It seems more likely that the maximum level is maintained at least between 20 and 30 weeks. The pattern of change before mid-pregnancy is not clear. Palmer and Walker found the high plateau of cardiac output to have been reached in their earliest measurements, during the 3rd month, and Hamilton's data also show a steep rise in early pregnancy with the plateau reached by about 16 weeks. Many more data are needed to complete the picture.

There seems no better way of summarizing than by averaging the results of the three studies by Palmer and Walker, Hamilton and

Bader *et al.* (Table 2.1; Figure 2.1). These average figures show that cardiac output rises early in pregnancy from a mean of about 4.5 litres per minute before pregnancy to about 5.5 litres by the 3rd or 4th month. Thereafter, cardiac output changes relatively little; it rises to about 6.0 litres per minute before mid-pregnancy and remains at that level until about the last 2 months during which there is a steady decline to between 5.0 and 5.5 litres per minute at term. This general picture of a plateau about 1.5 litre per minute above the non-pregnant average from before mid-pregnancy to about 32 weeks, followed by a decrease to term has been confirmed in a still unpublished study by Dr W. Walters at the Postgraduate Medical School, London. But, in early pregnancy, before 12 weeks, where few observations have been made, Walters recorded the highest values. One might be tempted to dismiss these high values as possibly due to emotional excitement in women having their first measurement made, but the pulse rates were not unduly high which suggests that excitement did not contribute to the high outputs.

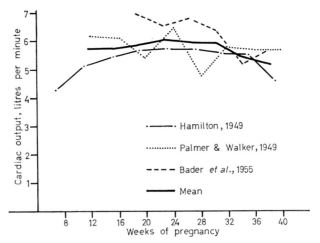

FIGURE 2.1. Cardiac output during pregnancy. The results of three studies where the direct Fick method was used.

To confirm the early rise and to determine its timing it would be necessary to study a number of women from before pregnancy. These figures, it must be emphasized again, refer only to the pregnant woman completely at rest. The effect of exercise will be considered later in this chapter.

The increase in cardiac output is brought about both by an increased heart rate and an increased stroke volume.

Heart rate

Burwell in his textbook (Burwell and Metcalfe, 1958) shows a graph of increasing pulse rate which suggests that the rate rises steadily during pregnancy to a maximum at about 30 weeks which is, on average, some 10 beats per minute above a non-pregnant average of 78; thereafter there is a decline in rate until the end of pregnancy. These figures are based on a serial study of 4 women, one of whom had heart disease, and whose pulse rates varied considerably from one observation to the next; none followed the pattern of the average curve and one woman had a pulse rate in pregnancy which was consistently lower than her post-partum control value (Burwell et al. 1938).

As can be seen from the data collected in Table 2.2, a mean maximum increase of 10 beats per minute is almost certainly an underestimate. The non-pregnant level found by most observers is about 70 per minute, a figure which is well supported by a considerable body of physiological data. There appears to be a marked increase in rate early in pregnancy with four studies giving an average of about 78 for the end of the first trimester (Hamilton, 1949; Brehm and Kindling, 1955; Gemzell, Robbe and Ström, 1957; Ihrman, 1960c). Thereafter, the rate rises more gradually to a maximum of about 85 or a little more in late pregnancy, giving an overall increase in rate of at least 15 per minute. There is little convincing evidence of a fall in rate in late pregnancy although a fall was suggested by the data of Hare and Karn (1929) and Widlund (1945). It is difficult to explain the almost complete absence of change in the women studied by Hare and Karn, but the high non-pregnant value would indicate that these subjects, at least, were not in the basal state. The same can be said of the women whose cardiac output was measured by Bader, Bader, Rose and Braunwald (1955).

Like cardiac output, heart rate can be temporarily raised by a great many minor stimuli, and standardization of conditions is vital for a study of changes during pregnancy. It cannot be said that any of the published investigations is entirely satisfactory from this

TABLE 2.2 Changes in Heart Rate in Pregnancy

Authors	Heart rate per minute — Time in pregnancy	1 month or more post-partum	Non-pregnant	Remarks
Hare and Karn (1929)	*Weeks 5–20* 82.2$_0$; *21–24* 81.3$_0$; *25–28* 84.72; *29–32* 86.86; *33–36* 84.07; *37+* 82.91	—	83.4	Women lying down for 20 minutes. From 54–107 subjects in each group
Landt and Benjamin (1936)	*Months 3* 82; *4* 85; *5* 87; *6* 89; *7* 93; *8* 96; *9* 92	76		Nineteen subjects. From graph—no figures published
Widlund (1945)	*Months 3–4* 72.7; *5* 76.0; *6* 78.3; *7* 82.4; *8* 85.0; *9* 84.7; *10* 82.3	70.8	69.8	157 subjects observed from 1–9 times during pregnancy. Subjects fasting and lying down for 30 minutes
Hamilton (1949)	*1st trimester* 78; *2nd trimester* 78; *3rd trimester* 82	—	68	A cross sectional study of 68 women having cardiac output measured. Fasting and resting

TABLE 2.2. (continued)

Authors	Heart rate per minute — Time in pregnancy	1 month or more post-partum	Non-pregnant	Remarks
Brehm and Kindling (1955)	*Months 2* 76, *4½* 80, *6½* 78, *8* 86, *9* 86, *10* 86	69		256 estimations on 72 healthy women, mostly primigravidae. 30 mins. resting but not 'basal'
Bader, Bader, Rose and Braunwald (1955)	*Weeks 17–20* 87, *21–24* 98, *25–28* 94, *29–32* 91, *33–36* 91, *37–40* 95			A cross sectional study of 46 women having cardiac output measured. 'Basal', post-absorptive
Gemzell, Robbe and Ström (1957)	*Weeks 13.5* 78.2, *20.3* 79.1, *29.8* 86.4, *36.0* 88.9	69.3		A serial study of 20 women. No information about conditions except 'resting in the supine position'
Ihrman (1960c)	*Weeks 9–13* 78.2, *18–21* 79.9, *25–29* 81.1, *35–37* 85.3	64.7		A serial study of 50 women

point of view and a careful longitudinal study of the pulse rates of even a few sleeping pregnant women would be of great interest.

Stroke volume

Since the mean cardiac output in pregnancy rises from $4\frac{1}{2}$ litres per minute to a maximum of about 6 litres per minute, an increase of one third, and the heart rate rises by only about one fifth, from 70 to 85 per minute, it is clear that the amount of blood expelled by the heart at each beat, the stroke volume, must increase also.

A measure of stroke volume can be obtained only from those studies in which cardiac output is estimated and the heart rate counted simultaneously, but almost no such data are available. Adams (1954), without presenting his figures, states that the increase in cardiac output is due primarily to an increased stroke volume; from 84 cc in the non-pregnant woman, to 98 cc at the maximum cardiac output at 28 weeks. As far as can be calculated with figures derived from his graphs the proportionate rise in pulse rate must have been at least as great. Both Hamilton (1949) and Palmer and Walker (1949) counted the heart rate in their subjects, but the information is not published in a form to allow calculation of the stroke volume. Bader et al. (1955) give figures for stroke volume which show little indication of change during pregnancy except for a terminal fall coincident with the fall in cardiac output. Since these workers found unusually high heart rates, it is not easy to interpret the findings.

Arterio-venous oxygen difference

The increase in cardiac output in pregnancy is proportionately greater than the increase in oxygen consumption, particularly in early pregnancy when cardiac output has risen considerably and oxygen consumption relatively little (Chapter 3), so that more oxygen is returned to the heart from the venous circulation and the arterio-venous (A-V) oxygen difference is smaller.

Palmer and Walker found the A-V oxygen difference to be least in early pregnancy, averaging 33 ml per litre in the 3rd month and not reaching the average non-pregnant level of about 45 ml per litre until the 10th month. Apart from curiously aberrant findings in the 7th month all the A-V differences before 34 weeks are below the non-pregnant level. The findings of Bader et al. are similar.

In their series, the A-V differences rose from about 34 at mid-pregnancy to 44 ml per litre at term.

Hamilton's figures are less striking but tell much the same story: the mean A-V differences were 41.57 ml per litre in the first trimester, 43.94 in the second and 48.4 in the third; the non-pregnant average was 46.75.

INTRAVASCULAR PRESSURE

Arterial blood pressure

Arterial blood pressure, 'blood pressure' in the ordinary clinical sense, is generally measured in the brachial artery by indirect means using an inflatable cuff connected to a mercury manometer. Bordley *et al.* (1951) in a report to the Scientific Council of the American Heart Association discussed the errors and inaccuracies of this apparently simple method and made recommendations for the standardization of technique. They begin by saying 'It should be clearly recognized that arterial pressures cannot be measured with precision by means of sphygmomanometers'. When compared to direct measurement of blood pressure the standard method of sphygmomanometry gives a reading for systolic pressure which is 3 to 4 mm Hg too low and a reading for diastolic pressure which is about 8 mm Hg too high. The error of a single measurement is about ±8 mm Hg. For the literature on arterial blood pressure in pregnancy one has to assume a reliable technique; it is seldom possible from the description to know what precautions have been taken. Minor differences of technique may explain some of the differences of findings in apparently similar studies.

The measurement of arterial blood pressure in late pregnancy may be complicated by the so-called 'supine hypotensive syndrome'. Howard, Goodson and Mengert (1953) found that 18 of 160 women at term (11.2 per cent) had a fall of at least 30 mm Hg in systolic blood pressure after lying on their backs for 3 to 7 minutes, and describe a woman in whom the fall was so profound as to resemble surgical shock. The phenomenon is attributed to pressure of the uterus on the inferior vena cava obstructing the return of blood to the heart. Quilligan and Tyler (1959) in a study of 196 women in late pregnancy found a less striking effect. Only 6 (3 per cent) of their subjects showed a fall of systolic blood pressure of 30 mm Hg or more when they lay on their backs; after two minutes there was a mean drop of 3 mm in the pulse pressure of the group.

In almost every investigation of cardiovascular physiology in pregnancy the arterial blood pressure has been recorded, but there have been relatively few systematic studies of large numbers of normal pregnant women. What has been published has been bedevilled by the fact that as blood pressure rises in pregnancy it is increasingly associated with pre-eclamptic toxaemia (for example, MacGillivray, 1961). Many obstetricians regard a blood pressure above a limit of 140 mm Hg systolic, 90 diastolic, or even as low as 130/80, as abnormal in itself. An outstanding example of this un-fortunate prejudgement is provided by Andros (1945). In his study, 300 women each had eleven serial readings of blood pressure made during pregnancy and, perhaps uniquely, most of them had at least one record of blood pressure made before pregnancy. The general conclusion that 'systolic blood pressure does not vary at any time during normal pregnancy from the level for a normal and healthy young woman who is not pregnant' is invalidated by the arbitrary condition that 'a systolic pressure of 140 or a diastolic pressure of 90 at any time during the pregnancy eliminated the patient from this study even in the absence of any other sign or symptom of toxemia.' For the subjects who did not exceed those limits the mean systolic blood pressure varied little more than 1 mm on either side of about 115 mm Hg, but the diastolic pressure was lower in the first two-thirds of pregnancy, about 69 mm, than in the final trimester when it rose to about 72 which was the non-pregnant mean. The pulse pressure, the difference between systolic and diastolic pressures, was therefore higher than normal until the last trimester.

Henry (1936) studied 618 women at a Montreal ante-natal clinic, but he included in his analysis 'a number . . . whose blood pressure was moderately elevated but did not show any other signs or symptoms of toxaemia'. He did not present figures, only a graph from which it appears that the mean systolic pressure was between 115 and 120 mm Hg until the last three weeks of pregnancy when it rose slightly to about 125. The diastolic pressure was close to 65 mm Hg until about seven months when it rose slowly to about 70 to 75 mm. Pulse pressure remained consistently about 50 mm Hg. Henry concluded that the systolic pressure was slightly lower than in the non-pregnant woman and the diastolic pressure quite a lot lower. Pulse pressure was about 10 mm Hg above the average non-pregnant figure. There was no difference between primigravidae and multigravidae. Henry's description is similar to the findings of Hare and Karn (1929), Burwell *et al.* (1938) and Brehm and Kindling (1955).

In summary, the evidence suggests that the systolic arterial blood pressure in pregnancy is probably a little below the non-pregnant level, rising in late pregnancy, and the diastolic pressure is considerably below non-pregnant levels from early in pregnancy until the last 2 or 3 months when it rises towards non-pregnant levels. Pulse pressure, for at least the first two-thirds of pregnancy appears to be raised above non-pregnant. This description is pictorial rather than numerical because the actual readings, which vary considerably from study to study, are probably influenced by the techniques of measuring blood pressure and there would be nothing to gain from attempting a grand average. There is no way of knowing to what extent the figures are influenced by other things; for example the age structure of the population studied might have a marked effect because there is abundant evidence that the arterial blood pressure rises with age, at least in primigravidae (MacGillivray, 1961).

PERIPHERAL RESISTANCE

The peripheral resistance of the circulation is calculated from the cardiac output and the mean arterial blood pressure. Since cardiac output is raised in pregnancy and arterial blood pressure is not, it follows that the resistance to flow, the peripheral resistance, must be decreased. Bader *et al.* (1955) made the calculation from their data and showed that the total peripheral resistance was considerably below normal in mid-pregnancy, 986 dynes sec cm^{-5} in the period 14–24 weeks, and rose progressively towards a normal non-pregnant figure of about 1250 at term.

Venous pressure

Compared to arterial blood pressures, changes in venous pressures during pregnancy can be relatively dramatic. It seems to be established that the pressure in the veins of the arm is not altered by pregnancy (Thomson *et al.* 1938; Bickers, 1942; McLennan, 1943). But pressures in the femoral and other leg veins are high. McLennan (1943) reviewed the evidence and presented the results of a large scale investigation of his own; some of his data are shown in Figure 2.2.

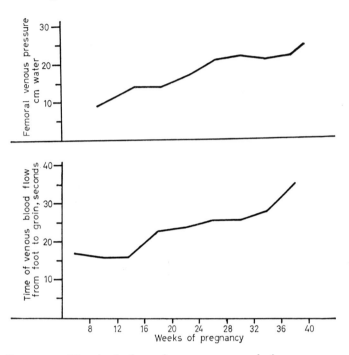

FIGURE 2.2. The rise in femoral venous pressure during pregnancy (MacLennan, 1943) compared to the slowing of venous flow in the lower limb (Wright, Osborn and Edmonds, 1950)

The femoral veins lead directly to the inferior vena cava and the heart without intervening valves, so that with the subject horizontal venous pressures from the legs to the heart are normally similar. The pressure in the right atrium of the heart is not raised in pregnancy (Palmer and Walker, 1949; Hamilton, 1949) and as Ferris and Wilkins (1937) pointed out, a rise in femoral venous pressure without a rise in right atrial pressure must indicate venous obstruction between the two points. In pregnancy there are two possible causes for the obstruction: simple mechanical pressure by the weight of the uterus on the iliac veins and inferior vena cava and by the pressure of the foetal head on the iliac veins; and hydro-dynamic obstruction due to the outflow of blood at relatively high pressure from the uterus. There is evidence for both of those mechanisms. The high pressure in the femoral veins drops abruptly after delivery. McLennan (1943) for example, found that at caesarean section femoral venous pressure dropped abruptly when the foetus was removed and before removal of the placenta. He describes the change as similar to that seen after removal of a big pelvic tumour and interprets it as indicating that obstruction in pregnancy is mechanical and not due to the 'arterio-venous' shunt of the placenta discharging blood at a higher pressure into the pelvic veins. Wright, Osborn and Edmonds (1950) found confirmatory evidence in that venous blood flow in the legs was greatly reduced after the foetal head had engaged in the pelvic brim.

On the other hand there is evidence that blood at relatively high pressure does leave the uterus, particularly when it contracts. Palmer and Walker (1949) showed a striking rise in right atrial pressure associated with painless uterine contractions in late pregnancy, and Hendricks (1958) calculated that 250–300 ml of blood is expelled from the uterus during a contraction in labour. Bickers (1942) measured venous pressure in both femoral veins and showed convincingly that when the pressures were dissimilar, the placenta, which he localized by passing his hand into the uterus after delivery, was always implanted on the side of the higher pressure. In eleven such cases the mean pressure on the side of implantation was 199 mm of water; on the other side it was 172 mm of water, a difference of 27 mm. In twelve cases where the placenta was on the anterior or posterior wall of the uterus the difference in pressures between the two femoral veins never exceeded 12 mm and the mean difference was 3 mm. Where ankle oedema was greater on one side than the other, the greater oedema was on the side of implantation.

As would be expected with a pressure rise due to obstruction, the rate of blood flow in the leg veins is also considerably reduced. Wright, Osborn and Edmonds (1950) injected saline labelled with [24]Na into a vein on the dorsum of the foot and timed its appearance at the groin with a Geiger counter. The increase in time taken is parallel to the rise in pressure shown by McLennan (Figure 2.2): the speed of flow is approximately halved and the venous pressure doubled by the end of pregnancy.

While it seems likely that obstruction by the weight of the uterus and by the uterine blood both play a part in raising venous pressure in the legs, the pure weight effect is probably the more important.

Varicose veins of the legs and vulva, and haemorrhoids, may appear in pregnancy and are usually accentuated by pregnancy if they were present beforehand. It would be reasonable to assume that the heightened intravenous pressure would contribute to their development. But while some women develop huge tortuous veins in pregnancy, the majority of women have no visible varices which suggests that other influences may be at least as important. McCausland et al. (1961) showed by an ingenious finger plethysmographic method that distensibility of veins, their degree of dilatation for a given pressure, increased by about half during pregnancy and returned quickly to non-pregnant levels in the puerperium. In women with varicose veins the increase in distensibility of the finger veins was much greater than in women who had none. The reason for the increase in distensibility and for the difference between the two groups of women is unknown but McCausland et al. suggest that it may be hormonal.

Another difference was found in women with varicose veins by Veal and Hussey (1941). Pressure in the popliteal vein of a standing woman was measured before and after the exercise of rising on tiptoe 20 to 30 times per minute. In women with varicose veins, but not in others, there was a rise in pressure after exercise.

LOWER LIMB OEDEMA

This is an appropriate place to consider oedema of the legs. Pitting oedema of the lower limbs is noted in the routine clinical records of about 30 per cent of primigravidae who have no sign of preeclampsia; and in about 5 per cent there is clinical evidence of more generalized skin oedema, causing for example undue tightness of rings or puffiness of the face. These incidences, especially of generalized oedema, are considerably raised when associated with hypertension in late pregnancy. It is reasonable to attribute the gravitational oedema of the legs to the increased venous pressure. The evidence by Bickers (1942) that femoral pressure was greater in oedematous legs, and where there was oedema in only one leg was greater on that side, supports the view. It is also well recognised clinically that the oedema usually goes away when the legs are raised for a few hours and is greatly accentuated by periods of standing. Further research may show that in normal pregnancy the water content of the skin is raised, and that this phenomenon should be differentiated from the gravitational type of oedema which is of mechanical origin.

The overall picture in late pregnancy of gravitational oedema, falling plasma volume, falling cardiac output, increased pulse rate and increased diastolic arterial blood pressure is similar to the acute effect of gravity which is well known from experiments on non-pregnant subjects on a tilting table (Turner, Newton and Haynes, 1930). At least part of the fall in cardiac output in the last weeks of pregnancy may be attributed to the slowing of circulation in the lower limbs from venous obstruction. If something of the order of one litre of blood per minute is pumped through the lower limbs in early pregnancy, then the reduction of blood flow caused by venous obstruction may be about half a litre per minute. Although this is an attractive explanation of the fall in cardiac output we have only suggestive evidence that blood flow through the lower limbs is reduced; flow rate is undoubtedly less but could be compensated by an increased size of veins so that volume of flow was maintained. The supine hypotensive syndrome (see p. 61) is an exaggeration of the same mechanism. Zimmermann (1950) showed an immediate rise in cardiac output, following removal of the placenta and baby at caesarean section.

Pulmonary blood pressure

Angelino *et al.* (1954) and Bader *et al.* (1955) showed that the pressure in the right ventricle, the pulmonary artery and the pulmonary 'capillaries' remained at the normal non-pregnant level throughout pregnancy as would be expected since the pulmonary circulation is known to have a great capacity for absorbing high rates of blood flow without pressure change. It can do this only by decreasing resistance to flow, probably by dilatation of the vascular bed, so that when cardiac output is increased the volume of the pulmonary circuit also increases. The characteristic radiographic appearance of 'increased vascularity' and enlarged pulmonary vessels which is almost invariable in pregnancy supports this view.

Unfortunately, no satisfactory measurement of pulmonary blood volume has been published. Adams (1954) found the 'central blood volume', which he calculated from his dye indicator curves, to be increased in pregnancy but he sampled his arterial blood from the femoral artery after injecting dye into an arm vein and the volume measured therefore included all the blood between injection and collection, much more than pulmonary blood volume. On the other hand Lagerlöf et al. (1949) in a dye dilution study found the mean pulmonary blood volume in eight pregnant women to be below the non-pregnant average.

CIRCULATION TIME

We have shown above that blood flow in the lower limbs is slowed in late pregnancy, but there is no convincing evidence of a change in the speed of blood flow elsewhere in the body. Speed of blood flow is generally expressed as circulation time, the shortest time a particle of blood takes to go from one point to another, and in practice this is measured between the arm and either the lung or the tongue. If a substance such as saccharin or decholin is injected into an arm vein its arrival at the tongue, indicated by a sweet or bitter taste, can be timed. The arm-lung time can be similarly estimated with paraldehyde or ether which is detected when it reaches the breath. More modern methods depend on radioactive tracers or dyes which can be detected objectively but they have not been used in pregnancy.

Theoretically, if a small labelled section of blood travels directly from the point of entry to the point of detection, circulation time is equal to the volume of the vessels between the two points divided by the flow. In fact, the labelling substance inevitably spreads by mixing and if there are big differences of vessel bore *en route* not all the blood will travel at the same speed as the label. The measurement is therefore only semi-quantitative and changes are difficult to interpret since they may be due to either a volume change or a change of flow or both. A big change in blood flow with a parallel change in the volume of the vascular system would result in no alteration of circulation time.

The measurements of circulation time which have been made in pregnancy are contradictory. Spitzer (1933) and Landt and Benjamin (1936) who both measured the arm-tongue circulation time with decholin found no trend in pregnancy and all values were within the normal non-pregnant range. Greenstein and Clahr (1937) used saccharin for arm-tongue times and ether for arm-lung times. They found 13 pregnant subjects to have times which were within the normal non-pregnant range, but claimed that the average times increased during pregnancy, from 11 seconds at 18 weeks to 15 seconds at the end of pregnancy for arm-tongue time and from 4 seconds to 5.5 seconds for arm-lung time. There was considerable individual variation and several exceptions to the average trend.

Manchester and Loube (1946) made a similar investigation of 48 women, with calcium gluconate and paraldehyde and came to the opposite conclusion. The mean arm-tongue time fell from 12.4 in the first trimester to 10.2 in the 3rd and the mean arm-lung time fell from 6.6 to 5.0 seconds.

It seems reasonable to conclude that if the circulation time does change, the change is trivial. Since a great increase in blood flow through the lungs is undoubted, that conclusion strengthens the indirect evidence of a parallel increase in pulmonary blood volume.

CHANGES IN HEART SIGNS
Size of the heart

Physicians in the nineteenth century believed, on the basis of physical examination of the chest, that the heart enlarged in pregnancy. They were almost certainly led to the conclusion by a change in the position of the heart to the left, but modern methods of stereoscopic radiology have confirmed their belief, and a great many studies have been made. Interest has been aroused again recently by Räihä and his colleagues (Räihä et al. 1957; Räihä, 1959) who have suggested that women with small hearts are more liable to have premature babies.

Gemzell, Robbe and Ström (1957) found the mean heart volume of 20 healthy pregnant women to rise from 671 ml at 14 weeks to 746 ml at 36 weeks, an increase of 75 ml, and Ihrman (1960d) described a similar increase of 78 ml from 611 ml at 9–13 weeks to 689 ml at 35–37 weeks in a group of 50 women. Räihä (1959) described a relation between heart size in the mother and the birth weight of her baby, but heart size shows also a close correlation with the body size of the subject (Ihrman, 1960d) and one would therefore expect to find a relation to birth weight. Hytten et al. (1963) showed that a very small correlation between the heart volume at 30 weeks of pregnancy and the size of the baby at

F

birth disappeared completely when the effect of maternal height was taken into account.

Calculation of heart volume from a few linear measurements which are themselves subject to considerable observer error, involves a number of assumptions, the bases of which are not necessarily constant in the changing conditions of pregnancy; but even allowing the validity of the calculations it is not clear what the increase in size of the X-ray shadow of the heart represents. Some of it must be attributable to increase in diastolic filling associated with the greater stroke volume, but Ihrman (1960d) found the size to be still increased two months after delivery and concluded that hypertrophy must also have occurred. In the series studied by Gemzell *et al.* the mean heart volume had returned to the non-pregnant average one month after delivery.

Position of the heart

A large number of studies agree that the heart is pushed upwards by the elevation of the diaphragm and rotated forwards. This, together with the enlargement of the heart, produces a characteristic and well-recognized X-ray picture. In a careful study by Hollander and Crawford (1943) for example, 10 of 18 women showed indentation of the anterior wall of the oesophagus in the right anterior oblique position; in two there was straightening of the upper left cardiac border, and in three prominence of the pulmonary conus.

Electrocardiographic changes

The main changes in the ECG are attributed to the changed position of the heart. Many studies agree that there is a deviation to the left in the electrical axis of the heart. In the series studied by Hollander and Crawford (1943) the average maximum shift was 15°, the highest individual 28°. The movement was reversed a little in late pregnancy. In many women the T wave becomes negative or flattened in lead III (Landt and Benjamin, 1936; Hollander and Crawford, 1943; Zatuchni, 1951; de Bettencourt and Fragoso, 1952; Gemzell, Robbe and Ström, 1957) with occasional depression of the S–T segment in both chest and limb leads (Oram and Holt, 1961). Other changes described include low voltage QRS complexes and deep Q waves, and the occasional occurrence of U waves. Zatuchni (1951) discusses the evidence for hypertrophy of the heart, a subject of considerable debate in the literature; he could find no cardiographic evidence of it, although de Bettencourt and Fragoso (1952) thought the evidence in some of their subjects suggested hypertrophy.

The X-ray and ECG changes described briefly above are variable, both in their occurrence and extent, and taken with the common finding of a systolic murmur over the base of the heart are liable to mimic minor degrees of heart disease. These problems are discussed by Burwell and Metcalfe (1958).

REGIONAL DISTRIBUTION OF INCREASED BLOOD FLOW

The uterus

The uterus can be regarded as the central target of the increased circulation of pregnancy, but the measurement of uterine blood flow is particularly difficult and relatively few observations have been made.

TECHNIQUES OF MEASUREMENT

Ideally, what is wanted is a direct measure of uterine blood flow, but even in animals where direct-reading flow meters can be introduced into vessels measurement is by no means easy because the uterus is supplied by a number of arterial channels and it is not possible to know how much of the total supply is destined for the placenta.

An electromagnetic flowmeter has been used by Assali, Rauramo and Peltonen (1960) to measure uterine blood flow in a few women in early pregnancy but for late pregnancy no use of flowmeters has been made and the results are all based on indirect methods. Two groups of American workers have used techniques based on an application of the Fick principle (see p. 51) with nitrous oxide, a method originally developed by Kety (1948) for cerebral blood flow.

Techniques of applying this principle to the human uterus have been described by Assali *et al.* (1953a) and Romney, Reid, Metcalfe and Burwell (1955). Only one term in the equation can be found with confidence, the arterial concentration, because it can be measured in samples from any convenient artery such as the brachial. By contrast, it is difficult to sample uterine venous blood at all and it may be impossible to get a representative sample because the plexus of veins which drains the uterus drains also the vagina and other structures, and blood predominantly from the placental site is unlikely to be the same as blood from elsewhere in the uterus. A vein may be cannulated directly, at caesarean section for example, and both teams have done that although the veins tear easily and it is not as simple as it might first seem. Moreover the subject must be kept under anaesthesia with the abdomen open for as long as it takes the nitrous oxide to equilibrate with the uterine contents, at least half an hour, possibly much longer.

Assali has used a second method of sampling the uterine venous blood by passing a long Cournand catheter through the basilic vein to the heart, through the right atrium, the inferior vena cava and the iliac veins to the uterine venous plexus. This technique is not only unsuccessful in many cases; it is difficult to justify it on other grounds. Assali says that the procedure 'does not involve serious risk', but cardiac arrhythmia is common and pulmonary embolism apparently occurs, albeit 'rarely'. Perhaps the greatest hazard is the prolonged use of X-ray fluoroscopy to see where the catheter is during the long manipulative process. Assali says 'we have not seen serious radiation effects' but 'patients who are apprehensive or sensitive to radiation should be eliminated.'

The next difficulty is the estimation of the amount of the nitrous oxide in the uterus and its contents. Romney et al. assume that the myometrium is in equilibrium with maternal arterial blood after 30 minutes and assume an average weight of 1 kg for the uterus. They assume also that the foetus and placenta are in equilibrium with umbilical arterial blood although, as Assali recognized, the body fat of the foetus, which may be a considerable though variable quantity at term, dissolves relatively much more nitrous oxide than the rest of the foetus. The concentration in liquor amnii can be measured; its volume has to be assumed but errors in assessing liquor volume would have a relatively small effect on the final sum.

Huckabee (1962) criticized the use of nitrous oxide because of its prolonged equilibration time. Instead he injected 4-amino antipyrine in an application of the Fick principle to uterine blood flow and claimed that it diffused quickly into the uterus and foetus, reaching equilibrium in 15 to 20 minutes.

It must be clear from this brief summary that estimates of uterine blood flow rest on elaborate and difficult, even hazardous techniques which involve a number of assumptions some of which may lead to substantial errors.

One other method of estimating blood flow in the placental site itself has been used by Browne (1959). The chorio-decidual space can be approached directly, if the placenta is implanted anteriorly, by putting a needle through the abdominal and uterine walls; Browne claims that this presents no technical difficulty but a recent study by Fuchs, Spackman and Assali (1963) [see p. 198] suggests that there are considerable problems. When the space has been

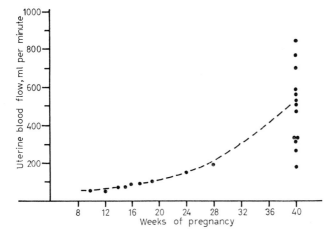

FIGURE 2.3. Uterine blood flow in pregnancy. Figures before 30 weeks are from Assali, Rauramo and Peltonen (1960); those at term are from Romney *et al.* (1955) and Metcalfe *et al.* (1955)

found a tracer dose of ^{24}Na is injected and its disappearance from the space is followed by a Geiger counter placed over the site of injection. If the size of the pool into which the sodium is injected is known then the blood flow through it can easily be calculated from the slope of disappearance of the radiation. Unfortunately the size of the pool cannot be known. Browne suggests that 250 ml would be 'a not unreasonable figure' but the same could be said of an estimate of 150 ml which would almost halve the estimate of blood flow. Some sodium will disappear across the placenta and Browne estimates this as about $7\frac{1}{2}$ per cent, but the disappearance of most of it must surely depend on where in the placental pool the injection is made. If the sodium is placed immediately over a venous outflow the disappearance may be very much quicker than if it were at a

TABLE 2.3. Uterine Blood Flow in Pregnancy

Author	Period of gestation	Foetal weight g	Uterine blood flow ml/min
Metcalfe *et al.*	Term	3.5	590
(1955)	,,	3.1	535
	,,	3.0	330
	,,	3.2	560
	,,	3.1	480
	,,	3.6	510
	,,	3.7	315
	,,	3.7	840
	,,	2.9	255
	,,	3.2	770
	,,	3.5	700
	,,	3.9	335
	,,	3.3	175
	,,	Twins $\begin{cases} 3.5 \\ 3.5 \end{cases}$	1150
	wk		
Assali, Rauramo	10	No data	51.7
and Peltonen	12	,,	56.7
(1960)	14	,,	62.2
	15	,,	66.0
	16	,,	75.6
	16	,,	73.6
	16	,,	72.8
	17	,,	90.5
	19	,,	98.0
	24	,,	153.0
	28	,,	185.0
Huckabee (1962)	Term	No data	'700–800'

more distant part of the system. Certainly the range of values found in normal subjects was very wide: half-times of disappearance of 15 to 30 seconds in 8 illustrated cases.

Browne claims a considerable difference in clearance rates between a group of normal pregnant women and a group of hypertensive pregnant women and, if the finding is confirmed, it might in that context be a useful clinical tool. The uncertainties and possible errors are too big for it to be considered seriously as a physiological technique.

It is to be hoped that new methods may eventually provide

better estimates of uterine blood flow. The electromagnetic flow-meter has yet to be tried in late pregnancy and its application to a uterine artery at term would be technically difficult. The thermo-electric probe described by Prill and Götz (1961) which exploits the principle that the greater the blood flow, the more rapid the transference of heat, may offer a more profitable line of approach.

ESTIMATES OF BLOOD FLOW

For early pregnancy we have only the few observations of Assali, Rauramo and Peltonen (1960). They measured the uterine blood flow in twelve women at operation for hysterotomy, both by the electromagnetic flowmeter and by the nitrous oxide method. The flow could be estimated by flowmeter in only the one uterine artery. The resultant value was doubled to give an estimate of blood flow to the uterus and the estimates were similar to those cal-culated from the nitrous oxide method. The subjects were from 10 to 28 weeks pregnant (Table 2.3, Fig. 2.3). Considering the technical difficulties of the procedure, the curve is astonishingly smooth.

Estimates at term were made by the Boston group (Romney et al. 1955; Metcalfe et al. 1955), using the nitrous oxide method, and these are much more widely scattered (Table 2.3, Fig. 2.3). Faced with this spread we can do no more than agree with the authors that 'the uterine blood flow is in the order of magnitude of 500 cc per minute'. The figures are discussed again in relation to oxygen transport in Chapter 8.

Huckabee's (1962) technique with 4-amino antipyrine has been applied mostly to studies in ruminants, but he quotes, without any detail, the finding that blood flow through the human uterus at term is 700 to 800 ml per minute. Details of this work will be awaited with interest and it is to be hoped that confirmatory studies with this superior tracer will follow.

MECHANICS OF UTERINE BLOOD FLOW

For obvious reasons there is little experimental evidence about the mechanics of blood flow in the human pregnant uterus. We have only the exceedingly elegant experiments, mostly with the monkey, by Ramsey (for example Ramsey (1959)) as a guide to what happens. The picture is well described by Ramsey et al. (1959):

'Arterial blood enters the placenta [intervillous space] from the endometrial arteries under a head of maternal pressure sufficiently higher than that prevailing in the vast, amorphous lake of the inter-villous space so that the incoming stream is driven high up toward the chorionic plate. Gradually this force is spent and lateral dis-persion occurs, aided by the villi which, acting as baffles, promote mixing and slowing and, by their own pulsation, effect a mild stirring. Eventually the blood in the intervillous space falls back upon the orifices in the basal plate which connect with maternal veins, and, since there is an additional fall in blood pressure between the intervillous space and the endometrial veins, drainage is accomplished. The pressure differential is further enhanced by the intermittent myometrial contractions (Braxton Hicks) which compress the thin-walled veins, temporarily preventing escape of blood from the placenta [intervillous space] and raising the inter-villous pressure. When the myometrium relaxes, the elevated inter-villous pressure produces rapid drainage.'

The mean uterine arteriolar pressure is probably not much less than the mean peripheral arterial pressure, between 80 and 100 mm Hg. Pressure in the intervillous space is probably about 15 mm Hg in the relaxed uterus (Alvarez and Caldeyro-Barcia, 1954), some 5 mm Hg above the pressure in the amniotic fluid. In measurements on two subjects not in labour Prystowsky (1958) recorded inter-villous space pressures of 3.2 mm and 5.7 mm Hg but in 2 'resting' uteri during second stage labour pressures were 10.5 and 19.8 mm Hg. Hellman, Tricomi and Gupta (1957) found in 8 women at laparotomy a mean pressure of about 13 mm Hg, with a range of from about 10 to 20 mm. During uterine contractions the pressure is much greater, and remains above the pressure of the amniotic fluid. For 5 of Prystowsky's subjects in the second stage of labour the mean pressure was 38.2 mm Hg and in one subject after a pitocin-induced contraction Hellman et al. found a pressure of about 35 mm Hg. Hendricks (1958) calculated from the increase in cardiac output that 250 to 300 ml of blood are squeezed from the uterus during a contraction in labour.

There is little information about uterine venous pressure. The impression at caesarean section when these veins are tapped is of a considerable pressure but Alvarez and Caldeyro-Barcia (1954) suggest that it is normally only 8 mm Hg. Burwell et al. (1938), in pregnant bitches, showed that uterine venous pressure exceeded the pressure in the femoral veins, and if the same is true of women, that would explain at least in part the rise in femoral pressure in late pregnancy, although the weight of evidence suggests it is due chiefly to mechanical compression (p. 64). There is need for much more work on intravascular pressures in the uterine circulation.

ARTERIO-VENOUS SHUNTS

There is some evidence of direct arterio-venous anastomoses in the uterus. Heckel and Tobin (1956) injected glass spheres of about 200 μ diameter into the arterial system of pregnant and non-pregnant uteri which had their vascular system washed out after removal at operation. In twelve of 21 non-pregnant uteri and each of the 4 pregnant uteri, the spheres were found in the veins, suggesting that there are connecting channels of at least 200 μ diameter, as big as a moderate sized arteriole. Nothing is known of these shunts, or of any mechanism which might control them, although they could obviously divert a great deal of blood from the placental site if they were open. They might, for example, short circuit the uterine blood flow after the placenta is delivered.

Much has been made in the past of Burwell's suggestion that the intervillous circulation is similar in its effects to an arterio-venous fistula (Burwell, 1938). Among suggested similarities are the increased cardiac output and pulse rate with a low diastolic blood pressure, a bruit over the site of the fistula and a relatively high oxygen content in blood leaving the area of high blood flow. But uterine venous blood does not have a particularly high content of oxygen and the other signs common to pregnancy and an arterio-venous fistula cannot be attributed to flow through the placental site. Cardiac output and pulse rate increase most rapidly in early pregnancy when uterine blood flow is trivial. It might more convincingly be argued that the sudden increase in renal blood flow in early pregnancy simulates an arterio-venous shunt.

INTRA-ARTERIAL CUSHIONS

An interesting suggestion has been made by Fourman and Moffat (1961). When an arteriole gives off a branch at right angles, blood in the branch generally has a smaller proportion of cells than the parent vessel because it takes its blood from the periphery of the main vessel while the cells tend to stream in the centre (p. 5). Uterine arterioles give off many right-angled branches and yet, in the rat, the proportion of red cells in the branches exceeds that in the parent vessel. Fourman and Moffat explain this by showing that the branches leave the main vessel from the centre of an intra-arterial cushion which raises the mouth of the branch into the centre of the axial stream. The branches therefore skim the red cells. It would be of the greatest interest to know whether this mechanism operates in the human uterus.

The kidneys

Renal blood flow is fully discussed in Chapter 4. It rises in early pregnancy to about 400 ml per minute above non-pregnant levels by the beginning of the second trimester and declines slowly to about 300 ml per minute above non-pregnant levels by 32 to 36 weeks. Then, within a few weeks of term, it falls quite sharply until the increase is only about 100 ml per minute at the end of pregnancy.

The skin

There is abundant clinical evidence that blood flow in the skin, particularly in the forearms, hands and feet, is greatly increased in pregnancy. The skin is characteristically warm and the hands clammy. The women themselves feel warm and they often complain of the heat but feel more than usually comfortable in cold weather.

A few measurements of blood flow in the extremities have been made with a water-filled plethysmograph which records the change in volume caused by the inflow of blood over a given time, when the venous outflow is obstructed. The method is simple in principle but the temperature of the water can have a considerable influence on the results. Ideally, the conditions of an ordinarily clothed limb should be simulated. Barcroft and Edholm (1945) showed that, for the forearm in non-pregnant subjects, a water temperature of 35 °C maintains the deep muscle temperature but causes skin temperature to rise so that blood flow is overestimated. At a water temperature of 33 °C skin temperature remains constant but the temperature of the deeper tissue falls and blood flow in the forearm is under-estimated. They concluded that the best temperature was probably about 34 °C.

No study using this temperature has been made in pregnancy and it is therefore difficult to interpret the two published investigations which have been made with widely different temperatures.

Burt (1950) used a water temperature of 35°; Abramson, Flachs and Fierst (1943) a temperature of 32°C. Abramson, Flachs and Fierst conducted their experiments at a relatively high room temperature, 25 to 27°C. They claimed that the blood flow in the forearm and leg did not change during pregnancy from non-pregnant control levels, but rose in the hand from about 7 ml per 100 ml of hand volume per minute before pregnancy to about 20 ml per 100 ml in the last trimester of pregnancy.

The study by Burt (1950) is technically more satisfactory. She showed that forearm blood flow rose from about 2 ml per 100 ml per minute in non-pregnant women to about 3.5 ml in late pregnancy but findings were not published to show the pattern of change during pregnancy. A graph shows that flow in the hand was about 2 ml per 100 ml per minute before pregnancy and rose little before 13 weeks, after which it increased to about 7 ml per 100 ml per minute between 13 and 24 weeks, to 10 ml per 100 ml at 29 to 36 weeks and to 13 ml per 100 ml at term; there was a wide individual scatter. The room temperature for Burt's experiments was cool: 17°C, so that there was no likelihood of reflex vasodilatation.

A large scale study of peripheral blood flow in pregnancy was reported by Herbert, Banner and Wakim (1958). They made 5660 determinations of forearm and leg blood flow in 58 normal pregnant women, and 3750 determinations in 25 non-pregnant women. The study appears to have been conducted with great care, but almost no technical detail was published and it is not possible to compare it with the studies described above. Few findings are presented. Blood flow in the forearm rose from a mean of 4.56 ±0.10 ml per 100 ml of tissue in the non-pregnant subjects to 8.73 ±0.48 ml at 36 weeks. In the leg the increase was from 1.87 ±0.10 to 3.18 ±0.29 ml per 100 ml. All the increase took place after mid-pregnancy and there was a tendency for leg flow to fall in the last month of pregnancy.

These data show a similar order of change to that described by Burt but the absolute estimates of flow are widely different in the two studies and it would be pointless to attempt a compromise estimate for the basis of a calculation of the increase in skin flow. We will use the more extensive and more recent data of Herbert, Banner and Wakim (1958). If we assume that the volume of the two forearms is 1200 ml, and of the two legs 4000 ml, then blood flow in forearms and legs together rises from a non-pregnant rate of about 130 ml per minute to about 230 ml per minute at 36 weeks, an increase of 100 ml per minute. Burt found blood flow through the hands to rise much more than that through the forearms. If a similar order of increase occurs in the feet, then hands and feet with a combined volume of about 1500 ml may account for as much as 150 ml per minute, a total maximum increase in blood flow through the extremities of about 250 ml per minute.

Although Herbert, Banner and Wakim found no increase in skin blood flow before 20 weeks, this may have been due to the environmental temperature which appears, from their recorded skin temperatures (see below) to have been much higher than the 17°C in which Burt conducted her experiments. In Burt's subjects, blood flow increased throughout the second trimester, and clinically there is little doubt that the skin feels warmer than usual quite early in pregnancy. It is not likely that the skin of the distal extremities alone participates in the increased blood flow, and indeed subjectively the whole of the skin seems warmer in pregnancy. It may be then that something of the order of an extra 500 ml per minute is circulating in the skin in late pregnancy, which is not an extravagant estimate. In a warm atmosphere the increase will be greater; Burt, for example, showed that blood flow in the forearm rose from 3.5 ml per 100 ml per minute during the control period to 5 or 6 ml per minute after the feet had been immersed in warm water (43.5°C) for thirty minutes. We have suggested above (p. 67) that total blood flow through the lower limbs is probably reduced in the last weeks of pregnancy by mechanical obstruction. Burt (1950) found little change in the skin temperature of the toes during the last trimester, but this is no more than an indirect indicator of flow. In any case, skin flow could be maintained while the total flow through the limb fell.

SKIN TEMPERATURE

The increased blood flow in the skin causes a considerable increase of skin temperature. Burt (1949) showed that the skin temperature of the fingers which were exposed to a room temperature of 17°C for 30 minutes rose steadily from about 22°C before pregnancy to about 34°C at term. For toes the rise was from about 20°C to 27°C. The rise was apparent before the 13th week although Burt considered that there was no real change until the second trimester. Herbert, Banner and Wakim confirm the change. In their subjects finger skin temperature rose from 34.2 ± 0.35 °C in the non-pregnant subjects to 35.9 ± 0.04 °C at 36 weeks and toe skin temperature from 29.1 ± 0.55 °C to 31.7 ± 0.54 °C. The difference in levels suggests that in that study the environmental temperature was much higher than in Burt's study. The finger temperature in late pregnancy is close to the physiological maximum and is similar to the temperature reached in non-pregnant subjects when reflex vasodilatation is caused by immersing the feet in hot water. In late pregnancy little or no increase occurs with such reflex heating.

OTHER EVIDENCE OF PERIPHERAL VASODILATATION

Melbard (1938) examined microscopically the capillaries of the nail bed in 58 pregnant women and found capillary dilatation in two-thirds of them. At term there was an average increase of about 16 per cent in the number of capillaries. Bean, Dexter and Cogswell (1947) observed vascular spiders and palmar erythema in about 60 per cent of white women at an ante-natal clinic.

The vasodilatation in pregnancy apparently obliterates any tendency to arteriolar spasm and Raynaud (1862) noticed the effect when he originally described the syndrome which bears his name. The following translated extract from Raynaud's thesis is taken from his description of a case.

'Mme. X., aet 26 years, has never been ill; but she has been the subject since childhood of an infirmity which makes her an object of curiosity to her acquaintances.

Under the influence of a very moderate cold, and even at the height of summer, she sees her fingers become ex-sanguine, completely insensible, and of a whitish yellow colour. This phenomenon happens often without reason, lasts a variable time, and terminates by a period of very painful reaction, during which the circulation is re-established little by little and recurs to the normal state.

Mme. X. has no better remedy than shaking her hands strongly, or soaking them in lukewarm water. The index of the left hand presents a susceptibility greater than all the other fingers, and is often affected alone. The feet, more impressionable even than the hands, are regularly attacked at meal times and whilst digestion is going on.

Menstruation does not appear to have any influence upon the

appearance of the phenomenon, but it is a remarkable fact that the complete disappearance of attacks of local syncope has always been noted by this lady as the first index of a commencing pregnancy.'

The increased blood flow to the hands may explain the phenomenon of increased fingernail growth observed by Hillman (1960).

Another area where blood flow is apparently increased during pregnancy is the nasal mucous membrane. Congestion of the mucosa over the turbinates occurs in association with the menstrual cycle, with sexual excitement and in pregnancy (Fabricant, 1960). If we assume, as seems reasonable, that the peripheral vasodilatation is for the purpose of dissipating heat from the foetus, then one would expect the nose to participate, since it apparently serves this purpose in many mammals (Scott, 1954). In human pregnancy the vasodilatation does little more than provoke nose bleedings, and where the nasal passages are narrow, an irritating blockage; husbands complain that their wives snore during pregnancy.

Other sites

Little more is known about regional changes in the distribution of blood. Munnell and Taylor (1947) measured hepatic blood flow by the Fick principle with bromsulphthalein in 15 non-pregnant women and 15 pregnant women; there was no difference.

McCall (1949) measured cerebral blood flow by the Fick principle with nitrous oxide and similarly found no difference in rate between pregnant women and men.

It is possible that spleen size increases during pregnancy but the evidence is fragmentary. Sheehan and Falkiner (1948) found spleen size above average in 40 per cent of 163 'unselected routine obstetric necropsies', and stated that the average spleen size increased with length of gestation. It is arguable whether any pregnant woman coming to necropsy can be taken as normal and spleen weights were correlated with hyperplasia of marrow in the femur and conditions such as anaemia, accidental ante-partum haemorrhage and gross puerperal infection. Rupture of the spleen, although rare, seems to be somewhat more frequent in pregnancy and has been described in apparently healthy women following slight exertion or quite trivial trauma (Sparkman, 1958). At present we must reserve judgement on whether or not splenic enlargement is usual in normal pregnancy.

There are other possible sites of increased vascularity. The breasts are certainly engorged in early pregnancy and changes which are probably vascular, a sudden enlargement and a sensation of heat and tingling, may be one of the first signs in pregnancy. Dilated veins on the surface of the breast suggest a greatly increased blood supply throughout pregnancy.

The gut may function with more than usual efficiency in pregnancy (Chapter 5). It is possible that it too has an increased blood supply.

SUMMARY

It should now be possible to describe the increased cardiac output of pregnancy in terms of regional increases in flow. In Figure 2.4 we have attempted to do so. The uterine and renal blood flows can be put in with moderate confidence; the rest is tentative. We have

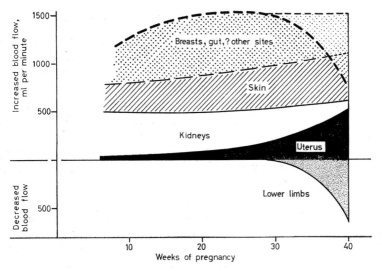

FIGURE 2.4. The distribution of increased cardiac output in pregnancy

kept blood flow in the skin to a maximum during the last trimester of about 500 ml per minute, although it may very well be higher than this in the warm hospital atmospheres where cardiac output is measured. The rest of the cardiac output cannot be accounted for with any certainty. Some undoubtedly goes to the breasts, and some is likely to go to the gut; there may be other areas of increased flow.

Except for renal blood flow there is no evidence that any other site suffers a progressive diminution as pregnancy proceeds. The relatively rapid terminal decrease in cardiac output must be attributed to the fall in blood flow to the lower limbs because of rising venous pressure.

Two points are worth making: first, that many of the regional increases in blood flow start early in pregnancy; uterine blood flow is an exception; second, that two of the major sources of increased blood flow, those to the kidneys and to the skin serve purposes of elimination, the kidneys of waste material, the skin of heat. Both processes require plasma rather than whole blood which gives point to the 'disproportionate' increase of plasma in the expansion of the blood.

CONTROL OF VASCULAR CHANGES

The mechanisms controlling the regional changes in blood flow in pregnancy are unknown. Inevitably the steroid sex hormones have been blamed, but almost nothing is known of their effects. What little is known is discussed in Chapter 6.

The studies by Assali's group on ganglion blocking agents is of considerable interest (for example, Assali *et al.* 1952). An intravenous injection of 400 mg of tetraethyl ammonium chloride (TEAC) was given to normal non-pregnant and pregnant women; the drug blocks the autonomic system at the ganglia. In the non-pregnant subjects there was little effect on blood pressure; the systolic pressure fell on the average by 8 per cent, the diastolic by 4 per cent. In pregnant women the effect was striking and increased throughout pregnancy until in the 3rd trimester the mean fall of systolic blood pressure was 40 per cent and of diastolic, 37 per cent. Two or three days after delivery the effect was found to have disappeared. Assali *et al.* were interested primarily in the fact that this did not occur in women with pre-eclampsia, or indeed in women who did not develop clinical pre-eclampsia until some weeks later, and they suggest that the vessel tone in pre-eclampsia is therefore maintained by a humoral agent. That vessel tone in normal pregnancy is so much more dependent on sympathetic control than before pregnancy, suggests that the autonomic nervous system is correcting for the effect of an active vasodilator substance, perhaps the agent responsible for increasing blood flow in the skin and abolishing Raynaud's disease. It would be of great interest to know what it is.

PHYSIOLOGICAL RESPONSE TO EXERCISE

All that we have said above about cardiovascular adaptations in pregnancy refers to the 'basal' state, or at least to women at rest. Subjectively, the average pregnant woman becomes progressively less able to perform physical exercise. The ordinary daily round of housework and shopping is more tiring; she finds herself cumbersome and awkward, and climbing stairs and boarding buses is more difficult. This is hardly surprising since her weight is much increased and the distribution of added weight alters her normal balance.

How the pregnant woman responds to exercise is the subject of a diffuse and unsatisfactory literature which fails to answer the important questions: is a pregnant woman handicapped in her ability to perform tasks and is she able to work as efficiently as before pregnancy?

Some of the earlier studies, for example those of Hare and Karn (1929) and Krukenberg (1932), showed no difference during pregnancy in the pattern of pulse rates and blood pressure after standard step tests. Gemzell, Robbe and Ström (1957) used a test which consisted of measuring the 'steady state' pulse rate, the plateau of pulse rate reached between the second and sixth minutes of exercise at a given rate of work. Their series of pregnant women worked at rates of 200, 400 and 600 kg-m per minute on a bicycle ergometer; there was no change in the steady state pulse rate during pregnancy at any of these work rates, a curious finding in view of the fact that the resting pulse rate rose progressively during pregnancy.

Harris (1958) in a discussion of exercise tolerance tests in general stated that the relation of heart rate to exercise is poorly understood and that these tests are difficult to interpret. He felt that the most promising measure of exercise tolerance was the oxygen cost. Only Widlund (1945) has attempted such a measure in pregnancy. He measured the 'oxygen debt', the oxygen consumption between two and five minutes after step tests in which the woman lifted her

G

body 7, 13 and 17 metres per minute. As far as can be calculated from his data, they show that in late pregnancy the increase above basal oxygen consumption per minute for the easiest test was 46 cc compared to 48 cc for non-pregnant women, for the middle test the figures were 80 and 78 and for the hardest test 156 and 143 cc. That is, the pregnant woman, for a moderate amount of work uses a little more oxygen. Inasmuch as she would be raising a bigger body weight, differences in this direction are to be expected. It is not possible to deduce from Widlund's data whether, for a *given amount of work* the pregnant woman incurred a greater oxygen debt.

Bader *et al.* (1955) found that the increase in cardiac output was proportional to the increased oxygen uptake in pregnant women pedalling an ergometer while lying on their backs.

What we should like to know is whether a given task, preferably one to which the women are accustomed, costs more in pregnancy; that is, whether her efficiency is lower or whether she simply feels less efficient. Measurements of oxygen consumption over hours in which the woman did, say, a standard amount of walking and climbing, might answer the question. Modern techniques with, for example, the Woolf Integrating Motor Pneumotachograph (IMP) make it reasonable to suppose that such experiments may be made.

CHAPTER 3

Respiration

Principles and Definitions

The main purpose of breathing is to acquire oxygen and to eliminate carbon dioxide in amounts closely related to the needs of the body. To that end the rate and depth of breathing must be exactly controlled. The mixing and effective distribution of gases in the lungs depend on that control. More remotely, tissue respiration and the metabolic activities of the body generally make demands on gas exchange, and the whole is subject to central nervous control. Not all of those aspects of respiratory function have been studied in pregnancy.

A detailed discussion of the methods of investigation is not necessary to an understanding of the results which follow and we will give here no more than a reminder of the divisions of lung volume and a few definitions. Comroe *et al.* (1955) give an outstandingly clear exposition of this subject, and one on which we have drawn in part for this introduction.

Four lung 'volumes' and four 'capacities' are recognized and commonly measured in respiratory physiology (see Fig. 3.3, p. 95).

The four volumes, which do not overlap, are:

(1) *The tidal volume*, the volume of gas inspired or expired in each respiration. Obviously tidal volume will vary with needs, but when not otherwise defined the term refers to quiet respiration at rest. The position of the chest at the end of quiet expiration, when the respiratory muscles are inactive, is known as the resting end-expiratory position.

(2) *Inspiratory reserve volume* is the maximum amount of air which can be inspired, *beyond* the normal tidal inspiration.

(3) *Expiratory reserve volume* is the maximum amount of air which can be expired from the resting end-expiratory position.

(4) *Residual volume* is the volume of gas remaining in the lungs, not including the anatomical dead space of the trachea and bronchial tree, at the end of maximal expiration.

The four 'capacities' each include two or more of the 'volumes' defined above.

(1) *Total lung capacity* includes them all; it is the total amount of gas in the lung at the end of a maximum inspiration.

(2) *Vital capacity* includes all but the residual volume; it is the maximum volume of gas which can be expired after a maximum inspiration.

(3) *Inspiratory capacity* is tidal volume + inspiratory reserve volume; that is it is the maximum volume of gas which can be inspired from the resting end-expiratory position.

(4) *Functional residual capacity* is expiratory reserve volume + the residual volume; that is the amount of gas which remains in the lungs at the resting end-expiratory position, and the volume of gas with which the tidal air must mix.

Except for the residual volume and the lung capacities which contain it, these spaces can readily be measured by direct spirometry. The residual volume must be estimated by a more elaborate gas dilution technique.

Average volumes and capacities for normal healthy women are given in standard physiological texts. Since they vary a little with the technique of measurement, in order to compare pregnant and non-pregnant women measurements should be by the same investigators. We will therefore give normal non-pregnant values later when we discuss the findings for pregnant women.

Ventilation, the volume of air breathed and indices derived from it form the basis of many measurements of lung function for which data have been collected in pregnancy. The *minute volume* is the amount of air inspired and expired in a minute, or the tidal volume multiplied by the rate of respiration. From a functional viewpoint this simple measure is insufficient. Some of the tidal air merely fills the anatomical dead space and makes no contribution to gas exchange, and the important measure is *alveolar ventilation* which roughly approximates to tidal volume minus the volume of the anatomical dead space. It should be clear therefore, that, for a given minute volume, a fast respiratory rate with a small tidal volume gives a smaller alveolar ventilation than a slow respiratory rate with a correspondingly bigger tidal volume.

The *ventilatory equivalent* for oxygen is the number of litres of ventilation for each 100 ml of oxygen taken up by the body.

TESTS OF VENTILATION

Two tests are commonly employed:

(1) The *maximum breathing capacity* (MBC) or maximum voluntary ventilation, is the maximum amount of air which can be inspired and expired by forced voluntary breathing over 15 seconds. The test may be by expiring into a bag whose contents are subsequently measured in a gas meter, or through a recording gas meter or respirometer. When the test is performed conscientiously it is extremely exhausting and requires considerable co-operation from the subject. It correlates closely (Needham, Rogan and McDonald, 1955) with a less exacting test:

(2) The *timed vital capacity*, usually expressed as the proportion of the vital capacity which can be exhaled in a given time from a maximum inspiration. Normally, over 80 per cent of the vital capacity can be exhaled in 1 second and 100 per cent in 3 seconds. The *air velocity index* defined as

$$\frac{\text{percentage of predicted MBC}}{\text{percentage of predicted vital capacity}}$$

is sometimes used, but as Comroe *et al.* have said, it is open to mis-interpretation because a ratio of unity can result from a proportionate reduction of both numerator and denominator. If the subject is breathing maximally, as in a test of maximum breathing capacity, and the gas movements are recorded on a high speed kymograph, the rate of gas flow at various times in the respiratory cycle can be calculated and so inspiratory and expiratory breathing 'resistance' may be separated. One other test of function has been investigated in pregnancy: the *intrapulmonary mixing index*, which measures the adequacy of distribution and mixing of inspired gas in the alveoli. It depends on the speed with which nitrogen can be flushed out of the lungs when pure oxygen is breathed.

The diffusion of gases between the alveoli and the pulmonary blood has not been studied in pregnancy. Changes in pulmonary blood flow are discussed in Chapter 2. There are, by contrast, many studies of alveolar and blood gas content, and of blood pH.

RESPIRATORY FUNCTION IN PREGNANCY
Lung volumes and capacities
VITAL CAPACITY

The only fraction of lung volume which has received repeated attention is vital capacity. Cugell, Frank, Gaensler, and Badger (1953) made a most detailed and comprehensive serial study of respiratory function in 19 women during normal pregnancy and again between two and six months post-partum. They found no difference between the vital capacities, measured at term and post-partum both in the upright and supine positions, and there was no real change during the course of pregnancy. Rubin, Russo and Goucher (1956), on the other hand, found the mean vital capacity at term in eight healthy women to be 294 ml below the mean vital capacity measured in the same women 7 to 14 weeks post-partum. This difference was statistically significant although of the eight women three, all primigravidae in whom the foetus had moved down in the abdomen, showed no real difference. Rubin *et al.* reviewing the literature, claim a majority as supporting their findings but they agree that the fall of vital capacity may be terminal, as suggested for example, by Alward (1930). Most authors have shown little or no trend during pregnancy, or if any-thing, a slight increase of vital capacity, as for example Root and Root (1923) in a detailed study of one woman, Cohen and Thomson (1936), Landt and Benjamin (1936), Widlund (1945), and Ihrman (1960b). Usually, where the vital capacity in pregnancy has been shown to be below that of non-pregnant controls, the studies have been cross-sectional and the non-pregnant control groups were not necessarily comparable in physique to the pregnant subjects. For such a study to be valid pregnant and non-pregnant subjects should be carefully matched.

There is no final proof that vital capacity is reduced in pregnancy and until more repeat measurements have been made in the same subjects, we will accept the findings of Cugell *et al.* that vital capacity is unchanged.

TIDAL VOLUME, RESPIRATORY RATE, AND
MINUTE VENTILATION

Tidal volume rises throughout pregnancy (Plass and Oberst, 1938; Widlund, 1945; Cugell *et al.* 1953). In the study by Cugell *et al.* the mean tidal volume at term was 678 ml compared to 487 ml post-partum, an increase in pregnancy of 191 ml or 39 per cent. In nine subjects measured each month from the 3rd month, the tidal volume was already raised by nearly 100 ml at the 3rd month, and rose progressively thereafter until term (Figure 3.1).

The respiratory rate rises relatively little in pregnancy, if at all. In the nine women studied serially by Cugell *et al.* there was no

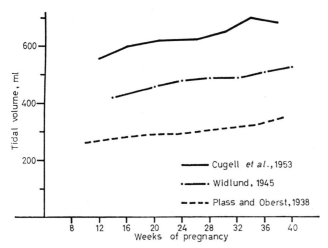

FIGURE 3.1. Respiratory tidal volume in pregnancy

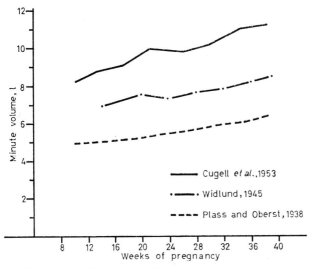

FIGURE 3.2. Respiratory minute volume in pregnancy

change in rate from an average of 16 per minute and Widlund (1945) also found a constant rate of about 16. Landt and Benjamin (1936) showed a small rise of rate in 19 women, from 16 to about 18 per minute at term, and the average for all 19 of the subjects studied by Cugell *et al.* was 16 at term and 15 some months post-partum. Since there is little or no increase in respiratory rate the minute ventilation rises in proportion to the increased tidal volume. In the 19 subjects studied by Cugell *et al.* the mean minute ventilation was 10.34 litres at term compared to 7.27 litres post-partum, a rise in pregnancy of 3.07 litres or 42 per cent. A similar proportionate increase both in tidal volume and minute ventilation was found by Plass and Oberst (1938) and Widlund (1945), but as shown in Figures 3.1 and 3.2 there are big differences in the absolute values recorded by what should be a technically simple measurement. There is in fact a strong secular trend more likely to be referable to improvement in the apparatus used than to change in the test subjects.

The pregnant woman, then, increases ventilation by breathing more deeply and not more frequently. Since her anatomical dead space is not likely to be altered by pregnancy, the minute *alveolar ventilation* will be increased even more than overall minute ventilation. If we assume a constant dead space of 140 ml, then tidal alveolar ventilation will, on the average figures of Cugell *et al.* be 538 ml (678–140) at term compared to 347 (487–140) post-partum, and minute alveolar ventilation at term will be 8.6 litres, an increase above 5.2 litres of about 65 per cent. We will discuss minute ventilation again (p. 100) when gas exchange is considered.

INSPIRATORY CAPACITY

The inspiratory capacity (tidal volume + inspiratory reserve volume) is increased in late pregnancy. Cugell *et al.* found a mean increase, from 2625 to 2745 ml; 120 ml, or 5 per cent of the non-pregnant capacity. Thirteen of their nineteen women showed an increase and two showed no change. Rubin, Russo and Goucher (1956) claimed, on the basis of their study of nine subjects, that there was no change in inspiratory capacity. Nevertheless, four of the women showed an increase and one no real change, and the apparent absence of change was largely determined by one subject with a very small capacity in pregnancy and an increase of 700 ml at the post-partum measurement. Cugell *et al.*, in their nine subjects, measured serially, found the increase to occur only from about the 6th or 7th month of pregnancy.

EXPIRATORY RESERVE

In the Cugell study the mean expiratory reserve was 555 ml at term and 655 ml post-partum, a decrease in pregnancy of 100 ml or 15 per cent. Again this change developed only in the last half of pregnancy. Rubin et al. also found a low expiratory reserve in pregnancy.

RESIDUAL VOLUME, FUNCTIONAL RESIDUAL CAPACITY

We have only the main study of Cugell et al. for these volumes. Mean residual volume was 770 ml at term and 965 post-partum, a fall of 195 ml or 20 per cent; functional residual capacity was 1325 ml and 1620 ml, a fall in pregnancy of 295 ml or 18 per cent. Both changes were progressive from about mid-pregnancy.

The conspicuous fall in the functional residual capacity makes the increased tidal volume and alveolar ventilation even more impressive; the increased volume of tidal air is required to mix with a much smaller residual volume of air in the lungs.

The changed lung volumes of pregnancy have been likened by Patton et al. (1953) to induced pneumoperitoneum where total lung volume and vital capacity are unchanged but inspiratory capacity is increased at the expense of expiratory reserve and residual volume.

ANATOMICAL CHANGES

Anatomical changes in the chest during pregnancy have been recognized for many years and pregnant women themselves are well aware that their lower ribs flare and do not always fully recover their original position after pregnancy. Thomson and Cohen (1938) found the subcostal angle to increase progressively from about 68° in early pregnancy to 103° in late pregnancy. The changes were noted long before there was any possibility that they could be attributed to mechanical pressure. In his series the angle had returned to normal within a few weeks of delivery. Thomson and Cohen noted also, in X-ray studies, that the level of the diaphragm rose in pregnancy by a maximum of about 4 cm and that the transverse diameter of the chest increased by about 2 cm. A similar picture was shown by Klaften and Palugyay (1926, 1927). McGinty

(1938) in a comprehensive review of the literature found that the idea of the diaphragm being 'splinted' and its action obstructed by pregnancy had been current since the early 19th century, with few dissentients. He made a careful X-ray study of two pregnant women and found the excursion of the diaphragm during breathing, whether sitting or lying down, to be greater in pregnancy than in the puerperium, and he concluded that breathing in pregnancy is more diaphragmatic than costal.

Omatsu (1957) quotes the work of a colleague, Takano, who found by electromyography that the abdominal muscles have much less tone and are less active in pregnancy.

Lung markings are always found to be increased in radiographs taken during pregnancy, partly because of the more collapsed state of the lungs in expiration and partly because there is more blood in the lung vessels (see Chapter 2).

Summary. The volume of air breathed each minute increases considerably during pregnancy and the increase is brought about by an increase in tidal volume with little or no increase in respiratory rate. Because of this, alveolar ventilation is increased proportionately more than total ventilation. The vital capacity is probably unchanged by pregnancy but there is a rearrangement of its components; the inspiratory capacity increases at the expense of the expiratory reserve so that the lung is relatively more collapsed at the end of a normal expiration. The residual volume, and with it the total lung volume, is reduced. These changes are summarized in Figure 3.3.

Tests of pulmonary function

MAXIMUM BREATHING CAPACITY (MBC)

Maximum breathing capacity, the maximum rate of ventilation the subject can achieve by forced voluntary breathing for 15 seconds, seems to be little affected by pregnancy. Cugell *et al.* (1953) found the mean rate to be 96 litres per minute in late pregnancy and 102 litres per minute some months after delivery; the difference of 6 per cent was barely significant statistically. There was no change during the course of pregnancy. Rubin, Russo and Gaucher (1956) found the MBC to be 59.9 litres per minute per square metre of body surface in late pregnancy and 54.9 post-partum, a difference which was not significant. In the study of Ihrman (1960b) the MBC in late pregnancy, 91.0 litres per minute, was the same as the

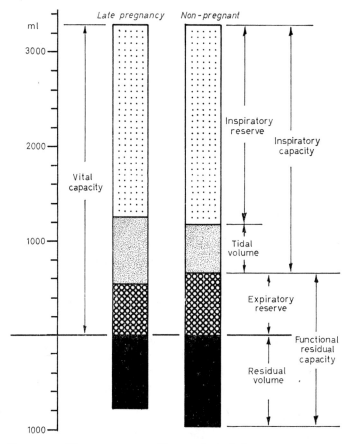

FIGURE 3.3. The components of lung volume in late pregnancy compared with those in the non-pregnant subject

MBC two months after delivery, 90.6 litres. Ihrman found a marked increase during pregnancy, from about 70 litres per minute in the first trimester. The increase might be due to training as Ihrman hints in his discussion. It is not possible to interpret the much larger difference in his study between the pregnant women and a group of non-pregnant women who had a relatively large MBC of 120 to 140 litres per minute, a breathing capacity which could be regarded as a good mean for young men (Comroe *et al.* 1955).

TIMED VITAL CAPACITY

Timed vital capacity is not appreciably altered by pregnancy. In the women studied by Cugell *et al.* (1953) the average proportion of the upright vital capacity which could be expired in the first second was 82 per cent in pregnancy and 84 per cent post-partum. The subjects studied by Rubin, Russo and Gaucher (1956) performed the test semirecumbent and recorded 73.1 per cent when pregnant and 80.3 per cent post-partum.

Rates of gas flow, both average and maximum, during inspiration and expiration are little altered in pregnancy as might be predicted from the unchanged MBC and timed vital capacity (Rubin, Russo and Gaucher, 1956). But it was also shown by these workers that the pressure required to achieve these flow rates in pregnancy was less than in the non-pregnant subject. They measured 'alveolar pressure' by the method of interrupted flow described by Otis and Proctor (1948), a technique criticized by Comroe *et al.* (1955) but still useful for a comparative study.

It is difficult to explain why, for a given pressure of air in the alveoli, gas flow to and from them should be greater, because it is by no means clear what influences affect the resistance to breathing. The major part may be resistance to flow through the tracheobronchial tree but resistance in the lung tissue itself is also involved. Rubin, Russo and Gaucher attribute the change in resistance to relaxation of smooth muscle in the airways, possibly due to relaxin.

GAS DISTRIBUTION IN THE LUNGS

As would be expected from the greatly increased alveolar ventilation, mixing and distribution of gas in the lungs is more efficient in pregnant than in non-pregnant subjects. Cugell *et al.* (1953), in their larger group found the 'pulmonary mixing index', the percentage of nitrogen remaining in the lung after 7 minutes of breathing pure oxygen, to be 0.46 in late pregnancy and 0.56 some weeks after delivery; in the 9 women studied serially there was a progressive fall from about 0.60 in early pregnancy to about 0.40 at the end.

Gas exchange

OXYGEN CONSUMPTION

Published studies of basal metabolism in pregnancy are almost all

Table 3.1. Oxygen Consumption in Pregnancy

Author	Oxygen consumption: ml per minute			Difference between late pregnancy and		Remarks
	First trimester	Late pregnancy	More than one month post-partum	First trimester	Post-partum	
Stander and Cadden, 1932	No data	267	212	—	55	One of seven cases, data incomplete for other six
Plass and Oberst, 1938	232	269	210	37	59	A study of 45 women during pregnancy and 21 post-partum
Widlund, 1945	230	267	216	37	51	157 normal pregnant women, 84 primigravidae
Hamilton, 1949	198	251	No data	53	—	75 normal pregnant women
Cugell et al., 1953	No data	266	201	—	65	19 normal pregnant women
	217	238	196	21	42	9 women measured serially
Omatsu, 1957	170	220	173	50	47	An intensive study of one woman, Ht 153 cm; Wt 51 kg

unsatisfactory. Many give results as percentage changes only; for example Sontag, Reynolds and Torbet (1944) found a difference of about 14 per cent, Sandiford, Wheeler and Boothby (1931) in a careful intensive study of one woman, 25 per cent, and Naranjo Vargas, Cornejo and Bermeo (1953), who studied 40 normal pregnant women in Quito, Ecuador, 48 per cent. Few are serial studies from early pregnancy, and few have adequate control measurements. The more promising studies where measurements near term could be compared with measurements either in early pregnancy, or some weeks post partum in the same subjects, are summarized in Table 3.1.

There is no study in which a large number of women has been studied serially and it is clear from the table that such a study is badly needed. All that can be said from the array in Table 3.1 is that the increment of oxygen consumption at the end of pregnancy appears to be between 50 and 60 ml per minute above the non-pregnant level.

All work on basal metabolism has to face the difficulty of making sure that the subject is in the post-absorptive state and completely relaxed. It is less easy for a woman in late pregnancy to relax, especially since the supine position may be uncomfortable for her, and the foetus may be restless. Under such conditions an error of 10 per cent, or even more, would not be unexpected. There is no reason to suppose that the metabolic rate of maternal tissues is raised.

In Chapter 8 we discuss oxygen supply to, and consumption by the foetus. It is argued there that the oxygen consumption of the foetus is not likely to be higher than that of the mother because the foetus itself does not have to maintain its body temperature. We have computed the probable increment on the assumption that the metabolic rate of the foetus is the same as that of the non-pregnant woman under basal conditions, and that the placenta and extra maternal tissues have the metabolic rates found *in vitro*. Direct measurements of the oxygen consumption of the pregnant uterus at term are in substantial agreement. The result is shown in Table 3.2 and Figure 3.4. The total is 27.6 ml giving a percentage increment of 14 over the calculated oxygen consumption of the non-pregnant woman. That agrees with the estimate of Sontag, Reynolds and Torbet (1944).

An increment of 14 per cent is in excellent accord with the

TABLE 3.2. The Extra Components of Oxygen Consumption in Pregnancy

Source of extra energy output	Increment at weeks of pregnancy				Estimated cost: ml O_2 per minute	Increment of O_2 consumption: ml per min, weeks of pregnancy				References
	10	20	30	40		10	20	30	40	
Cardiac output l/min	1.0	1.5	1.5	0.75	About 20 at 4.5 litres per minute Increase pro rata.	4.5	6.8	6.8	3.4	Chap. 2, Best and Taylor, 1961
Respiration l/min	0.5	1.75	3.0	3.75	1.0 per litre ventilation	0.5	1.8	3.0	3.8	Fig. 3.2, p. 91
Uterine muscle g	135	585	810	900	3.7 per kg	0.5	2.2	3.0	3.3	Chap. 11
Placenta g { Wet	20	170	430	650	3.3 per 100 g dry weight	0	0.5	2.2	3.7	Chap. 10
Placenta g { Dry	2	17	65	110						
Foetus g	5	300	1500	3300	3.65 per kg	0	1.1	5.5	12.0	Chap. 10
Breasts g	45	180	360	410	3.3 per kg	0.1	0.6	1.2	1.4	Chap. 7, Hoover and Turner, 1954
Total, ml per min						5.6	12.9	21.6	27.6	

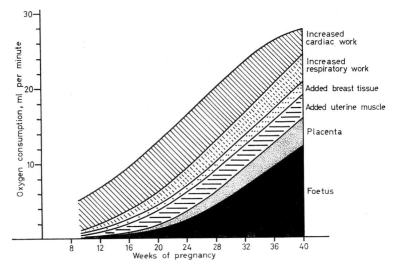

FIGURE 3.4. The components of increased oxygen consumption in pregnancy

increment in oxygen carrying capacity of the blood, estimated in Chapter 1 (p. 22) at 18 per cent, giving a difference which will account for the reduced arterio-venous oxygen difference.

With oxygen consumption increasing by less than 20 per cent and minute ventilation increasing by more than 40 per cent, it is clear that there is considerable 'hyperventilation'. This is all the more pronounced in view of the more effective ventilation of pregnancy; alveolar ventilation increases by probably 65 per cent, more than twice the increase of oxygen consumption. In the series studied by Cugell *et al.* (1953) the ventilatory equivalent for oxygen was 3.3 litres [of ventilation] per 100 cc [of oxygen consumed] at term compared to 3.0 litres per 100 cc some weeks after delivery, an increase of only 10 per cent, which undoubtedly minimises the true extent of the overbreathing.

CARBON DIOXIDE OUTPUT

Measurement of carbon dioxide production by the body is difficult. While oxygen is taken up from minute to minute in response to needs, the minute to minute output of carbon dioxide depends on much more than its rate of production. The body has a considerable capacity for storing CO_2 in the blood, largely as bicarbonate, and the amount breathed out by the lungs in a short interval will be influenced to a considerable extent by storage, or release of CO_2 from stores, with changes of blood pH. For this reason the ratio of carbon dioxide breathed out, to oxygen breathed in, the respiratory quotient (RQ), cannot be reliably interpreted when estimated from a short observation period such as most investigators have employed for the measurement of oxygen consumption. A meaningful measure of RQ would require collection of expired gas for some hours under carefully controlled conditions. Such evidence as there is, for example that of Spiga-Clerici (1937), Burwell *et al.* (1938), or Plass and Oberst (1938) shows no systematic change of RQ during pregnancy. Only Omatsu (1957) in his careful intensive study of three women describes a fall from about 0.95 in the early months to 0.9 or less at the end of pregnancy. He remarks on the great day-to-day variation of the measurement.

ALVEOLAR CARBON DIOXIDE

Overbreathing in pregnancy causes carbon dioxide to be washed out of the lungs and the alveolar concentration of CO_2 is lower than in the non-pregnant subject. This has been demonstrated repeatedly. For example Plass and Oberst (1938) showed that the percentage of CO_2 in expired air was 2.83 in late pregnancy and 3.31 in the non-pregnant. Expressed in more modern terms, Bouterline-Young and Bouterline-Young (1956) found the pCO_2 to fall to a mean value of 30.9 mm Hg by the end of the second trimester and to remain at that level until delivery; the mean was 37.3 mm in non-pregnant subjects. At high altitudes, where pCO_2 tends to be lower because of increased ventilation, the reduction due to pregnancy is added to the altitude effect. Hellegers *et al.* (1959), who studied women living at an altitude of 14,500 feet in Peru, found the mean alveolar pCO_2 to be 27.9 mm in non-pregnant women and 22.9 mm in pregnancy.

The reduction of alveolar, and therefore of arterial, carbon dioxide tension affords an illustration of the general truth that adaptations in pregnancy occur in advance of the need for them. Goodland and Pommerenke (1952) showed that alveolar pCO_2 fell from about 36–37 mm at ovulation to about 32–33 mm immediately before menstruation and Bouterline-Young and Bouterline-Young (1956) found alveolar pCO_2 to average 36.3 mm

H

in the 15 days before menstruation and 37.8 mm at other times in the cycle. It is almost certain therefore that the decline in pregnancy starts even before the fertilized ovum embeds.

The reduction of pCO_2 may be induced by progesterone. Goodland et al. (1953) reduced alveolar pCO_2 in male medical students by about 2.5 mm Hg by injecting progesterone and Tyler (1960) induced hyperventilation with a dramatic fall of pCO_2 in patients with emphysema and hypercapnia. Tyler demonstrated also that the effect was not common to all so-called 'progestational' compounds. Progesterone itself had a pronounced effect, but anhydrohydroxy-progesterone, 1,2-dehydroprogesterone and 19-norethinyl testosterone were ineffective. The site of action of progesterone is unknown.

The reduced maternal pCO_2 will slightly increase pO_2 and presumably helps the foetus to dispose of CO_2, which may be important since the newborn infant, and presumably also the foetus, is more sensitive than the adult to CO_2 (Cross, Hooper and Oppé, 1953).

The cost of ventilation

The work of breathing becomes proportionately greater with increasing rates of ventilation, and in pregnancy the effect is accentuated. Bader, Bader and Rose (1959) had a group of eleven women in late pregnancy breathe at a fixed rate of 20 per minute and vary their minute volume by varying only tidal volume; carbon dioxide was added to the mixture in sufficient quantities to prevent discomfort. The rise of oxygen consumption with ventilation rate was much steeper for the pregnant women than for three non-pregnant controls. For example at a ventilation rate of 15 litres per minute, the non-pregnant women used additional oxygen at a rate of between 1.4 and 2.2 ml per litre of ventilation, and a typical pregnant woman needed 3.3 ml of oxygen per litre. Judged from the information given by Bader et al., about 3 ml oxygen per litre of ventilation would be a reasonable average over the range of resting ventilation found in late pregnancy.

Bader, Bader and Rose suggest that the cost is likely to be less for more natural, slower rates of ventilation and their figures may be more appropriate for respiration after exercise than for respiration at rest. They are certainly much above the averages found by Campbell, Westlake and Cherniack (1959) for young men who used only 0.65 ml of oxygen per litre of ventilation in the range 9 to 22 litres per minute, a level which agrees with most other published studies. Until the study by Bader, Bader and Rose has been repeated and extended we are unwilling to accept their very high figures. The possibility that ventilation in pregnancy costs more than before pregnancy seems reasonable, but it would be surprising if it were much above about 1 ml of oxygen per litre of ventilation.

The effect of exercise

Tests of capacity for exercise are not entirely satisfactory but Harris (1958) in a review suggests that oxygen debt after standard exercise may be the most reliable indicator.

Widlund (1945) measured oxygen debt as the amount of oxygen consumed between the 2nd and 5th minutes after three grades of step test which involved lifting the body 7, 13 and 17 metres per minute. Apart from the fact that it is difficult or impossible to standardize the performance in step tests, it is not easy to interpret his results since measures of oxygen consumption by two methods, Krogh spirometer and Douglas bag, correlated poorly. Absolute measures are not given, only percentage increases, but working back to absolute figures it appears that the extra oxygen uptake for the first test was 47.6 ml in the non-pregnant controls and 45.6 ml at the end of pregnancy, for the second test 78.4 and 80.5 ml and for the hardest test 143.0 and 156.4 ml. That is, only for moderately hard exercise is it likely that the pregnant woman incurs a bigger oxygen debt than the non-pregnant woman. Such a difference might be expected; the pregnant woman has more weight to lift and the cost of her increased ventilation is probably greater. There is no evidence to suggest reduced efficiency in pregnancy.

Widlund found no difference in the relative increase in minute volume between pregnant and non-pregnant women after exercise. In terms of resting levels of ventilation, minute volume increased by about 50 per cent for the easiest test, 80 per cent for the second and 150 per cent for the hardest. Oxygen debt was not proportional to resting oxygen consumption because the pregnant woman had similar increments of oxygen consumption with exercise but increasingly higher levels of resting oxygen consumption. Ventilation therefore appears, in this study, to rise by more than the increase in oxygen debt; hyperventilation is accentuated. Cugell et al. (1953), on the other hand, found no hyperventilation with exercise.

Dahlström and Ihrman (1960) showed no change in respiratory frequency during pregnancy either at rest or at various levels of activity on a bicycle ergometer.

Dyspnoea

The normal person is ordinarily unconscious of the automatic process of breathing, and even when moderate exercise increases the ventilation rate, the change is usually unnoticed. When the need to breathe becomes conscious, there is 'shortness of breath', which is one of the commonest causes of complaint by the pregnant woman. The symptom in pregnancy is not necessarily related to exercise and, paradoxically, it may be present when sitting down but not when walking about. Moreover, it adds confusion in a situation where there may be other misleading signs, usual in pregnancy, but otherwise regarded as abnormal, such as a low haemoglobin concentration, or equivocal signs of heart disease (see p. 71).

Dyspnoea is common when ventilation is mechanically restricted or when there is airway resistance; neither of these causes accounts for the symptom in pregnancy; on the contrary resistance to breathing is less. Cugell *et al.* (1953) showed that dyspnoea, which was a complaint of 13 of their 19 subjects, was not related to maximum breathing capacity, oxygen uptake, ventilation, vital capacity or any of the subdivisions of lung volume. Two of the women with a definite reduction of maximum breathing capacity had no dyspnoea; two others with considerably increased maximum breathing capacity were short of breath even at rest. Eighteen of the 31 women studied by Thomson and Cohen (1938) complained of dyspnoea, but its appearance was capricious; it might be present one month and not the next. Its appearance was not related to vital capacity. Bader, Bader and Rose (1959) suggested that the extra cost of ventilation might contribute to the sensation of dyspnoea.

An ingenious theory has been developed by Moran Campbell (Campbell and Howell, 1963) to explain the sensation of dyspnoea: he believes that it arises when the ventilatory response is 'inappropriate' to the demand, which must imply that some centre is continuously relating the demand for ventilation to the actual ventilation. Although Comroe *et al.* (1962) have claimed a number of exceptions to the theory, it appears to cover most situations.

As we have seen, there is overbreathing in pregnancy so that, in one sense, ventilation is inappropriate to demand. A recent study by Gilbert, Epifano and Auchincloss (1962) supports the suggestion that it may be the basis of dyspnoea. They studied the ventilatory adjustments of 14 normal pregnant women during mild exercise. Five of the subjects complained of dyspnoea during the exercise and dyspnoea occurred when alveolar pCO_2 was lowest. Moreover these 5 women had a higher pCO_2 than the others before pregnancy and the authors suggest that their sensations of breathlessness might be due to their unfamiliarity with low tensions of CO_2. For a woman habituated to breathing with an alveolar pCO_2 of over 40 mm Hg, the compulsion to breathe in pregnancy with an alveolar pCO_2 of perhaps 30 mm Hg may very well seem, in Campbell's phrase, inappropriate.

CHAPTER 4

Renal Function

Principles and Techniques of Study

For the direct study of function the kidney is not accessible. The composition of blood perfusing it must in general be inferred from the composition of blood in peripheral vessels, and the urine secreted is available for examination only after it has spent an unknown time in the renal pelves, ureters and bladder. For these reasons elaborate techniques of study have been developed which must be applied with great care to give trustworthy results. Most of the development of recent methods has been in Homer Smith's laboratories in the United States and much of what follows is derived from his text-book on the kidney (Smith, 1951). No more can be given here than an outline of broad principles sufficient for the interpretation of data obtained during pregnancy.

Renal clearances

The concept of blood 'clearance' to indicate the rate at which the kidney excretes a substance, was first used by Möller, McIntosh and Van Slyke in 1929 in reference to urea; it has now achieved universal acceptance as the basis for measurement of the excretion of other substances. For any substance X, if U is the concentration in the urine in mg per ml and V is the rate of urine formation (ml per minute), then the rate of excretion of X is UV mg per minute. If P is the concentration of X in the plasma (mg per ml), then UV/P is the amount of plasma required to supply the quantity of X excreted each minute, or is in effect the volume of plasma completely cleared of X in one minute. The plasma clearance, UV/P, is fundamental to many measures of renal physiology, and the practical difficulties of most studies lie simply in the accurate estimation of the three terms, U, V and P.

The value of renal clearance techniques has extended beyond their use as a measure of excretion of substances such as urea and creatinine which are normally excreted by the kidney. For example, if a substance were to be completely filterable at the glomerulus and neither reabsorbed nor excreted by the tubules then the clearance of such a substance would equal the volume of plasma filtered each minute by the glomeruli, the glomerular filtration rate (GFR). A number of substances have been suggested as fulfilling the criteria for a completely filterable substance and it is generally conceded that the polysaccharide inulin is the most satisfactory. Thiosulphate clearance is normally only a little higher than inulin clearance; the difference seems to be greater in pregnancy (Lambiotte, Blanchard and Graff, 1950). Endogenous creatinine clearance also is used by some as a measure of GFR and is clinically convenient, but some creatinine is known to be excreted by the tubules in man and therefore gives a larger estimate of GFR than inulin does. It is undoubtedly inferior to inulin as a tool in research. Renal clearance of inulin is taken as equivalent to GFR although, as Dicker (1956) pointed out, that they are equivalent is 'a working hypothesis rather than a revealed truth.' There is certainly no proof of their equivalence in pregnancy.

Other substances are excreted by the tubules in addition to being filtered by the glomeruli, and their excretion will exceed the GFR by an amount equal to the tubular clearance. Obviously there is an upper limit to possible clearance because the kidneys cannot excrete more of a substance in any period than is brought to them by the blood. The maximum possible renal clearance is therefore equal to the total plasma flow through the excretory tissues of the kidney, the 'effective' renal plasma flow (RPF). Since the mid 1940s, effective RPF has been estimated almost always by the clearance of *para*-amino hippurate (PAH). If the blood in the renal veins is sampled directly by, for example, cardiac catheter, then it can be shown that about 92 per cent of the PAH which enters the renal artery is removed in its passage through the kidney. That percentage is termed the extraction ratio. It is assumed that the discrepancy of 8 per cent is accounted for by the fact that some blood must perfuse the perirenal fat and other inert supporting structures in the kidney and that extraction is close to 100 per cent where the blood perfuses functional renal tissue. The PAH clearance, uncorrected for the extraction ratio and therefore representing an average of about 92 per cent of renal plasma flow is sometimes called the 'effective' RPF, but recently just RPF. Smith (1951) suggests that the simplification should be accepted as convenient and that where the correction is made for extraction ratio the term used might be 'total renal plasma flow'.

Whole blood flow is sometimes calculated simply as:

$$\frac{\text{Effective renal plasma flow (PAH clearance)}}{(1—\text{haematocrit})}$$

The ratio of glomerular filtration rate to renal plasma flow GFR/RPF is termed the filtration fraction.

Much of the earlier work on renal plasma flow used diodrast (3,5-di-iodo-4-pyridone-N-acetic acid) as the clearance substance. Diodrast has clearance characteristics which are probably identical with those of PAH, but PAH has many advantages in practice. A minor disadvantage of PAH is that it forms a complex with glucose which is not cleared efficiently by the kidney, although it is measured as PAH in plasma. For this reason PAH should not be infused in glucose solution.

The clearance of a substance is calculated from its concentration in urine and in arterial plasma and the rate of formation of urine. Accuracy can be achieved only if the concentration in the plasma during the period of measurement is known and if the whole amount of urine, and only that amount, formed by the kidneys during the period of clearance can be recovered for measurement and analysis.

It is essential for accuracy to have an almost constant concentration of the test substance in the plasma, which is achieved by a priming dose to give the desired concentration followed by intravenous infusion to maintain it. Provided the volume of distribution does not change, the rate of excretion will eventually equal the rate of infusion. Some workers have claimed that a single dose administered subcutaneously, so that it is released slowly, is as good as a constant infusion; it is undoubtedly more convenient. Michie and Michie (1951) showed that, with inulin and PAH, the time required to reach clearance equilibrium was 20 to 30 minutes *from the attainment of constant plasma levels*. The delay is due to the time required to wash away completely the urine formed before the constant plasma level is reached. It follows that if the plasma concentration is changing, as it is bound to change after a single injection, then concentration in urine will never be in equilibrium with concentration in plasma.

Urine should be collected by catheter, with suprapubic pressure and, to ensure complete emptying, the bladder should be washed out with sterile water. The error will be less if a moderately high flow of urine is induced, say 2 ml per minute or more. Since the passage of a catheter into the bladder may introduce infection, especially liable to affect the urinary tract in pregnancy, it may be difficult to justify studies of renal function involving this procedure in healthy pregnant women.

It is never possible to be sure that only the urine is collected that leaves the kidneys during the period of clearance. The time taken by urine to reach the bladder, the 'delay time', varies, and the allowance of $2\frac{1}{2}$ to 5 minutes usually made for the time elapsing between the sampling of peripheral blood and the arrival in the bladder of urine formed from that blood is arbitrary.

Many workers appear to have interpreted the 'delay time' as the time taken for a solid front of new urine carrying the test substance to appear in the bladder. As ordinarily used, 'delay time' covers only the time taken between injection of the test substance and its *first appearance* in the bladder. Urine containing the test substance is then mixed with 'old urine' and, with a urine flow of about 2 ml per minute, complete washing out of old urine takes 20 minutes or more. The dead space of the kidney and renal tracts is calculated from the rate of urine flow and the delay time. If the urine is flowing at the rate of 2 ml per minute and a substance takes 3 minutes to appear in the bladder after injection into the blood, then the dead space is 6 ml. The figure quite clearly has no real meaning because, as we have explained, the first appearance of the substance does not mean that the urinary dead space is uniformly filled with it. McSwiney and de Wardener (1950) have called this estimate the 'minimal dead space' and for calculating 'maximal' dead space use the delay time from injection of the substance until its appearance at maximum concentration. Michie and Michie (1951), on the basis that 20 minutes were needed for equilibration between blood and urine, calculated the 'dead space' of the kidneys to be about 40 ml.

The true anatomical dead space presumably lies somewhere between the two extremes. In pregnancy the anatomical dead space certainly increases; there is obvious dilatation and kinking of the ureters. From pyelograms in a large number of women and post mortem examination of 84 women who died after the seventh month of pregnancy, Baird (1935) described in detail the anatomical changes in the ureters. Dilatation of the tract occurred in all. It begins as early as the 10th week, on both sides and uniformly throughout the length of the ureters, presumably as part of the general atony of smooth muscle. Later, the right side becomes more dilated than the left with involvement of the renal pelvis, although there may be no dilatation below the pelvic brim; on the left side, the ureter more typically tapers from renal pelvis to bladder. Kinking, which may be acute, occurs on both sides. The changes sometimes decrease after the sixth month, particularly on the left side.

In Baird's series primigravidae were affected more than multigravidae. At autopsy the volume of the ureters was measured by filling them with water. In 32 primigravidae 22 had a right ureter volume of more than 20 ml and in 2 it exceeded 50 ml; on the left side ureter volume exceeded 20 ml in 13 and exceeded 50 ml in 2. In 52 multigravidae volumes in excess of 20 ml occurred on the right side in 14 and on the left side in 9.

Longo and Assali (1960), from the first appearance time of PAH calculated the equivalent of McSwiney and de Wardener's 'minimal dead space'. They showed it to rise from about 6 ml at 10 weeks to about 10 ml at 30 weeks, and they claim a reduction of the dead space between 30 and 40 weeks which the data do not support; the range of dead space is much increased and values between 7 and 12 occur throughout the last 10 weeks. Longo and Assali's findings were made at a wide range of rates of urine flow and were adjusted in some way to a constant urine flow of 2 ml per minute. The mathematical manipulations are not given and this attempt to measure the dilatation of the urinary tract is to some extent unsatisfactory. In any event, the use of delay time to estimate the concentration in blood at the time when the collected urine was filtered by the kidney gives an entirely spurious impression of accuracy, as Michie and Michie have shown. For reliable estimates of renal clearance there can be no effective substitute for a constant level of the test substance in the blood. A study, such as that by Michie and Michie to demonstrate the time taken to establish clearance equilibrium, is needed for pregnancy.

The difficulties of measuring renal clearances are not all solved by the accurate measurement of the terms U, V and P. There are physiological changes which make the procedure difficult to standardize. For example, Miles and de Wardener (1953) have shown that minor emotional disturbance may increase GFR and Smith (1951) has said that pain and fright both may reduce RPF and GFR. Posture has an important effect: Sims and Krantz (1958) found no systematic difference in GFR between women lying on their backs and the same women lying on their sides, but Pritchard, Barnes and Bright (1955) found that when a pregnant woman lies on her back, urine flow, electrolyte excretion, GFR and RPF are all considerably lower than when she lies on her side, and Buttermann (1958) got lower clearance values in women with 'atonic ureters' when lying on their back than when lying on their sides. Smith (1951) sums up by saying 'some subjects make much better experimental guinea pigs than others. For critical experiments it is wise to use a subject who is accustomed to the clearance procedure'.

It should be clear that the pregnant woman, with dilated ureters, unable to lie comfortably on her back, more emotionally labile than normal, and unlikely to be accustomed to renal clearance measurements is a disheartening subject for the physiologist, and published results must be viewed in that light.

Tubular function: tubular excretion

Any substances whose clearance from the blood exceeds that of inulin may be assumed to be excreted by the tubules in addition to being filtered by the glomeruli. The clearance of PAH described above as an index of renal plasma flow also gives a measure of tubular excretion. The difference between the amount of PAH filtered at the glomeruli, which can be calculated from GFR or inulin clearance, and the total PAH excreted, is excreted by the tubules. Tubular excretion of PAH is limited to a constant and reproducible maximum rate which 'may be used to characterize the quantity of tubular excretory tissue in health and disease' (Smith, 1951).

The dye, phenol red (phenolsulphonphthalein, PSP), historically important because of its use in an early test of renal function, was the first substance for which tubular secretion was demonstrated. It has a clearance of about 60 per cent of the diodrast or PAH clearance. It is no longer used.

Tubular function: tubular reabsorption

Many substances of small molecular weight which are filtered by the glomeruli are normally absent from the urine, and it follows that they must be reabsorbed by the tubules. These substances are characteristically nutrients which are important to the economy of the body and include glucose, amino acids, phosphate and vitamin C. Reabsorption is against a higher concentration in blood and transfer from the filtrate back to the blood is limited by a maximum capacity characteristic of each substance reabsorbed.

Glucose, for example, appears in the urine when the quantity filtered exceeds the maximum reabsorptive capacity of the tubules. Maximum rates of tubular transport are conventionally indicated by Tm, with a suffix to indicate the solute concerned; the maximum rate of glucose reabsorption is Tm_G. For normal women Tm_G is about 300 mg per minute (Smith, 1951) with a standard deviation of about 55. With a normal non-pregnant filtration rate of 117 ml per minute, that load would theoretically be reached at an arterial plasma level of about 260 mg per 100 ml; but as Smith points out, appearance of glucose in the urine can be expected at any level above about 60 per cent of that, because of unevenness of glomerular function.

The Tm values for amino acids are greatly in excess of the load normally presented to the tubules although constant small quantities of amino acids are lost by the normal person. The loss varies for different amino acids and is greatest for histidine where 5 to 10 per cent of the filtered load is excreted (Cusworth and Dent, 1960). Soupart (1960) found the clearance rate for histidine in 5 non-pregnant women to be about 10 ml per minute.

Urea and uric acid, both metabolic end products, are also reabsorbed to some extent. The amount of urea which diffuses back from the glomerular filtrate depends on urine flow. At rates above 2 ml per minute, urea clearance is approximately 60 per cent of inulin clearance. Urate clearance is less than 10 per cent of inulin clearance.

Excretion of water and electrolytes

We do not intend to summarize here what is known about how the kidney handles water and electrolytes. Huge amounts of both are filtered each day and all but a very small fraction is reabsorbed, electrolytes under the influence of hormones from the adrenal cortex, water under the influence of antidiuretic hormone from the posterior pituitary gland. Even minor disorders of control can cause disastrous losses or accumulations of water and electrolytes, so that the small variations of water or electrolyte balance which might be seen in pregnancy would require only minute changes of control, too small to be demonstrated by present techniques. Response to abnormal loads of water and electrolyte can be studied but the results must be interpreted with caution. Anti-diuresis, in particular, can result from such influences as emotional disturbance, discomfort or physical exercise and, in late pregnancy, from lying supine (Pritchard, Barnes and Bright, 1955). Diuresis, also, has been shown by Miles and de Wardener (1953) to follow emotional disturbance.

Correction for body size

So that individual subjects of different body size can be compared, it is conventional practice to express renal clearances in terms of body surface area. Correlation with area is better than with either height or weight alone. It is generally recognized that the only logical basis for comparison of clearance values would be either kidney weight or the number of glomeruli and, at least in animals, kidney weight is closely related to body surface area. McIntosh, Möller and Van Slyke (1929) derived from medico-actuarial tables an average surface area of 1.73 m² for 25-year-old men and women, and since that time 1.73 m² has been almost universally accepted as the basis to which clearance values are referred. While it is possible to defend this arbitrary correction for comparisons of subjects of differing body size, it seems totally illogical to extend it to the comparison of clearances at different times in the same adult subject. For example if a woman of 160 cm height weighs 60 kg before pregnancy her calculated surface area will be 1.61 m². In late pregnancy her weight is likely to be about 73 kg and her cal-culated surface area would be 1.75 m². Expressed in conventional terms her renal plasma flow may change from 600 to 800 ml per minute per 1.73 m² between these two points. But this is not simply a change of plasma flow of 200 ml per minute, because the absolute plasma flow would be about 560 ml per minute before pregnancy and 810 ml per minute in late pregnancy, an actual change in plasma flow of 250 ml. Since there is no evidence of a change in kidney weight or in number of glomeruli in human pregnancy, then logically, the actual change of 250 ml per minute is more meaning-ful than the apparent change of 200 ml per minute when clearance is related to a changing surface area. Unfortunately data about surface area are seldom published and it is usually impossible to calculate the real change in clearance values.

CHANGES DURING PREGNANCY
Renal blood flow

In a recent review Chesley (1960), who was one of the earliest investigators in this field, generously admits that he 'got the subject off on the wrong foot' in concluding that pregnancy had no effect on renal blood flow. In the early paper referred to (Chesley and Chesley, 1939) the diodrast clearance in nine normal women in the last four weeks of pregnancy was found to be 610 ml per minute per 1.73 m^2 body surface area, compared to 518 in eleven non-pregnant women. The calculated renal blood flows were 879 and 836 ml per minute. Welsh, Wellen and Taylor (1942) found a similar mean plasma flow for 21 women, mostly during the last four weeks of pregnancy: in relation to surface area 631 ml per minute compared to 525 for a control group. The blood flows were 970 and 858 ml per minute. The differences between pregnant and non-pregnant groups in these two investigations are not negligible, particularly when it is remembered that the pregnancy figures have been artificially diminished by reducing the actual plasma flow to a standard body surface area. And yet both groups concluded that pregnancy had no effect on renal blood flow. Dill, Isenhour, Cadden and Schaffer (1942) in a technically unsatisfactory study of eight women in the last month of pregnancy found a mean renal plasma flow of 637 ml per minute compared to 630 for a group at an unstated time after delivery. The blood flows were calculated to be 950 and 980 ml per minute.

In the first reported study of renal blood flow throughout pregnancy, Bonsnes and Lange (1950) stated, in a very short note, that the PAH clearances were significantly elevated in early pregnancy, but fell towards term. They gave no figures and appear never to have published the information in detail. A number of studies followed and confirmed the general pattern. Bucht (1951) found an average PAH clearance of about 775 ml per minute per 1.73 m^2 up to the 4th month and about 617 ml per minute in the 9th and 10th months compared to 557 ml for a non-pregnant control group. Similar patterns were described by Lanz and

Hochuli (1955), Sohar, Scadron and Levitt (1956), Buttermann (1958), de Alvarez (1958), Sims and Krantz (1958) and Gylling (1961). Assali's group have described a continuously increasing renal plasma flow in pregnancy (Dignam, Titus and Assali, 1958; Assali, Dignam and Dasgupta, 1959) and Brandstetter and Schüller (1956) in a cross-sectional study of 44 women in pregnancy and the second week of the puerperium found renal plasma flow to increase continuously, but only slightly, above the non-pregnant level; renal blood flow throughout pregnancy was no different from the non-pregnant rate. Brandstetter and Schüller state that their clearances are expressed in terms of the standard body surface. Assali and his collaborators make no statement about this and their findings, which are so conspicuously out of line with the generally agreed trend, may be affected by their not applying this traditional correction. Most of these studies are technically unsatisfactory and there is little point in attempting a synthesis of their findings. For example, most of the studies were cross-sectional with few subjects; Bucht (1951) and Gylling (1961) used a single injection of PAH; and Lanz and Hochuli (1955), de Alvarez (1958) and Assali gave PAH infusions in dextrose solutions. Few studies publish all the data.

The study by Sims and Krantz (1958) is exceptional. The technique appears to have been impeccable, the data are fully reported and the twelve subjects were studied serially. They were all healthy women of between 19 and 35 years who had normal pregnancies. Parity ranged from one to five. The control group were healthy non-pregnant women, 21 to 33 years old with an average parity of 1.1. What follows is derived wholly from this paper.

Figure 4.1 and Table 4.1 show the average effective renal plasma flow (C_{PAH}) for the 12 subjects at 5 stages in pregnancy and 4 periods post-partum. It is expressed in two ways: as Sims and Krantz themselves calculated it, in the conventional terms of a constant body surface of 1.73 m² (Figure 2 in their paper) and recalculated by us as the actual measured clearances before manipulation. Plasma flow, and blood flow which we have calculated in the usual way from the published haematocrit figures are clearly above the non-pregnant level during the whole of pregnancy. The widely accepted pattern of plasma flow falling to within the non-pregnant range at term is apparent in the published figures and is consistent for all subjects, but the average is still about 75 ml per minute above the non-pregnant mean, when the absolute flow figures are used, as logically they should be. The fall in the post-partum period is curious but consistent. We have used the final figure at an average of about a year post-partum as the non-pregnant level.

TABLE 4.1. Mean effective Renal Plasma Flow (C_{PAH}) Calculated from the Data of Sims and Krantz (1958)

Mean week	No. of Subjects	Mean effective renal plasma flow (C_{PAH}): ml per minute			
		per 1.73 m^2	SD	Actual measurement	SD
Pregnancy					
15.4	12	769	90	726	104
25.2	12	761	74	734	80
30.6	9	680	146	672	156
33.7	7	716	170	723	179
37.8	10	589	113	577	130
Puerperium					
5.8	6	462	112	434	100
12.5	8	490	85	449	92
25.7	6	462	79	412	70
60.0	5	549	122	504	124

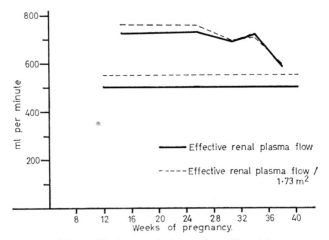

FIGURE 4.1. Mean effective renal plasma flow (C_{PAH}) in pregnancy. From the data of Sims and Krantz (1958)

During pregnancy, the individual plasma flows showed considerable irregularity of pattern, so that we must accept a mean curve with some caution, but until more figures are available, collected with equal care from many more women in a longitudinal study, it is reasonable to conclude that effective renal plasma flow is raised by about 225 ml per minute, from about 500 to 725 ml, an increase of about 45 per cent, from at least the beginning of the second trimester, until about a month before term when it falls to less than 100 ml per minute above the non-pregnant level.

Effective renal blood flow has a similar pattern to plasma flow, but because of the decreasing haematocrit level, tends to fall slightly throughout pregnancy before the final, more rapid decline near term (Figure 4.2; Table 4.2). Early in the second trimester the average effective renal blood flow was about 1200 ml per minute (almost 1300 ml per 1.73 m²) falling to about 1100 ml at 34 weeks and about 900 ml near term. The non-pregnant mean was 885 ml per minute (965 ml per 1.73 m²).

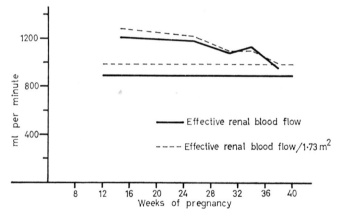

FIGURE 4.2. Mean Effective renal blood flow in pregnancy. From the data of Sims and Krantz (1958)

It is not known when the increase of renal blood flow is first apparent in pregnancy; it is obviously one of the earliest phenomena. Sims and Krantz report one woman whose effective renal plasma flow was 557 ml per minute before pregnancy and 805 ml per minute in the ninth week of pregnancy. That is a dramatic change and more data are needed to confirm it.

TABLE 4.2. Mean Effective Renal Blood Flow Calculated from the Data of Sims and Krantz (1958). Numbers of Subjects differ from those in Table 9.1 because the Haematocrit Value was not always stated

Mean week	No. of Subjects	Mean Effective renal blood flow: ml per minute			
		per 1.73 m²	SD	Actual measurement	SD
Pregnancy					
15.4	9	1280	161	1214	178
25.2	11	1216	108	1161	142
30.6	8	1098	271	1071	286
33.7	7	1116	268	1127	281
37.8	10	941	186	922	213
Puerperium					
6.4	5	886	270	816	252
12.5	8	841	153	770	162
25.7	6	825	165	737	157
60.0	5	965	272	885	265

Glomerular filtration rate

Investigations of glomerular filtration rate can be divided into two classes: those where GFR was found to be raised in early pregnancy and to fall towards, or to, normal non-pregnant levels at term; and those where GFR was found to be raised throughout pregnancy. The rise and fall class is represented by Bonsnes and Lange (1950), de Alvarez (1958), Buttermann (1958) and Gylling (1961). The second class by Bucht (1951), Lanz and Hochuli (1955), Sohar, Scadron and Levitt (1956), Brandstetter and Schüller (1956), Sims and Krantz (1958) and Dignam, Titus and Assali (1958).

Except for Lanz and Hochuli who used thiosulphate, all investigators measured the inulin clearance, but again Sims and Krantz provide the most satisfactory data and we will rely on them. Figure 4.3 and Table 4.3 show the average glomerular filtration rates (C_{inulin}) in the same way as renal plasma flow was shown in Figure 4.1 and Table 4.1. There is no doubt that the inulin clearance is considerably raised throughout pregnancy, and it remains consistently at a high level at the end of pregnancy when renal plasma flow is apparently declining. In Sims and Krantz's subjects the non-pregnant level was about 90 ml per minute (about

100 ml per minute per 1.73 m²) while throughout pregnancy it remained at a level of about 145 ml per minute, an increase of 55 ml per minute or about 60 per cent.

TABLE 4.3. Mean Glomerular Filtration Rate (C_{inulin}) Calculated from the Data of Sims and Krantz (1958)

Mean week	No. of Subjects	Glomerular filtration rate (C_{inulin}): ml per minute			
		per 1.73 m²	SD	Actual measurement	SD
Pregnancy					
15.4	12	157	18.4	148	26.3
25.2	12	152	21.0	147	27.0
30.6	9	147	20.3	145	27.2
33.7	7	163	24.1	165	29.9
37.8	11	146	22.3	144	29.1
Puerperium					
5.8	6	98	7.7	92	7.8
12.5	8	95	16.8	88	20.7
25.7	6	100	13.5	90	18.1
60.0	5	97	11.4	89	10.1

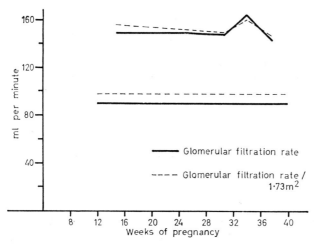

FIGURE 4.3. Mean Glomerular filtration rate (C_{inulin}) in pregnancy. From the data of Sims and Krantz (1958)

Filtration fraction

Since glomerular filtration is raised in pregnancy by a proportion greater than that of renal plasma flow, the proportion of the plasma flow which is filtered, the filtration fraction, is raised above the non-pregnant level. In late pregnancy when renal plasma flow shows a relative fall, the filtration rises still further. We have estimated filtration fractions from the calculated absolute measurements of renal plasma flow and glomerular filtration rate in Tables 4.1 and 4.3. The average non-pregnant filtration fraction is about 0.18; during most of pregnancy it is about 0.20 and it rises to about 0.25 during the last two months.

Creatinine clearance

Creatinine clearance has been used as a measure of glomerular filtration rate, but creatinine is known to be excreted by the tubules and its clearance should therefore exceed the inulin clearance. Published results are confusing. For example, Brandstetter and Schüller (1956) found creatinine clearance to be almost identical to inulin clearance and with the same variance throughout pregnancy, while de Alvarez (1958), who used 24-hour specimens of urine to calculate creatinine clearance, and Buttermann (1958) found it to be slightly but consistently lower than the inulin clearance. Bucht (1951) on the other hand found it to be considerably above the inulin clearance in non-pregnant women and in early pregnancy, but the same as inulin clearance in late pregnancy. Sims and Krantz (1958) confirmed Bucht's finding and found creatinine clearance to be much more variable than inulin clearance.

Whatever its relation to inulin clearance, there is no doubt that the absolute clearance is raised in pregnancy and plasma levels of creatinine are lower than normal as a result. Sims and Krantz found the mean blood level in pregnancy to be 0.46 mg ± 0.13 compared to 0.67 mg ± 0.14 per 100 ml of serum for non-pregnant controls.

There are many technical difficulties in the estimation of creatinine, and its clearance, and since it is now no longer considered a serious rival to inulin as a measure of glomerular filtration rate, there is nothing to be gained by a critical assessment of these contradictory findings. Nor are they of any particular physiological interest; we include them simply because they hold a prominent place in the literature.

Urea clearance

Urea clearance has an important place in the history of renal function tests and is still widely used as a clinical test of renal competence. It was for urea that the concept of plasma clearance was first suggested by Möller, McIntosh and Van Slyke in 1929. A high urea clearance was demonstrated in pregnancy before measurements of glomerular filtration rate with inulin had been made; it depends upon and follows glomerular filtration rate (Nice, 1935; Chesley and Chesley, 1939). Bonsnes and Lange (1950) first showed urea clearance to be raised in parallel with inulin clearance. The raised urea clearance leads to the well known low blood level of urea in pregnancy. For example, Sims and Krantz (1958) found the plasma urea nitrogen to be 8.7 mg ± 1.5 from the 15th week of pregnancy to term compared to 13.1 mg ± 3.0 for non-pregnant subjects.

Uric acid clearance

Uric acid clearance also is raised in pregnancy. For the non-pregnant person, estimates vary widely but Smith (1951) says that normal may be taken as about 12 ml per minute. Hayashi (1956) found uric acid clearance to be 18.4 ±4.9 before 32 weeks of pregnancy and 13.0 ±4.0 after 32 weeks. Blood uric acid averaged 3.2 and 3.0 mg per 100 ml for the two periods, compared to an average value of about 6 mg per 100 ml for the non-pregnant (Smith, 1951). Different chemical methods of estimating urate may give widely different results and a careful study of pregnancy with adequate non-pregnant control subjects is needed.

Excretion of sodium

In normal pregnancy, the concentration of sodium in body fluids is maintained at normal non-pregnant levels and one would not expect any change in the renal excretion of sodium; but there is a widespread belief that oedema is associated with excessive retention of sodium, particularly in pre-eclamptic toxaemia, and dietary restriction of sodium is commonly advised in antenatal clinics. In view of this, the dearth of published information about the renal excretion of sodium in pregnancy is surprising. Since the glomerular filtration rate is raised, the load of sodium presented to the tubules for reabsorption is similarly raised, but for a substance of such importance to the osmotic integrity of the blood it would be likely that the extra load would be well within the reabsorptive capacity of the tubules. Chesley, Valenti and Rein (1958), who loaded pregnant and non-pregnant women with a 3 per cent intravenous infusion of NaCl containing 410 mEq of sodium, found that the reabsorption of sodium was unaltered in pregnancy. In two hours from the beginning of the infusion, which took 20 minutes, the non-pregnant woman had excreted 20 per cent of the injected sodium compared to 18.6 per cent by the normal pregnant woman; the difference was not significant.

It is difficult to draw physiological conclusions from an experiment which involved such an abnormally large load, but it is clear that at least under these conditions the enhanced filtration of sodium in pregnancy is matched by an equally enhanced ability to reclaim sodium from the filtrate.

Pritchard, Barnes and Bright (1955) showed that there was a considerable reduction of sodium excretion, averaging 44 per cent, when pregnant women at term changed from lying on their sides to lying on their backs. They attributed the difference to compression of the renal veins by the pregnant uterus.

Excretion of water

While much has been written about body water in pregnancy, and particularly about excessive retention in pre-eclampsia, surprisingly few investigations seem to have been made of the way the kidney handles water in pregnancy.

Frequency of micturition is one of the commonest and earliest symptoms and recurs in late pregnancy. It is often attributed to irritability of the bladder, first by pelvic congestion and later by pressure from above, yet it has never been clearly established whether or not the frequency is associated with an increased quantity of urine.

In 1932 Janney and Walker showed that the ability to excrete an oral water load declined as pregnancy progressed and the disability was said to be more pronounced in pre-eclampsia (McManus, Riley and Janney, 1934). Theobald and Verney (1935) suggested that the effect might be mechanical from accumulation of water in the lower limbs. They further suggested that the familiar nocturia of pregnancy might be due to mobilization of the accumulated water after lying down.

Recently, Hytten and Klopper (1963) gave water loads of 1 litre by mouth to healthy pregnant women and measured the urine passed at 15 minute intervals between 9 a.m. and 12.30 p.m. Apart from trips to the toilet to pass urine the women were sitting at rest. The normal non-pregnant woman in these circumstances reaches a mean maximum urine flow of about 16 ml per minute (240 ml in 15 minutes) and in two hours has excreted an average of about 950 ml. During the second trimester of pregnancy there was considerable improvement on the non-pregnant performance. Peak urine flows were as high as 30 ml per minute and almost all were well above the non-pregnant average; the amount of urine excreted in 2 hours after the load was similarly enhanced and ranged from 900 to about 1500 ml. During the last trimester there was a dramatic decline in the ability to excrete water, so that at term most women were well below the non-pregnant average. One woman reached a maximum flow of only 4 ml per minute and had excreted less than 200 ml in two hours. These results are shown in Figures 4.4 and 4.5.

It is not clear what physiological conclusion can be drawn from these results since they represent the response to an abnormal stimulus. The woman with the maximum urine flow of 4 ml per

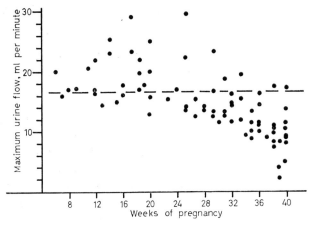

FIGURE 4.4. The maximum rate of urine flow after drinking one litre of water in pregnancy (Hytten and Klopper, 1963)

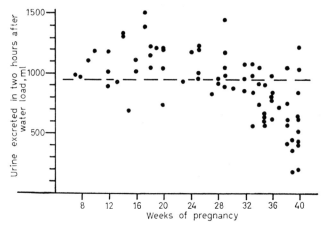

FIGURE 4.5. The volume of urine passed in two hours after drinking one litre of water in pregnancy (Hytten and Klopper, 1963)

minute, for example, would not have drunk a litre of water in the ordinary course of events. In early pregnancy, on the other hand, thirst is one of the commonest symptoms and many women will volunteer the information that they are continually drinking water, which they never did before pregnancy. It was established that the enhanced ability to excrete water in early pregnancy was not due to a sodium diuresis, but a diuresis of 'free' water. Much more information is needed in this field.

Excretion of other substances

Sugar. Pregnancy may reveal a latent diabetes mellitus (see chap. 6) but benign glycosuria is commonplace in pregnancy and its incidence, according to Chesley (1960) may be up to 35 per cent. The presence of glycosuria after glucose loading was once used as a test for the diagnosis of pregnancy. The excretion of sugar is probably no more than the result of increased glomerular filtration: more glucose is filtered and presented to the tubules per minute than they can reabsorb. Christensen (1958) showed that the maximum rate of reabsorption of glucose by the tubules (Tm_G) was not altered by pregnancy. For 6 women in the 3rd and 4th months, average Tm_G was 353 ± 66 mg per minute compared to 331 ± 74 for a non-pregnant control group; for two women in late pregnancy the figures were 278 and 527. Although we may accept this evidence as suggesting an unaltered Tm_G, a much larger number of pregnant women must be investigated in detail before it can be accepted with confidence that there is no change.

The mammary glands probably make lactose from blood glucose throughout most of pregnancy, and some of it passes back to the blood and is excreted in the urine. It may be the source of galactose and fucose for the manufacture of glycoproteins and glycolipids in the foetus.

Amino acids. The pregnant woman excretes more amino acids in her urine than the non-pregnant woman. The excretion of histidine, which suffers the major loss in urine, has been studied particularly. Page, Glendening, Dignam and Harper (1954) calculated the histidine clearance in ten normal pregnant women to be 28 ml per minute compared to about 8 ml per minute for the same women in the puerperium. Inulin clearance, measured simultaneously, showed that the glomerular filtration was raised by 64 per cent in pregnancy, but even with the somewhat higher blood levels of histidine in pregnancy, this explained only about half the increased loss in urine. Since the ability of the tubules to reabsorb histidine is greatly in excess of the load presented to them in pregnancy (Smith, 1951) their failure to reabsorb is a mystery. Page *et al.* concluded that there was an inhibition of the reabsorption mechanism in pregnancy and Petersen and Frank (1958), quoted by Chesley (1960), came to a similar conclusion, but there is no direct evidence of inhibition.

Wallraff, Brodie and Borden (1950) in a study of twelve women, mostly in late pregnancy, described increased renal excretion of a number of amino acids and this has been confirmed by Christensen, Date, Schønheyder and Volqvartz (1957). Wallraff, Brodie and Borden found, for example, that while the non-pregnant woman excreted an average of 112 mg of histidine in 24 hours, the pregnant woman excreted 371 mg, a difference of 259 mg (see also Chapter 13).

Other nutrients. Amino acids and sugar are not the only nutrients squandered by the kidney in pregnancy as an inevitable consequence of the increased GFR. Inorganic iodine is also lost in greatly increased amounts: renal clearance of iodine rises from an average non-pregnant figure of about 30 ml per minute to over 60 ml per minute in late pregnancy, reducing the plasma level of inorganic iodine to less than half its normal value. That change is almost certainly responsible for the goitre of pregnancy (see Chapter 6). There is also a greatly increased clearance of folic acid from the blood in pregnancy (Chanarin *et al.*, 1959; Hansen and Klewesahl-Palm, 1963). These workers injected 15 μg per kilogram body weight intravenously and sampled the blood 15 and 30 minutes later. The change during pregnancy was negligible compared to the difference between pregnant and non-pregnant values. (see Figure 13.1). For example, in the women described by Chanarin *et al.* the normal non-pregnant subjects 15 minutes after the injection had a serum folic acid concentration of 43 mμg per ml; at 12 weeks of pregnancy it was 28 mμg per ml and fell only to about 22 in late pregnancy, a difference which might be largely explained by increased dilution in the bigger plasma volume. Chanarin *et al.* explain these changes in terms of increased competition for folic acid from the uterus and its contents but the picture is much more likely to result from the increased renal clearance. The wastage may predispose to megaloblastic anaemia in pregnancy.

There are almost certainly other examples of nutrients being spilled through the kidneys in pregnancy; it is a fertile field for research. The subject is discussed again in Chapter 13.

Response to acidosis

Assali, Herzig and Singh (1954–55) studied the effect of giving 15 g of ammonium chloride daily for 3 or 4 days to six normal pregnant women. Detailed results were not published but the general conclusion was that 'the pattern of renal response was qualitatively similar to that of non-pregnant subjects.'

MECHANISMS FOR THE CHANGES IN RENAL FUNCTION

Almost nothing is known of the way in which the changes in renal function we have described are brought about. The effect, if any, of the steroid sex hormones on renal function in pregnancy is unknown partly because it is wellnigh impossible to produce in non-pregnant subjects the very high concentrations of hormones reached in pregnancy. Dignam, Voskian and Assali (1956) gave a single intravenous dose of 25 or 50 mg of oestradiol-17β, or 8 mg by intramuscular injection for 3 to 6 days, to a group of menopausal women, without altering either renal plasma flow or glomerular filtration rate. Sodium excretion fell and some water was retained. Preedy and Aitken (1956) on the other hand, found no change in sodium excretion in subjects to whom they gave daily intramuscular doses of 10 mg of oestradiol benzoate.

Both oxytocin and pitressin have been shown by Assali's group to reduce the free water clearance (Assali, Dignam and Longo, 1960; Abdul-Karim and Assali, 1961) pitressin (anti-diuretic hormone), but not oxytocin, reducing both the renal plasma flow and the glomerular filtration rate. It is possible that these posterior pituitary hormones are responsible for the terminal fall in renal plasma flow and the ability to excrete a water load, although it has been shown that the blood in pregnancy contains a substance which inactivates these hormones (Woodbury *et al.* 1946; Hawker, 1956).

Secretion and excretion of aldosterone increase greatly during pregnancy but the effects are not clear. It has been suggested that progesterone is an aldosterone antagonist and aldosterone production rises to combat the high progesterone production, but there is little firm evidence. These changes are discussed in detail in Chapter 6.

Filtration at the glomerulus depends to a large extent on filtration pressure in the glomerular capillaries. That pressure is the difference between the hydrostatic pressure of blood in the capillaries and the opposing colloid osmotic pressure of the non-filterable plasma proteins. It can be calculated from the changes in plasma protein concentration described in Chapter 1 that colloid osmotic pressure drops from about 25 mm Hg before pregnancy to as little as 16 mm Hg by the beginning of the second trimester, and this fall must greatly augment filtration rate.

It is difficult to see much biological sense in many of the changes we have described. While it might seem reasonable for the woman to increase her excretory powers to ensure adequate waste disposal for the foetus, even though the need must be small, it seems unreasonable to make the maximum adjustment in early pregnancy and then reduce it when one would have imagined the load to be greatest. It will be suggested later (Chapter 13) that the changes in composition of maternal blood which result, at least partly, from those renal changes may be related to the provisioning of the foetus.

CHAPTER 5

Alimentary Function

Upsets of gastro-intestinal function are perhaps the commonest cause of complaint by pregnant women but, although the gut is accessible compared with the heart or kidney, relatively few physiological measurements have been made.

APPETITE AND EATING HABITS

In an enquiry about appetite made by a dietitian at an Aberdeen ante-natal clinic (Taggart, 1961a) more than half the women reported an obvious increase of appetite, and increased thirst was even more common. For most of them the increase began in the first trimester; it might persist throughout pregnancy or decline in the later months. Change, or lack of it, in the sensation of hunger is not necessarily an accurate guide to change in food intake and we have the impression from a current study of weighed diet surveys in pregnancy that women may have a considerable increase of food intake without noticing any change of appetite. A bigger appetite in early pregnancy and a reduced capacity for large meals in late pregnancy leads to the more frequent eating of snacks between meals.

Qualitative changes in food habits are surprisingly common. A few women deliberately avoid certain things, notably fried or fatty foods, in an attempt to control heartburn, but preferences or cravings for, or aversions to certain foods without apparent reason occurred in two thirds of the series reported by Taggart. The most common craving was for fruit which was readily available and many women had a strong desire for highly flavoured or savoury foods, for example pickles, cheese or kippers. Aversions were almost as common, particularly to tea and coffee; fried foods and eggs also were disliked.

Harries and Hughes (1957) summarized information obtained by the British Broadcasting Corporation which had invited women to write about cravings after a broadcast programme on the subject. There were 514 letters, which provide a unique collection of anecdotal information, from writers not to be taken as a representative sample of pregnant women. Of 991 cravings reported, 261 were for fruit, 105 for vegetables and 187 for other foods, usually pickles or raw cereals. There were 193 instances of aversion, to tea, coffee and smoking. 'Many correspondents stressed the seriousness of these "cravings" during pregnancy and the lengths to which they went to satisfy them . . . many mentioned the sense of secrecy they experienced and how they kept their "cravings" secret even from their husbands'.

Pica also was reported by 88 of the BBC correspondents. In 35 the craving was for coal, in 17 for soap, in 15 for disinfectant and in 14 for toothpaste. These numbers almost certainly give an exaggerated picture of the incidence of pica although it is difficult to obtain information when many of the women who experience it are at pains to hide the fact. Of 800 Aberdeen women who discussed their diets at length with Taggart, none reported pica.

We have had personal experience of only one woman who showed no reluctance to discuss her pica. In the last few weeks of two otherwise normal pregnancies, this woman developed a strong craving for the chewing of pieces of coal and spent match heads, and for the sniffing of turpentine. She was fussy about the grade of coal she would eat and it seemed that texture rather than flavour was the criterion of quality; she preferred good quality coal which crunched in a satisfying way and ate about 2 dozen sweet-sized pieces daily. Soon after delivery she found the chewing of coal unpleasant.

Hansen and Langer (1935) have suggested that the desire for salted and spiced foods may be due to dulling of the sense of taste in pregnancy. In tests where 28 pregnant women were compared with 12 non-pregnant women, the threshold for all forms of taste, salt, sweet, sour and bitter, was raised in pregnancy.

THE MOUTH

The gums are often swollen and 'spongy' in pregnancy, and bleed easily and it is widely believed, both by dentists and the general public, that pregnancy damages the teeth; 'for every child, a tooth'. Yet scientific opinion is by no means unanimous in its support of this view. James (1941) reviewed the evidence and concluded that pregnancy has no effect on the teeth. The composition of the adult tooth, he said, is unaffected by even gross changes in metabolism, and he quoted an experiment in which a pregnant bitch was maintained on a calcium poor diet. At the end of the experiment the bones were so decalcified that they were almost invisible to X-ray and could be cut with a knife; yet the teeth showed no change either radiologically or by chemical analysis. Other studies, for example, by Deakins and Looby (1943) and Dragiff and Karshan (1943), confirmed by chemical analysis of human dentine that there was no demineralization during pregnancy.

That there is no demineralization of the dentine is no argument against possible deterioration of the surface of the teeth in pregnancy. There seems only to have been one small epidemiological study of the problem. Buhs (1959) found that there was a mean increase of 3.32 'carious surfaces' over a two month period in 50 pregnant women compared to 0.31 in 29 controls of similar age. The increase seemed to be greatest during the fifth to seventh months and was due largely to fissure caries. Buhs also analyzed the saliva. For the control women the average pH was 6.69, but it was 6.11 in early pregnancy, and reached a minimum of 5.98 in the eighth month. There was a negative correlation between the buffer capacity of the saliva and the incidence of new caries. The reduced pH of saliva in pregnancy was not confirmed by Rosenthal, Rowen and Vazakas (1959); they found the mean pH in pregnancy to be 7.0 compared to 6.5 in non-pregnant women. The measurement of pH in saliva is not simple. pH depends on both the pCO_2 and the bicarbonate concentration and loss of CO_2 after secretion raises the pH. The saliva must therefore be collected anaerobically; it must also be collected under standard conditions of flow since the flow rate also influences pH. In neither of these studies were these precautions taken. There is no theoretical reason why saliva should be more acid in pregnancy since both the pCO_2 and bicarbonate concentrations are affected proportionally by blood pCO_2 (Burgen and Emmelin, 1961).

The relationship of acidity in the mouth to the incidence of caries is not well understood and a more extensive investigation, both epidemiological and chemical, might be worth while.

Ptyalism, the excessive secretion of saliva, is quoted by all textbooks of obstetrics as a rare complication of pregnancy, almost always associated with nausea. Figures quoted by textbooks of obstetrics suggest that one to two litres of saliva may be secreted daily, but this would be accepted by physiologists (for example, Best and Taylor, 1961) as a normal volume. The confusion could arise simply because it may be difficult for the nauseated pregnant woman to *swallow* her saliva as she otherwise would; there is no real evidence of excessive secretion in pregnancy.

THE OESOPHAGUS

Many, otherwise normal, pregnant women suffer from heartburn, a subjective complaint characterized primarily by a painful retrosternal burning sensation. There has been no scientific study of the condition in pregnancy but Tuttle, Rufin and Bettarello (1961) who examined pressure and pH changes in the oesophagus, and the effect of introducing acid in men who had the symptom, gave convincing evidence that it is usually due to a reflux of gastric contents. If this is the mechanism in pregnancy, then a greater liability to reflux may be due to a general relaxation of the stomach, and with it of the cardiac sphincter (see below) particularly when intraabdominal pressure is raised. A study in pregnancy, similar to that of Tuttle, Rufin and Bettarello, would be interesting, although heartburn is seldom a serious disability and usually responds to antacids.

THE STOMACH

Although the stomach is a relatively accessible organ, it is far from easy to study it under normal working conditions. What we need to know is the response of the stomach to a normal meal, but food residues block the usual stomach tubes and complicate chemical analysis so that the procedures for studying gastric function have generally relied on the stimulation of secretion either by watery 'meals' or by histamine.

Studies of gastric emptying and patterns of motility can be made with normal meals by radiography, and some of the early work is based on such observations. But it would now be ethically difficult to justify such a study in normal women in view of possible radiation effects, and modern studies of gastric motility are based on the disappearance of standard watery 'meals'.

Methods of study and their interpretation are fully discussed in two recent monographs (James, 1957; Gregory, 1962).

Secretion

A satisfactory study of gastric secretion, where a large group of women has been studied serially in pregnancy, has yet to be made. Individual variation in gastric function is wide and cross-sectional studies with small numbers of subjects give unconvincing results. Nevertheless, there is striking consistency in the general finding that gastric secretion is reduced during pregnancy. Earlier work has been reviewed by Murray, Erskine and Fielding (1957). They themselves studied the effect of histamine on gastric secretion in fourteen pregnant women, using the augmented histamine test, 0.4 mg of histamine acid phosphate per 10 kg of body weight, which is said to provoke maximum gastric secretion. The undesirable side effects of such an amount of histamine were abolished by giving an antihistamine drug which does not influence the gastric effects, and care was taken that saliva did not contaminate the gastric contents. In aspirates of gastric juice collected for 45 minutes from fasting women, secretion of acid was found to be 79 ± 20 mg per 45 minutes in the first trimester, 36 ± 12 in the middle trimester and 107 ± 28 in the last trimester, compared to 63 ± 7.8 mg per 45 minutes for non-pregnant women. After histamine, the mean total acid rose to 249 ± 30 mg per 30 minutes in the first trimester, 262 ± 46 mg in the second trimester and 419 ± 52 in the last trimester, compared to 360 ± 44 in non-pregnant women. Hunt and Murray (1958) found a similar indication of reduced secretion in early or mid-pregnancy with a terminal increase, for both acid and pepsin in a small group of women who were given test meals of water or saline. The individual variation was so great, and the number of observations so few, that it is not possible to describe quantitative changes with any confidence.

The response to histamine is particularly difficult to interpret. Marks, Komarov and Shay (1960) have shown with dogs that the 'maximal histamine response' is highly correlated with the total number of acid-producing cells in the stomach, but when vagal tone is low it does not define the maximum secretory *capacity* of these cells. The reduced peptic activity and decreased motility (see below) of the stomach in pregnancy suggest that the vagal tone may indeed be low and this may be in part responsible for the reduced response to histamine.

A confirmation of the reduced peptic activity is given by

Gryboski and Spiro (1956) who measured the levels of pepsin in blood, taking these as reflecting gastric secretion. The blood levels were below the non-pregnant and post-partum levels until about the seventh month of pregnancy when they rose to approximately non-pregnant levels.

An attempt has been made in Figure 5.1 to summarize the pattern of change in gastric secretion shown by the studies we have

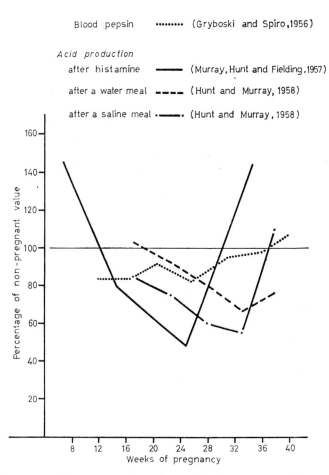

FIGURE 5.1. The pattern of gastric secretion in pregnancy. Measurements from three published studies are reduced to a comparable basis by expressing them as percentage changes from the non-pregnant mean

K

quoted above. To reduce these diverse results to a comparable basis they are shown in terms of percentage change; the non-pregnant or post-partum value is taken as 100 per cent. The results for pepsin secretion reported by Hunt and Murray (1958) are not included because they give no non-pregnant value.

The reduced secretory activity of the stomach may explain the well-known clinical observation that peptic ulcer is rare in pregnancy. For example, Clarke (1953) studied 118 women who had a total of 313 pregnancies while suffering from proven peptic ulceration. There was a clear remission of symptoms in about 9 out of 10 of the pregnancies, but the relief was short-lived and symptoms had returned in most cases by the third month after delivery.

Motility

It is generally assumed and has been confirmed by X-ray studies that gastric tone and motility are reduced in pregnancy. For example, Hansen (1937) described the stomach as hanging like a loose sack over the fundus of the uterus, and showed that the emptying time, judged from X-ray studies of radio-opaque meals, increased from a normal average of 50 minutes, to between 80 and 130 minutes in pregnancy. Boyden and Rigler (1944) in a study designed to find out whether slower emptying of the gall bladder in pregnancy might be due to slower emptying of the stomach, gave radio-opaque meals of egg yolk with barium sulphate to 35 primigravidae in the second and third trimesters of pregnancy. They claim little if any delay in emptying but the results are expressed in such a way that comparison with other studies, or with non-pregnant subjects, cannot be made. Normally, the rate of emptying of the stomach depends not only on its propulsive power, but on inhibitory mechanisms regulated from receptors in the duodenum and upper small intestine. Water and solid food both operate the duodenal 'brake' but solutions of about 100 mEq NaCl per litre of water leave the stomach very quickly, presumably because the inhibitory mechanism is not activated. Hunt and Murray (1958) gave test meals of both water and the saline solution to seven women in pregnancy. The performance of pregnant women in emptying a meal of 750 ml of water was little different from that of non-pregnant subjects; if anything, the emptying of the saline meal was more rapid than normal.

The evidence, on the one hand that motility is reduced and on the other hand that it is not, is not necessarily contradictory. If the secretion of gastric juice is reduced, then digestion may be slower and the emptying time of a normal, solid meal prolonged, even though a watery meal is emptied in a normal time. We need much more information.

A general lack of tone in the stomach during pregnancy would fit the picture of generalized relaxation of smooth muscle: of other parts of the gut, of the uterus, the ureters, the blood vessels. It might also explain the common tendency to nausea. Wolf (1943) showed that gastric relaxation and hypomotility were essential to the occurrence of nausea. He caused nausea by such provocation as caloric vestibular stimulation and the occurrence of nausea was associated with interruption of gastric contractions and decreased muscle tone of the stomach wall. If gastric tone and motility were maintained with prostigmine and atropine, nausea did not occur despite strong vestibular stimulation.

THE SMALL INTESTINE

Because of the anabolism of pregnancy, it might reasonably be expected that gut function would improve but, with most commonly eaten diets, there is not much scope to improve the percentage digestion of organic nutrients. Improvement is therefore more likely to be in the amount of food dealt with in a day, the rate of turnover. In perhaps the only published study of absorption of nutrients in human pregnancy, Hahn et al. (1951) showed that uptake of iron from a dose of ferrous sulphate labelled with ^{59}Fe increased progressively with advancing pregnancy. But this does not imply a changed ability to absorb iron; it is probably no more than an extension of the mechanism which operates in the non-pregnant subject: increased absorption when there is increased demand. There is no scientific evidence for or against improved efficiency of function, but there is clinical evidence, illustrated in a dramatic way by the following case reported by Montgomery and Pincus (1955).

A 23-year-old woman in three operations between the ages of 16 and 20, had the whole of her ileum and two feet of jejunum removed for stenosing ileitis, leaving only about three feet of small intestine. She was maintained with the help of testosterone in a somewhat precarious state of health, 10 to 15 lb underweight and passing 2 to 4 soft stools daily 'containing significant amounts of undigested fat and meat fibres as well as undigested vegetable material'. Mild infections resulted in considerable weight loss. Shortly after the start of the pregnancy only one stool per day was passed, more formed than usual, and which on microscopic examination appeared to contain less undigested food. She had an enormous appetite, eating a diet providing between 4000 and 5000 kcal daily and her weight gain in pregnancy was about 14 lb. She delivered a normal female infant weighing 6 lb.

Dr Montgomery tells us that she has had two more successful pregnancies with similar improvement in function and that her condition between pregnancies had returned to what it was before her first pregnancy. It is a great pity that an opportunity was not taken with this remarkable case to make balance studies.

THE LARGE INTESTINE

The colon may share in the general relaxation of smooth muscle structures; constipation is a common complaint.

THE LIVER AND GALL-BLADDER

The liver is deeply involved, during pregnancy as at any other time, with many metabolic processes and some of its functions are almost certainly running at a different level in pregnancy. There is no information.

The gall-bladder shares the general muscular sluggishness. Gerdes and Boyden (1938) showed by X-ray studies that the gall-bladder emptied poorly in pregnancy. For example, in five women studied before and after pregnancy the mean discharge of contents 40 minutes after an egg yolk and milk test meal was 38 per cent during pregnancy and 71 per cent 6 to 8 weeks after delivery. Huggins, Harden and Grier (1935) made a radiological study of the gall-bladders of 388 pregnant women and described some abnormality, usually gross enlargement or slow emptying in 208.

Potter (1936) examined the gall-bladder at 390 caesarean sections; 75 per cent had 'large, atonic, globular, distended gall-bladders' and the bile on aspiration was found generally to be thick, tarry and viscous. There seems to be no convincing evidence of any chemical change in the bile (Potter, 1936; Large *et al.* 1960). That childbearing predisposes to gallstones is widely accepted although well founded epidemiological evidence is lacking (Rains, 1961). Those who deny the relationship, for example Large *et al.* (1960), point to evidence that the chemistry of the bile is not altered, but with or without chemical change it seems reasonable that increased concentration of bile would favour stone formation.

In summary, we have little satisfactory information about alimentary function, but what we do know appears contradictory. Heartburn, nausea and constipation give the woman herself an impression of poor function and the physiologist has found evidence of depressed motor activity and reduced secretion. And yet there is a strong possibility that digestion and assimilation of foodstuffs is unusually efficient. There is a rich field here for research, and the use of isotopes and perhaps some imaginative new techniques should be capable of resolving this apparent paradox.

CHAPTER 6

Hormones

This section will deal both with those hormones which appear to play a specific role in pregnancy, such as the sex steroids, chorionic gonadotrophin, and some pituitary hormones; and those whose secretion, or the response to it, may be modified by the changing conditions of pregnancy; for example, thyroid, pancreatic and adrenal hormones.

For the first group, a voluminous and rapidly expanding literature is concerned mainly with the sex steroids, progesterone and a family of oestrogens, since they can be estimated chemically; much less has been written about those hormones whose estimation depends on more difficult animal assays. Although it is universally assumed that the sex steroids, at least, have important functions as chemical organizers of the physiological adaptations in pregnancy the mass of publications throw little direct light on their functions. We cannot attempt here, as we have in other chapters, to give a critique of methods. The details of both biochemical and animal assays are nevertheless of great importance to the understanding and interpretation of published results; they are the subject of a large volume of complex and often contradictory writings, and every worker in the field must bring considerable biochemical knowledge to bear on the minutiae.

Research has been mostly on the excreted end-products of hormones and more often from a clinical than a physiological interest. Though speculation provides a healthy stimulus to further work, it can fairly be said that a disproportionate amount of theory has been built on these results; there has been a tendency, as it were, to infer the whole theory and practice of the internal combustion engine from no more than a crude knowledge of the exhaust gases.

At the other extreme, a good deal is now known about the biochemical properties, *in vitro*, of some of the hormones; for example of their action in enzyme systems, although it is not known whether hormones have to be metabolized to exert their effect or whether they act as catalysts. And something is known of the physiological effects of administering hormones to man and animals usually by injection. For several reasons, interpretation of such experiments must be cautious: the action of a hormone given alone may be different from its action in the presence of other hormones; the site of administration may be sufficiently remote from the site of action for modification of the hormone to occur in transit; in many experiments a synthetic compound such as stilboestrol has been used and, while it may have certain powerful 'oestrogenic' effects, that does not necessarily help to an understanding of the action of natural oestrogens. We are obliged in this section to draw on many results from animal experiments simply because no evidence for man is available, but we must emphasize now that the actions of many hormones are known to vary from species to species and conclusions from animal evidence can be transferred to man only with great caution. The crucial information needed to understand hormone action still eludes the physiologist; namely the effects of different amounts and *combinations* of hormones *at their sites of action.* In some cases we do not even know the target organs or cells.

We propose to deal with the hormones individually, summarizing what is known about their sites of production, the amounts produced, their probable sites of action and their physiological effects. In the general sphere of the physiology of pregnancy, no subject of research is growing with the speed of endocrinology, and we are acutely aware that a general summary in a textbook of this sort may well be out of date before it is published. In the past few years there have been several excellent critical reviews which cover much of the ground and we will quote extensively from them. They provide comprehensive bibliographies for those who wish to penetrate the subject more deeply.

The sex steroids, progesterone, oestrogens and androgens, and the adrenocortical steroids are all closely related chemically and the biosynthesis of one may involve the manufacture of one or more of the others as intermediary products. Because of this, an excreted end-product may give an appearance of simplicity to what may have been an extremely complicated endocrine pattern.

PROGESTERONE

Sites of production

Progesterone, traditionally regarded as the hormone which preserves pregnancy, is produced in every menstrual cycle by the corpus luteum of the ovary, probably in the luteinized granulosa cells. After conception the corpus luteum continues to produce progesterone probably throughout pregnancy. The contribution it makes to total progesterone production during most of pregnancy is probably unimportant since pregnancy can continue successfully even if both ovaries are removed at an early stage, but in the first weeks of pregnancy ovarian progesterone may be vital (see also p. 162). Diczfalusy and Borell (1961) measured pregnanediol excretion before and after complete ablation of ovarian tissue in a pregnant woman 78 days after her last menstrual period and concluded that the ovarian contribution to total progesterone is negligible at that stage.

The main source of the hormone in human pregnancy is the placenta. Evidence for this is overwhelming and is discussed in detail in the review by Diczfalusy and Troen (1961). Deane and Seligman (1953) have shown histochemically that progesterone is produced in the syncytial cells of the trophoblast. The evolutionary movement from ovarian to placental control of pregnancy has been described by Medawar (1953) as 'towards a complete endocrinological self-sufficiency of the foetus and its membranes—in short, towards the evolution of a self-maintaining system enjoying the highest possible degree of independence of its environment'.

The maternal adrenal cortex also may produce some progesterone but the amounts are probably trivial; certainly adrenalectomized women who become pregnant show no evidence of reduced progesterone (Moses et al. 1959; Venning et al. 1959). The foetus itself may also contribute to the supply, possibly from its adrenal glands. Cassmer (1959), for example, showed a small but remarkably consistent fall in pregnanediol output in midpregnancy, after the foetus had been killed by tying the umbilical cord as a prelude to termination of pregnancy. These experiments will be discussed further below.

In summary, the major and possibly the only important source of progesterone during pregnancy is the syncytium of the placenta; small and physiologically unimportant amounts are produced by the mother's ovaries and perhaps her adrenal glands; and the foetus also may contribute small amounts.

The quantity produced

Most of our knowledge of progesterone production is derived from measurement of its characteristic, physiologically inert end-product, 5β-pregnane-3α:20α-diol (pregnanediol), excreted in the urine. Klopper and Michie (1956) computed the amount of pregnanediol excreted after intramuscular injection of 50 or 100 mg of progesterone in oil. In men and post-menopausal women recovery ranged from 5.1 to 16.8 per cent of the injected progesterone with a concentration of values around 13 per cent; both extremes of the range occurred in one woman. In one menstruating woman recoveries ranged from 6.4 to 14.5 per cent and in three women 15, 16 and 25 weeks pregnant, recoveries were 21.9, 12.8 and 11.0 per cent. There was no explanation for the wide range. Trolle (1955) found a somewhat smaller range, 10 to 14.8 per cent, in 3 women during different phases of the menstrual cycle and in one woman in early pregnancy.

The rate of secretion of progesterone (and of the oestrogens) has been estimated by dilution techniques. Progesterone labelled with ^{14}C or ^{3}H is injected into the subject and radioactive metabolites subsequently appear in the urine; the secretion of progesterone is reckoned to be related to the amount injected in the ratio of stable to radio-active metabolite excreted. Even if the inevitable errors, particularly of counting small amounts of awkward isotopes, be accepted, it is difficult to accept all the assumptions on which such a method is based. In making the calculation of secretion rate, for example, the injected progesterone must be assumed to mix with endogenous progesterone and to be metabolized in the same way; but progesterone is released from the placenta in two directions, to the maternal and foetal circulations, and the foetal fraction which the injected progesterone almost certainly cannot reach, is metabolized in quite a different way. Figures derived from such methods, which we will quote below, must be accepted only as first order approximations; so far they are the best available.

Pearlman (1957a) calculated the endogenous progesterone production by dilution of injected progesterone labelled with ^{3}H, and at the same time, the output of pregnanediol in urine. Three women at 25, 34 and 36 weeks of pregnancy (the last with twins) were estimated to be producing 275, 212 and 284 mg of progesterone per day with corresponding urinary excretion of pregnanediol of 16, 30 and 42 mg; i.e. recoveries were of 6, 14 and 15 per cent. In two non-pregnant women recoveries were of 14 and 27 per cent. Four other estimates of progesterone secretion in late normal pregnancy have been made with Pearlman's technique by Van der Wiele *et al.* (1960). The rates were 265, 370, 385 and 500 mg per 24 hours. Ejarque and Bengtsson (1962) made a similar study of one woman at 19 weeks of pregnancy with progesterone labelled with ^{14}C. They collected urine for only 24 hours after injecting the labelled hormone. The women produced an estimated average of 75 mg progesterone daily with a pregnanediol output of 17 mg, about 23 per cent.

Davis and Plotz (1958) injected ^{14}C-4-progesterone into 10 women between the 9th and 17th weeks of pregnancy. Recovery of radioactivity in the urine, presumably in breakdown products of progesterone but not necessarily all pregnanediol, varied from 15.3 to 61.7 per cent of the administered dose. Clearly we cannot with confidence derive progesterone production from pregnanediol output; the published range of recovery is from 6 to 27 per cent. Much more work is needed to confirm the range, to study possible reasons for the variation, and to see whether or not it changes during pregnancy; the issue is not only of great intrinsic interest, it is vital to a proper understanding of pregnanediol excretion. Not all the pregnanediol formed is excreted in urine; some appears in the faeces, probably excreted in bile (Klopper and Macnaughton, 1959). The full story of progesterone metabolism has yet to be written; other metabolities are known and may yet be found to provide a better picture of progesterone production. It is curious that so much research has been expended on polishing the technique for estimating pregnanediol and so little on discovering how faithfully it is likely to represent its parent hormone.

There have been many studies of the output of pregnanediol in urine. Most of these have been made for clinical purposes and the assay has enjoyed a vogue as a measure of placental function. Two recent studies in which the highly specific method of Klopper, Michie and Brown (1955) was used, and normal subjects were carefully selected, show closely similar average patterns of excretion (Shearman, 1959; Klopper and Billewicz, 1963). Their results are shown in Figure 6.1. The rise in output is continuous but the rate of increase falls off in late pregnancy and the shape of the curve has been likened to that of growth in weight of the placenta (Figure 10.5). The range about this normal average line is wide, with the highest value three or four times the lowest at all stages. To what extent the variation reflects differences in progesterone production cannot be known until more information is available about individual differences of conversion or excretion. Estimates of pregnanediol may give interesting information in an epidemiological survey, but it would seem unwise at present to read much into the results of measurements on an individual woman. Shearman found multigravidae to have a lower mean output than primigravidae but Klopper and Billewicz could not confirm

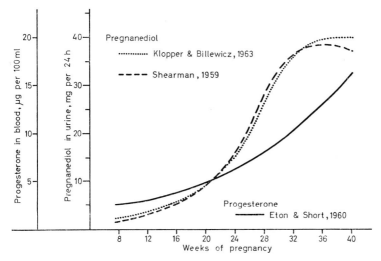

FIGURE 6.1. Excretion of pregnanediol in urine during pregnancy compared with the concentration of progesterone in blood

this. Shearman also showed a close correlation between the output of pregnanediol before delivery and the weight of the baby and of the placenta. He included abnormal pregnancies in his analysis and the coincidence of small babies delivered before term and low outputs of pregnanediol would greatly magnify such a correlation. For normal pregnancies with delivery at term, Klopper and Billewicz (1963) could find no relation between weight of the baby and pregnanediol output.

If we assume, for purposes of discussion, that the excretion of pregnanediol averages about 15 per cent of the progesterone produced and that rate of conversion is constant throughout pregnancy, then progesterone production at term will be about 300 mg daily. Just how much of it derives from the placenta is not known, but the ovarian output, which is likely to be the major nonplacental contribution of progesterone, is probably no more than 20–25 mg per 24 hours. The woman studied in mid-pregnancy by Ejarque and Bengtsson (1962) produced about 22 mg of progesterone after removal of the placenta, much the same level as one would expect in the luteal phase of the menstrual cycle when a peak of about 3 or 4 mg of pregnanediol is excreted in the urine.

Knowledge only of the rate of production contributes little to a useful picture of the physiology of progesterone in pregnancy. It seems well established that progesterone has a very short life, at least in the blood. For example, Pearlman (1957b) reported the 'turnover time' to be about 3 minutes and Short and Eton (1959) found the half life in the blood to be about 5 minutes. The liver appears to be the major site of degradation to pregnanediol but it may be that destruction takes place also within the cells where progesterone exerts its action; some disappears apparently unaltered into the tissues, particularly into depot fat (Davis and Plotz, 1958).

The development of techniques for measuring the very small quantities of progesterone present in samples of body fluids or tissues is at a relatively early stage and few results are available. The concentration in peripheral blood, where progesterone is carried mostly by plasma albumin (Haskins and Taubert, 1963), has been measured by a number of workers. Eton and Short (1960), for example, found the concentration in plasma to rise slowly from about 2 to 12 μg per 100 ml between the 9th and about the 35th week of pregnancy, and to rise more steeply thereafter to about 17 μg per 100 ml, but with individual values as high as 30 μg per 100 ml. Greig et al. (1962) used Short's method and found a similar picture, but they did not publish the data except as a graph; there was a wide scatter of results in late pregnancy. They noted that blood progesterone was more closely related to oestriol than to pregnanediol in urine. The pattern of blood progesterone is quite different from the pattern of pregnanediol excretion (see Figure 6.1) suggesting a changing rate of metabolism of circulating progesterone. But even the concentration in peripheral blood may be no more than an indirect reflection of what we need to know, namely the state of affairs at the site of action. In mid-pregnancy at least the concentration of progesterone in uterine venous blood is, on the average, about ten times that in peripheral blood (Fuchs, 1962).

We will discuss possible sites of action below but it can be said now that if the major action of progesterone is on the uterus then it may exert its action directly, by diffusion from the placenta, and any hormone which appears in the blood may be no more than an overflow. Progesterone secreted into the intervillous blood seems unlikely to exert much local effect on the uterus. The blood is swept past the myometrium in large venous channels without ever making intimate contact; the myometrium is supplied by the uterine arteries with peripheral blood. If it acts at a distance from its site of production, and some actions suggest that it does, then presumably the concentration in peripheral blood is relevant, and in that case a potent organizer is produced in extravagant amounts so that a small fraction which survives chemical annihilation by the liver can act effectively.

As might be expected, the placenta itself contains considerable quantities of progesterone but Zander (1959) has shown that, apart from very early pregnancy when the concentration is about 6 μg per g, the concentration remains relatively constant throughout most of pregnancy at about 2 μg per g.

Except for its affinity for adipose tissue, progesterone is not known to be selectively taken up by any tissue. Studies with the labelled hormone, for example, have shown it to have no special affinity for the myometrium or endometrium, two presumed sites of action. In a recent paper, Barnes, Kumar and Goodno (1962) describe a mean concentration of 0.63 μg per g in myometrium over the placenta and 0.31 μg in myometrium distant from the placenta, but individual results were inconsistent and more information is needed to confirm the difference.

In general, the body's endocrine secretions are under some central control, from the pituitary gland if not from the brain. But no such control has been demonstrated for the placenta and there is no evidence that its hormone production is regulated internally or from outside, according to need. In a case described by Little et al. (1958) the whole pituitary gland was removed because of carcinoma of the breast, at 26 weeks of pregnancy. The pregnancy continued until the 35th week with maintenance doses of thyroid hormone and cortisone. Excretion of pregnanediol in urine, measured unfortunately by a gravimetric method now known to be inaccurate, was much less than normal and failed to increase, but the child when delivered at 35 weeks weighed 5 lb and appeared healthy.

Another woman hypophysectomized at 12 weeks of pregnancy because of a chromophobe adenoma was described by Kaplan (1961). She was delivered of a 7½ lb baby by caesarean section at term and showed evidence of depressed progesterone production: her pregnanediol excretion near term was only 8 mg per 24 hours. That suggests the possibility of some pituitary control of progesterone production but obviously much more information is needed. The only other hint of a possible regulatory mechanism for progesterone is that of Landau and Lugibihl (1961) who suggested that progesterone causes sodium diuresis, less striking during pregnancy than in non-pregnant subjects, and that a high intake of dietary sodium provokes increased secretion of progesterone. A sodium-losing effect of progesterone could explain the rise in aldosterone excretion in pregnancy, the normal means of restoring equilibrium. The work has not been confirmed.

It is possible that some measure of control, at least of function, is imposed by other placental hormones, and we will be discussing below the likelihood that progesterone action is modified by other hormones, particularly the oestrogens.

Action of progesterone

In general, studies of the action of progesterone have been made at two widely separated levels: gross observable physiological changes which follow the administration of progesterone to intact animals, and biochemical reactions *in vitro*. At a deeper level a considerable literature is developing on the possible influence of progesterone on a number of intracellular enzyme systems. Such effects may eventually be shown to be the basis of hormone action, but their relevance to the physiological changes in pregnancy has not yet been demonstrated and we will not discuss them. Rather, we will examine briefly the evidence for attributing responsibility to hormones for some of the physiological changes characteristic of pregnancy.

THE UTERUS

It is generally believed that the main purpose of progesterone is to reduce muscle tone in the uterus and so to protect the foetus from the natural tendency of the uterus, like any other hollow muscular viscus, to expel its contents; an attractive hypothesis which makes good physiological sense, but its scientific basis is not yet solid. Many clinicians believe that progesterone will prevent abortion in women with a history of habitual abortion, or in cases of threatened abortion, but there has never been a controlled trial and the evidence is unconvincing.

A considerable amount of information on the effects of progesterone, and of oestrogens, on the uterus has been assembled, notably by Csapo and his group at the Rockefeller Institute in New York. They have used both intact animals and isolated uteri for their experiments and Csapo has recently reviewed some of the evidence (Csapo, 1961). The findings are complex, but the general conclusion is that progesterone reduces the excitability of the uterus, possibly by affecting the membrane potential of the myometrial fibres, particularly over the site of the placenta. Csapo has further found that some derivatives of progesterone, even pregnanediol, are capable of reducing electrical excitability of uterine muscle *in vitro*.

Growth of the uterus and changes in the vascularity and secretion of the cervix have also been attributed to progesterone (Fuchs, 1962).

OTHER SMOOTH MUSCLE

It has long been held that many of the changes in the functioning of smooth muscle in pregnancy may be due to the relaxing effects of progesterone, as described for the uterus. Such an effect might explain the atonic dilatation of the ureters, the reduced motility of stomach and colon and also the reduced vascular tone, all of which we have discussed in other chapters. Kumar (1962) has recently demonstrated, in experiments similar to those performed on uterine muscle by Csapo and his colleagues, that progesterone has an inhibitory effect on human smooth muscle from the ureter, the large bowel and the stomach. Unfortunately, both Kumar and Csapo used concentrations of progesterone which are likely to be far higher than physiological reality. It could be argued that concentrations of 5 μg progesterone per ml, which Csapo used, might be achieved in fluid bathing the myometrium near the placenta, but Kumar used solutions containing 12 μg per ml, and organs remote from the placenta, such as the ureters and stomach are being bathed by plasma which Short and Eton have shown to contain only about 0.02 μg per ml in early pregnancy when relaxation of smooth muscle is most apparent.

We need more evidence to establish a direct effect of progesterone on smooth muscle and a more simple hypothesis could explain all these phenomena equally well. If progesterone were needed to quieten the uterus it might achieve its effect by suppressing oxytocin secretion at its source in the hypothalamus. Such suppression would, *ipso facto*, reduce vasopressin secretion with consequent loss of tone in other smooth muscle structures, and could also help to explain the diabetes insipidus-like picture of water regulation in early pregnancy. It still remains to be explained why the uterus finally starts to contract, in labour, at a time when progesterone production is at its height; we shall see that at that time oestrogens which are said to oppose the action of progesterone on the uterus are also produced in large amounts.

A central site of action for progesterone would fit in with the observation by Trolle (1955) that male subjects given injections of progesterone complained 'of being tired, listless, sleepy and having difficulty in concentrating on their work' a picture which is familiar to many women in early pregnancy.

GENERAL METABOLIC EFFECTS

In most women the basal body temperature rises after ovulation in the normal cycle by about 0.5 to 1 °F, and if conception occurs, the raised temperature is maintained until about mid-pregnancy when it declines to normal levels (Davis, 1946; Buxton and Atkinson, 1948). Progesterone given to amenorrhoeic women causes a rise in body temperature (Palmer and Devilliers, 1939; Buxton and Atkinson, 1948), but the fever is now thought to be caused by derivatives of progesterone, primarily etiocholanolone but also pregnanediol (Kappas, Palmer and Glickman, 1961). Oestrogens are thought to oppose this action of progesterone and may be accountable for the fall of body temperature during late pregnancy (Palmer and Devilliers, 1939; Kaiser, 1955).

We have suggested in Chapter 11 that the extensive storage of depot fat in pregnancy could be governed by progesterone; no more than speculation at present but the finding of Galletti and Klopper (1962) that injected progesterone caused female rats to store fat supports the idea.

There is better evidence for the effect of progesterone in inducing overbreathing which reduces alveolar and arterial pCO_2 (Chapter 3). This striking pregnancy change has been duplicated in clinical practice by giving progesterone to emphysematous patients with hypercapnia (Tyler, 1960). The action may be central, possibly on the respiratory centres.

BREAST DEVELOPMENT

Both progesterone and oestrogens are generally assumed to be essential for breast growth, oestrogens alone causing mostly duct growth and the combined hormones, lobule-alveolar development. But in the monkey, for example, oestrogens alone can cause extensive growth of glandular tissue. The evidence has been recently reviewed by Benson *et al.* (1959). There is no experimental evidence for man and, in view of the species differences which are known to exist, the question remains open.

COMBINED ACTION WITH OTHER HORMONES

We will discuss the combined action of progesterone after we have discussed oestrogens since these are the hormones most often studied together. But it should be emphasized again that for many functions the action of one hormone is considerably modified by other hormones and in pregnancy, as distinct from most experimental situations, the large amounts of progesterone are always matched by large amounts of a number of other hormones.

THE OESTROGENS

The situation with regard to the oestrogens is even more complex than that of progesterone.

About eighteen oestrogens have so far been isolated from the urine in pregnancy. They are all related chemically, both to each other and to other steroid hormones such as progesterone and testosterone, and are probably derived from the metabolism of one or two primary compounds. Some of the pathways involved have recently been discussed by Klopper (1963). The three 'classical' oestrogens, oestrone, oestradiol-17β, and oestriol, occur in greatest profusion and are the only ones for which much information is available. Whether one of these is primary, in the sense that it is the only one made *de novo*, is not known; certainly oestrone and oestradiol-17β are readily interconvertible in the body. The many substances which are chemically classified as oestrogens differ in their physiological activity and a few appear to be inert. Differences

L

of action are likely to be subtle and almost nothing is known about them. It is usual to think of the oestrogens as separate pharmacological units, but perhaps we should pay more attention to the mixture itself; the level of one oestrogen may well affect the level of another, and the action of one may modify the action of another.

Sites of Production

Like progesterone, the oestrogens are produced cyclically by the ovaries of mature women, and by the adrenal cortex. In pregnancy the major site of production is the placenta, but whether the syncytial cells which produce progesterone also make oestrogens is not known. The evidence for placental production is detailed in the review by Diczfalusy and Troen (1961). They also review the evidence which suggests that, as with progesterone, the contribution of the ovaries and the adrenal cortex to oestrogen production in pregnancy is negligible. In one respect, the production of oestrogens by the placenta is curiously different from that of progesterone: it seems largely to depend on an intact foetal circulation. This particularly suggestive idea is being studied in Diczfalusy's laboratory in Stockholm and has recently been discussed in a review (Diczfalusy et al. 1961). Cassmer in that laboratory has described a series of experiments in which the umbilical cord was tied as a preliminary to termination of pregnancy (Cassmer, 1959). After the cord had been tied there was a precipitate drop in the maternal excretion of oestrone, oestradiol and oestriol to about half the pre-operative level, after which it declined slowly. Cassmer showed that the drop may be due, not to withdrawal of any contribution of hormone by the foetus, but simply to the absence of its blood circulation through the placenta. He perfused the foetal circulation with maternal blood for up to three hours while the placenta remained attached to the uterus and found oestrogen production almost completely restored. Cassmer has suggested that some of the enzymic reactions involved in the elaboration of oestrogens may be particularly sensitive to minor changes of oxygenation, but this is unlikely to be the whole story. Frandsen and Stakemann (1961) showed that in pregnancies where the foetus was anencephalic oestrogen excretion, but not the excretion of other hormones, was grossly depressed. It was suggested that the foetal adrenal gland, particularly the enlarged cortex, the 'foetal' zone, which is subnormal if not absent in anencephaly, may in some way be responsible for oestrogen production.

Quite clearly these findings conflict: Cassmer's that a blood circulation but not a foetus is necessary for oestrogen excretion by the placenta; that of Frandsen and Stakemann that a functioning foetal adrenal gland is necessary. More research is needed to resolve the conflict. In theory, the former arrangement would give the foetus, through control of its circulation, control over oestrogen supply to the mother, but there is no evidence at present to suggest that it does, in fact, exercise any such authority.

In addition to its role in maintaining suitable conditions for oestrogen synthesis, the foetus also metabolizes the oestrogens which flow back to it from the placenta, and much of what the mother finally excretes has been converted to oestriol and conjugated by her foetus to sulphates and glucosiduronates. We do not intend to pursue here the foetal side of this picture: briefly it seems that the foetus which might be embarrassed by the quantity of oestrogen presumably produced for the maternal requirements of pregnancy, is able, by its facility for conjugation, to live in an environment free from active oestrogens. Even that cannot be said with certainty; no one can say whether or not the conjugated hormones have any physiological activity. An alternative possibility is that the highly individual oestrogen environment of the foetus serves some purpose in promoting its growth.

The quantity produced

What we have said about the excretion of pregnanediol in relation to progesterone production, applies with even more force to the excretory end-products of the oestrogens. In one series of experiments in non-pregnant women, Brown (1959) showed that when oestradiol-17β was injected, 13–35 per cent of the dose was excreted as a mixture of oestradiol-17β, oestrone and oestriol, the last forming 44 ± 11 per cent of the total mixture. Whether the excretion of these three oestrogens gives a fair representation of oestrogen metabolism now seems doubtful, at least in non-pregnant subjects. Fishman (1963) has shown that 2-hydroxyoestrone, a metabolite which is readily lost in the usual methods of oestrogen isolation, may sometimes be a large fraction of oestrogen end-products.

Only the excretion of the three 'classical' oestrogens has been studied in detail during pregnancy, and in large numbers of subjects only oestriol. That oestriol has been singled out for special study is not because any special physiological function is known for it, although it probably dominates the particular oestrogen pattern of pregnancy, but because it occurs in great amounts and is therefore relatively easy to measure.

Figure 6.2 shows the rising curve of urinary excretion of the three classical oestrogens, measured serially by Brown (1956) on four normal pregnant subjects. The oestriol pattern has been confirmed by a number of other workers with other methods. That by Klopper and Billewicz (1963) for a large group of normal primigravidae is shown in Figure 6.3. The curve has an interesting shape; it does not follow the simple pattern of pregnanediol excretion but seems to be formed of two components, the second of which causes it to rise steeply in late pregnancy to levels of about 40 mg daily. Klopper

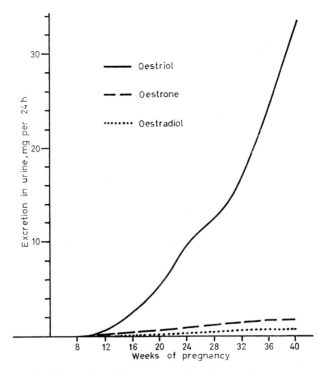

FIGURE 6.2. Excretion of the three major oestrogens in pregnancy. A serial study of four normal subjects (Brown, 1956)

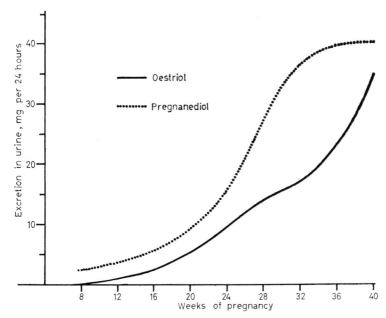

FIGURE 6.3. Excretion of oestriol in normal pregnancy (Klopper and Billewicz, 1963) contrasted with the excretion of pregnanediol (Shearman, 1959; Klopper and Billewicz, 1963)

and Billewicz suggest that the secondary rise may be due to the influence of the foetus on oestrogen metabolism, but we have no information. Coyle and Brown (1963) have shown that the amount of oestriol excreted is related to the size of the baby. Fishman *et al.* (1962) have measured the rates of secretion of the three main oestrogens by dilution after injecting labelled oestradiol. For three women in late pregnancy the secretion rates of oestrone, oestradiol and oestriol were calculated to be about 10, 11 and 222 mg per 24 hours.

Like pregnanediol, oestrogens are excreted in the faeces but they are also reabsorbed to some extent (Fuchs, 1962) and, as Diczfalusy and Lauritzen (1961) have shown, the partition between urine and faeces may vary. There are few estimates of oestrogen concentration in the mother's peripheral venous blood; they have been assembled in two recent publications (O'Donnell and Preedy, 1961; Roy, 1962). Most of the analyses have been made in late pregnancy and show a wide range. Oestriol, for example, ranges from 2.1 to 41.6 μg per 100 ml, oestrone from 1.5 to 43 μg per 100 ml and oestradiol-17β from less than 0.05 to 3.7 μg per 100 ml. There are not sufficient data to show what the pattern of change may be during pregnancy. Diczfalusy and Troen (1961) and Diczfalusy et al. (1961) gave some recent published figures for concentration of oestrogens in the placenta. These show a variable pattern but two important generalizations can be made. First, oestrone and oestradiol form a much bigger fraction of the total oestrogen than they do in body fluids, about half the free, unconjugated oestrogen; and second, while most of the placental oestrogen occurs in the free form, such conjugated oestrogen as there is, is predominantly oestriol. Little is known of the other oestrogens which have been identified in the placenta, and nothing of whether they are simply metabolic by-products of the major oestrogens or have some particular function of their own.

While much is now known of the concentration of oestrogens in a number of foetal organs, there is no information about oestrogen distribution in human maternal tissues. In a series of elegant experiments with rats, Jensen and Jacobson (1962) showed that injected oestradiol labelled with tritium appeared briefly in the blood and in organs such as the liver and kidney but was retained in the uterus and vagina. Injection of labelled oestrone resulted in the appearance of labelled oestradiol in the uterus.

Our knowledge of what might control manufacture in the placenta is as fragmentary for oestrogens as for progesterone. We have already suggested that the foetus may exercise some control, although there is no direct evidence that it does. There is also a little, largely indirect evidence, reviewed by Diczfalusy and Troen that human chorionic gonadotrophin (HCG) may play some regulating role, a possibility which would give the placenta an internal mechanism for control. The possibility also exists that the placenta may regulate its oestrogenic influence by altering the relative amounts of the various oestrogens produced, or even by in-activating them. The maternal pituitary apparently has little or no influence on the urinary excretion of oestrogen in pregnancy (Little et al. 1958), although the hypophysectomized woman des-cribed by Kaplan (1961) excreted little.

We have already mentioned the suggestion by Frandsen and Stakemann (1961) that the foetal adrenal gland exerts an important influence on oestrogen metabolism; it is also possible that the foetal pituitary gland may play a part, although in four out of five of their anencephalics the anterior hypophysis appeared, at least histologically, to be normal.

Action of oestrogens

For studies of the action of oestrogens there is the same unsatisfactory situation as for progesterone, except that the problem is even more complex because it is not yet known whether, when one oestrogen is converted into another, the action is attenuated, or even different. A lot of recent *in vitro* research has shown that the oestrogens may have a rate-limiting influence on intracellular enzyme systems, even those fundamentally concerned with energy exchanges (Hagerman and Villee, 1961; Laidler and Krupka, 1961). Another line of research has shown that oestradiol can stimulate tissue growth by speeding nucleic acid and protein synthesis (Mueller, Herranen and Jervell, 1958). The biochemical evidence for such synthesis is detailed and convincing but it is still a long way from explaining any of the physiological phenomena of pregnancy. The concentrations of oestrogen used in many experiments greatly exceed the likely concentration in real life.

We can do little more here than list the possible physiological changes in which oestrogens are thought to play a part. For many of their suggested functions they are thought to have a combined action with progesterone. Evidence, largely from animal experiments, for the interaction of the two hormones was thoroughly reviewed by Courrier (1950). The picture which emerges from the scanty evidence we have suggests that many processes such as development of breast and uterus are complex chains of events in which oestrogens and progesterone have influence at different points. Progesterone for instance might have no effect on a process unless it had been brought to a certain stage by oestrogen action. The two hormones should not be viewed as simple synergists or antagonists which can be titrated one against the other.

THE UTERUS

It is generally held that the major role of oestrogens is to control the growth and function of the uterus. Fuchs (1962) in a brief review discusses the development of the decidual lining of the uterus, the proliferation and growth of myometrial cells and the increased local blood flow, and attributes all these changes to the combined organizing effects of the oestrogens and progesterone. There is little direct evidence for what happens in human pregnancy; most observations have been made on the rat (Noall *et al.* 1957, Velardo, 1960).

Recent research, much of it in Csapo's laboratory, has concentrated on the antagonism by oestrogen to the myometrial relaxing effect of progesterone. Csapo believes, on the basis of *in vitro* studies, that oestrogen can affect not only the amount of contactile protein in the myometrium, but also its excitability: '. . . estrogen treatment of the immature animal brings the membrane potential of the myometrial cell into the "firing range", a prerequisite of normal excitability . . .' (Csapo, 1961).

Bengtsson (1962) in a recent summary of the views of that school of thought stated 'that oestrogen, by increasing the myometrial strength and reactivity, is of the utmost importance in labour in all mammals'. Clinical application of the idea has so far proved disappointing. In theory it should be possible to predict from the relative amounts of progesterone and oestrogen produced when the uterus will be sufficiently sensitive to go into labour. The 'safety catch' provided by progesterone domination of the myometrium should finally be released by the rising amounts of oestrogen, after which the uterus should react to oxytocin and proceed to expel the baby. Measurement neither of the urinary excretion of pregnanediol and oestrogens, nor of the blood levels of progesterone and oestrogen has revealed any ratio at which uterine contraction is certain, or offered any explanation of premature labour, prolonged pregnancy or uterine dysfunction (Bengtsson, 1962). Whether oestrogen in physiological amounts affects uterine contractility is undecided. In clinical practice, oestrogens are often given to assist induction of labour, but Klopper and Dennis (1962) in a well controlled trial could find no evidence that oestriol or stilboestrol shortened either the time between artificial rupture of the membranes and the start of labour, or the length of labour. On the other hand a recent preliminary communication by Pinto *et al.* (1963) suggests that in women with retention of dead foetuses oestradiol-17β intravenously at rates up to 400 μg per minute caused rhythmic uterine activity and increased uterine sensitivity to oxytocin.

It is an interesting possibility that oestriol, the predominant oestrogen produced in human pregnancy, may have a more potent antagonizing influence on the myometrial effect of progesterone than other oestrogens (Edgren, Elton and Calhoun, 1961), although it is generally regarded as a 'weak' oestrogen by other standards and some even consider it to be little more than an inert end-product. Borglin (1959) gave oestriol to post-menopausal women with uterine prolapse and found its action in increasing the thickness and vascularity of the vaginal and cervical mucosa, and in softening the cervix, to be at least as potent as that of stilboestrol.

BREAST DEVELOPMENT

As we have said above, both oestrogen and progesterone are thought to be necessary for development of both the duct and secretory systems of the breast. There is no direct evidence for man, but in the monkey oestrogen alone can cause extensive development of both ducts and alveoli (Benson et al. 1959). That cannot be the whole story since, as we shall show in Chapter 7, breast development in pregnancy is considerably influenced by maternal age, and oestrogen production appears not to be related to age (Klopper and Billewicz, 1963). Oestrogen may also influence nipple development. The nipples increase in both size and mobility (Hytten and Baird, 1958) and these effects have been obtained by local application of oestrogen to the nipples (Burrows, 1949). The effect on mobility may be by alteration of the connective tissue which normally binds the nipple close to the surface of the breast, as part of a general change in connective tissue which will now be discussed.

CONNECTIVE TISSUE

There is a good deal of evidence that oestrogens may alter the polymerization of acid mucopolysaccharides and thereby have a profound effect on the physico-chemical properties of the ground substances which, for example, act as the adhesive between fibres in collagenous tissue (Zachariae, 1959). The uterine cervix, which has a high collagen content and which in the non-pregnant woman is difficult to stretch, stretches with great ease in late pregnancy. The difference is clinically evident, but research on the human cervix is needed to confirm the work done by Harkness and Harkness (1959) and Zarrow and Yochim (1961) on the rat cervix. The hormone relaxin, which we discuss below, may also have some influence on the cervix, and on the generally greater mobility of the pelvic joints in pregnancy; and alteration of the connective tissue ground substance may be responsible for the increased mobility of the nipple.

One result of altering the polymerization of mucopolysaccharide is to increase its hygroscopic qualities and the effect of oestrogen, first described by Zuckerman (for example Zuckerman, Van Wagenen and Gardiner, 1938) in the sexual skin of the monkey, appears to have founded the belief that oestrogens are responsible for water storage. It might explain the common clinical finding in late pregnancy of generalized water retention in the skin. The face becomes slightly puffy and its shape alters; the fingers are swollen, rings are tight and there is a subjective impression of general swelling of the skin. This 'oedema' is probably distinct from the expansion of the extra-cellular space which also may occur in late pregnancy; there is no tendency for the water to gravitate to lower levels.

Other evidence that oestrogen provokes water storage is slight and unconvincing. Röttger and Hechenbach (1957) found that oestradiol valerianate or benzoate given to 30 postmenopausal women caused an increase in the thiocyanate space averaging 1355 ml; a striking effect which has never been confirmed. Dignam, Voskian and Assali (1956) found that oestradiol-17β given by intravenous or intramuscular injection reduced sodium excretion by the kidney, with consequent water retention, but experiments in Aberdeen (Klopper and Hytten, unpublished) have so far failed to confirm the finding.

OTHER EFFECTS

There can be few phenomena of pregnancy which have not, at one time or another, been attributed to the action of oestrogen. The evidence is generally negligible. Of some interest were the experiments reported by Freidlander, Laskey and Silbert (1935, 1936). Five castrated women were given oestrogen (injections of 'Amniotin') and their mean blood volume rose from 62.4 ml per kg to 84 ml per kg and returned to 62 ml per kg after treatment had stopped. There was no effect in two normal women. It is unlikely that blood volume can be induced to rise as an isolated phenomenon; it will increase only to fill an increase in demand, for example in the size of the vascular bed. What stimulus to increase blood volume was applied in these experiments is not known, but Edwards and Duntley (1949) produced vasodilatation in the skin of castrated women by administration of oestradiol benzoate or dipropionate; and progesterone reversed the effect. Unfortunately the doses of hormones used were so small that it is not possible to draw any conclusion.

HUMAN CHORIONIC GONADOTROPHIN (HCG)

Chorionic gonadotrophin is the only hormone, other than progesterone and oestrogens, which has been shown unequivocally to be produced by the placenta. No chemical method of assay is yet available for it, or for any other of the protein hormones, but many bioassays have been devised and there is a recent review of them by Loraine (1961). The international unit (IU) in which results are usually expressed is defined as the activity in o.1 mg of a standard preparation. An immunological method of assay may in time replace bio-assay in intact animals but one recently developed (Wide, 1962) was not specific for HCG and included pituitary luteinizing hormone.

Site of production

HCG is produced by the trophoblast and probably only by the trophoblast; the evidence has been summarized by Diczfalusy and Troen (1961). For example the hormone has been produced in transplanted placental tissue, in cultures of placental tissue and in perfused intact placentae. Histochemical techniques, which must be at the limit of their resolution with the small amounts of hormone present, suggest that HCG is present in both syncytial cells and the Langhan's layer (Zilliacus, Widholm and Pesonen, 1954), but such methods cannot distinguish sites of production from sites of storage and the exact place of manufacture is not known. Studies of tissue cultures have yielded equivocal results and Diczfalusy and Troen conclude that no more can be said than that the cytotrophoblast is 'probably the major if not exclusive source of HCG'.

The quantity produced

The quantities of HCG measured depend to some extent on the method of assay used, but the pattern of change in the placenta, the blood and the urine is not disputed.

In the placenta, the amount of HCG rises rapidly to reach a concentration of the order of 600 IU per gram wet weight in the second and third lunar month, after which there is an abrupt fall to a level which is consistently below 20 IU per gram from the fourth month onwards (Diczfalusy, 1953; Diczfalusy, Nilsson and Westman, 1958).

Concentrations of HCG in the blood serum and in the urine follow the same course. Albert and Berkson (1951) found HCG in the serum as early as the 23rd or 24th day of pregnancy, dated from the beginning of the last menstrual period, i.e. about 10 days after ovulation. A rapid increase started about the 40th day; there was a peak at about the 60th day and an abrupt fall about the 80th day to a level which is maintained throughout the rest of pregnancy. Loraine (1961) described the peak values as ranging from 20,000 to 100,000 IU per litre of serum, but concentrations as high as 1,000,000 IU per litre have been described. In the second and third trimesters the levels lie between 4,000 and 11,000 IU per litre and Loraine concluded that values consistently outside this range should be regarded as pathological. A similar picture has recently been drawn by Mishell, Wide and Gemzell (1963). The mean concentration of HCG in serum estimated by an immunological method is shown in Figure 6.4.

Excretion of HCG in the urine follows the same pattern as change

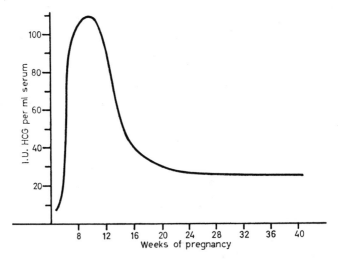

FIGURE 6.4. Concentration of chorionic gonadotrophin (HCG) in serum during pregnancy. From the data of Mishell, Wide and Gemzell (1963)

in the placenta and the blood. Again there is no unanimity about the actual levels and peak values between 20,000 and 500,000 IU per 24 hours have been reported (Diczfalusy and Troen, 1961). The period of high excretion probably does not exceed three weeks. In the last two trimesters of pregnancy excretion is fairly constant at from 5,000 to 10,000 IU per 24 hours.

The rate of manufacture of HCG cannot be stated with any assurance, but Diczfalusy and Troen concluded that about 10 per cent of the HCG produced appears in the urine. The amount excreted is not likely to be limited by the renal clearance of the hormone, which varies from 0.47 to 0.95 ml per minute (Loraine, 1961); the fate of the unexcreted fraction is not known. Bruner (1951) found that all the maternal tissues were permeated with HCG; the amounts in the foetal tissues were in much lower concentration. It is not known whether the placenta diverts more of the hormone to the mother than to the foetus or whether there are different rates of destruction on the two sides of the placenta.

There is no convincing evidence of a mechanism which might control either production or release of HCG.

Action of HCG

Diczfalusy and Troen sum up their review by saying that, although a great deal is known of the chemistry and pharmacology of the hormone, its role in human pregnancy is still unknown. 'The pharmacological action of HCG in different animal species, or in the human male or non-pregnant female—in instances in which the hormone does not normally occur—is relatively well understood. However its physiological actions on the mother, on the foetus and on the placenta are still obscure'.

The situation is not quite as bleak as they suggest. There can be little doubt that HCG is luteotrophic. Brown and Bradbury (1947) showed that daily administration of 5,000 to 10,000 IU of HCG to normal women considerably prolonged the menstrual cycle by maintaining the corpus luteum, and caused a decidual reaction in the endometrium. The same effect has been reported by a number of workers since (Segaloff, Sternberg and Gaskill, 1951; Fried and Rakoff, 1951; Palmer, 1957). In one of their subjects, Segaloff, Sternberg and Gaskill prolonged a menstrual cycle which was normally 28 days to 46 days by giving daily injections of 10,000 IU of HCG from the 24th to the 42nd day of the cycle. There was a well developed decidual reaction of the endometrium 'histologically indistinguishable from early pregnancy.' What hormone or combination of hormones prevents the usual menstrual shedding of the endometrium and prepares it for the embedding ovum is not clear. It may be no more than the prolonged effect of progesterone from the corpus luteum but it is also possible that HCG itself may have a direct effect.

It is true that gestation can continue without a corpus luteum, from an early stage. Tulsky and Koff (1957) removed corpora lutea at laparotomy between the 35th and 77th day in 13 women who were to have pregnancy terminated later. Abortion occurred in only two who had their 'luteectomy' on the 39th and 41st days. The remaining pregnancies, including that at 35 days, continued and pregnanediol output in urine seemed to be unaffected by the operation, although there were areas of focal necrosis in over half the endometria when the pregnancies were terminated 7 to 11 days later.

The peak of HCG secretion, at about 60 days of pregnancy, is therefore at a time when the corpus luteum it is thought to be maintaining is no longer essential to the pregnancy. Nevertheless, in the first few weeks of pregnancy, the functioning of the corpus luteum may well be vital and it is hard to escape the conclusion that it is HCG which maintains its function.

There remains to be explained the curious case of the Blažek twins described by Basch (1910). They were a well-known pair of conjoined twin sisters, joined in the region of the sacrum and having in common only the rectum and vaginal introitus. One sister became pregnant and delivered a normal male child and both experienced normal breast development and lactated. One apparently bizarre feature of the case was that the twin who was not pregnant was not prevented from regular menstruation by HCG produced in her pregnant sister.

Diczfalusy and Troen briefly examined the suggestion that HCG may stimulate the adrenal glands, both foetal and maternal, and concluded that there was no clear evidence of such a function.

Of more interest are the better founded suggestions (Troen and Gordon, 1958; Troen, 1961a) that HCG may influence oestrogen metabolism in the placenta. Much more evidence is necessary, but such a function for HCG might give the placenta an autoregulatory system.

For the clinician HCG may serve the useful purpose of confirming a diagnosis of pregnancy; most diagnostic tests for pregnancy are based on its action.

RELAXIN

Hall (1960) in an excellent review of the subject described relaxin as a 'hormone or hormone-complex produced during pregnancy in the ovaries and/or reproductive tracts of females of many species'. Relaxin is probably a polypeptide but little more than that is known and several polypeptides with relaxin activity have been separated from a commercial preparation (Frieden, Stone and Layman, 1960). Uncertainty about it as an entity is matched by uncertainty about its assay. Three bio-assays are used; all require preliminary priming with oestrogen and none is really satisfactory. The two most used are based on relaxation of the symphysis pubis of the guinea pig or mouse, and inhibition of spontaneous uterine contractions in the guinea pig, mouse or rat. These actions form the rationale of its clinical trial in human pregnancy.

The concentration of relaxin in blood has been shown to increase during human pregnancy, but with considerable irregularity, from 0.2 'guinea pig unit' (GPU) per ml of serum at 7–10 weeks to as much as 2 GPU per ml at 38–42 weeks (Zarrow et al. 1955). It has disappeared from the circulation 24 hours after delivery, which might suggest that it originates in the placenta or foetus, but it does not always occur in the placenta and Diczfalusy and Troen (1961) concluded that there was not sufficient evidence to decide its source in human pregnancy.

The principal source of commercial relaxin preparations, on which all evidence of action in women is based, is the ovary of the pregnant sow. It is not known whether the same hormone is produced in human pregnancy. Preparations from the sow appear to be only slightly antigenic, although several serious reactions have been reported (Hall, 1960).

Action of relaxin

There is a considerable literature on the effects of relaxin in a number of laboratory animals, but its action in human pregnancy, if any, is unknown. Two main claims are made: that the hormone may prevent or halt premature labour, and that it may assist labour by increasing cervical softening and relaxing pelvic joints. Both these situations are difficult to assess. Women go into and out of premature labour spontaneously, and cervical softening, 'ripeness', is still a subject of controversy among obstetricians from the point of view of diagnosis as well as prognosis. Because of these and other difficulties, experiments generally have been poorly planned and clinical trials of sow relaxin have been unconvincing. It would be best, at present, to keep an open mind about its role in human pregnancy and labour until a purer preparation is available and has been given a better trial.

THE PITUITARY HORMONES

The pituitary gland enlarges in pregnancy. Pearse (1953) examined 16 pituitary glands from women who died in pregnancy or the puerperium and found a 'great enlargement and increased granulation of the mucoid cells'. Sommers (1959) who examined a large series of pituitary glands said that the average adult pituitary gland weighs from 0.4 to 0.6 g, but that the weight was 'up to 0.8 g or more in women who have been pregnant'. Both acidophilic and basophilic cells have been reported as increasing during pregnancy, but the functional significance of changes in cell counts is not known. An increase in size is not, of itself, evidence of increased function. That the increase in size of the gland may start early in pregnancy is suggested by the case described by Kaplan (1961). A woman had her pituitary removed early in her fourth pregnancy for a chromophobe adenoma; but in her 3 previous pregnancies, two of which had ended with abortion at three months, she had headaches and blurring of vision from soon after missing a period until shortly after the end of pregnancy. Except for adrenocorticotrophic hormone and melanocyte stimulating hormone, now identified as polypeptides, the anterior pituitary hormones are proteins.

Pituitary gonadotrophins

Three gonadotrophic substances are thought to be secreted by the anterior pituitary gland: follicle-stimulating hormone (FSH), the interstitial cell-stimulating hormone or luteinizing hormone (ICSH or LH) and luteotrophin (LTH). LTH is probably the same as prolactin in the rat; the position in man is not known. A luteotrophic action of LTH has been demonstrated for the rat but not for man. Until recently, methods of assay have been unsatisfactory; newer methods involving better separation and immunological assay are likely to be more rewarding.

The effect of pregnancy on the secretion of pituitary gonado-trophins is not known. Their assay is at present made impossible by the huge amounts of chorionic gonadotrophin and more specific methods of measurement will be necessary.

Crooke and Butt (1959) claimed that FSH was excreted during human pregnancy, but Albert and Derner (1960) were critical of their method and claim, on good evidence, that the FSH activity measured can be attributed to HCG.

The administration of oestrogen to post-menopausal women causes a big reduction in excretion of gonadotrophin so that one might expect low outputs in pregnancy. Certainly successful pregnancy is possible, at least after the twelfth week, without pituitary gonadotrophins.

Adrenocorticotrophin or Adrenocorticotrophic hormone (ACTH)

It seems certain that secretion of adrenocortical steroids rises in pregnancy, and probably all come from the mother's adrenal cortex (see p. 168). It is generally assumed that the increase reflects production of the polypeptide hormone ACTH, but reports are contradictory; several workers have found increased amounts of ACTH in the plasma during pregnancy, others have failed to find any (Diczfalusy and Troen, 1961).

There have been many attempts to demonstrate that the placenta could be a source of ACTH in pregnancy. The hormone can un-doubtedly be isolated from placental tissue but in a detailed review of the evidence Diczfalusy and Troen concluded that no convincing case could be made for its production by the placenta; it may be stored or even concentrated there.

Thyrotrophin or Thyroid-stimulating hormone (TSH)

There is clear cut evidence of a change in thyroid function during pregnancy; the plasma inorganic iodine level is greatly reduced and the gland presumably 'works harder' to maintain a normal iodine uptake. This is discussed on p. 173. Whether TSH is involved in this change is not known. Assay is difficult and relatively unsatis-factory and there is almost no information about normal pregnancy.

M

Yamazaki, Noguchi and Slingerland (1961) measured TSH in maternal and umbilical cord blood serum at 10 deliveries. Concentration in maternal serum averaged 12.4 mU per 100 ml, foetal serum 11.2 mU per 100 ml. The difference was not significant and the conclusion was that TSH can cross the placenta or the foetus maintains a level equal to that of its mother.

Somatotrophin or Growth hormone (GH)

A few years ago, the idea developed that growth hormone and prolactin might be the same substance in man; more recent evidence suggests they are distinct. Little is known about GH in human pregnancy. It was once believed that over-production of growth hormone by diabetic mothers was responsible for their characteristically big babies. The idea is almost certainly not correct and another possible mechanism will be discussed below (p. 178).

Whether growth hormone is needed for foetal growth is not known; it seems unlikely. Certainly a foetus can grow satisfactorily without any maternal hormone (Little et al. 1958; Kaplan, 1961) and anencephalic foetuses can be well grown in the absence of a foetal pituitary gland. But the situation without either maternal or foetal pituitary has not been reported. There is no evidence that growth hormone can be produced by the placenta.

Melanocyte-stimulating hormone (MSH)

Changes in skin pigmentation are characteristic of pregnancy. The areola of the nipple and the linea nigra darken, naevi become more heavily pigmented and new ones appear, and there is occasionally a mask-like pigmentation of the face, chloasma. Similar, less marked, changes may occur in non-pregnant women in the premenstruum (McGuinness, 1961). These changes are probably brought about by melanocyte-stimulating hormone. MSH has now been identified as a polypeptide and synthesized (Li, 1962) but prior to the synthesis Lerner et al. (1954) had prepared a highly purified extract of pituitary which produced heavy pigmentation in experimental subjects without other effect. The normal level of this hormone in blood was shown by Shizume and Lerner (1954) to be about 1.3 unit per ml but in pregnancy it rose rapidly and by term concentrations as high as 200 units per ml were found.

MSH is chemically similar to ACTH (which itself has melanocyte-stimulating properties in frogs) and it was once difficult to separate them in pituitary extracts. They have other properties in common and may share a biosynthetic pathway; MSH, which appears to serve no useful purpose in pregnancy, may be a by-product of increased ACTH production.

Hormones of the posterior lobe of the pituitary

The two hormones, which come from the posterior lobe of the pituitary gland but originate in the hypothalamus, oxytocin and vasopressin (antidiuretic hormone, ADH) are chemically similar molecules of eight amino acids with a number of pharmacological actions in common. The main action of oxytocin is to stimulate milk-ejection and uterine contractions; vasopressin is both anti-diuretic and vasospastic. We do not know to what extent the manufacture and secretion of these two hormones is linked, but there is some evidence that secretion of one is inevitably accompanied by some secretion of the other. In men, for example, the need for ADH is met by secretion of both ADH and oxytocin, although oxytocin has no known function in the male.

Little is known about their secretion and activity in pregnancy. The concentration of oxytocin in the blood increases and appears to be matched by increase of an inactivator produced by the placenta (Hawker, 1956).

The role of oxytocin in the initiation of labour is obscure and it may eventually be shown to have little importance, although infused oxytocin does undoubtedly provoke labour in a majority of women tested at the end of pregnancy. The whole question of what makes a woman go into labour is still open and a tempting field for research. It has been argued (Little et al. 1958) that since a hypophysectomized woman can go spontaneously into labour oxytocin is not needed, but the posterior lobe of the pituitary is not necessary for the secretion of oxytocin; it acts merely as a store for hormone produced in the hypothalamus. There have been numerous observations of the performance in labour of women with diabetes insipidus and some but not all have had poor uterine action (Hendricks, 1954; McKenzie and Swain, 1955). A convincing example was described by Marañón (1947). The woman had severe diabetes insipidus from the age of 17 in 1921, before suitable preparations of pitressin were available. Pituitrin afforded relief but she did not persist with treatment and was content to put up with a urine output of about 20 litres per day. At the age of 29 she became pregnant. 'Parturition seemed to start several times but the pains stopped almost immediately. After 5 days without further pains she was delivered of a full term female child which was stillborn'. Three years later she was pregnant again but was given pituitrin when slight labour pains appeared and had a normal delivery. In a third pregnancy a year later she had no access to pituitrin and her first atonic labour was repeated with a further stillbirth.

Whether vasopressin has any role in pregnancy is not known. We have speculated that the conspicuous inability of the woman in late pregnancy to excrete a water load may be due to increased secretion of vasopressin (p. 127), but there may be some other anti-diuretic at work. Indeed this is suggested by the behaviour of the woman whose pituitary was removed at the 12th week of pregnancy (Kaplan, 1961). She developed diabetes insipidus after the operation and required vasopressin to maintain a reasonable output of urine. Progressively less was required as pregnancy progressed but the requirement increased again within 5 days of delivery. A diminishing need for vasopressin in pregnancy has been described also by McKenzie and Swain (1955). On the other hand other women with diabetes insipidus have deteriorated during pregnancy, and after reading the literature we are left with the impression that any pattern of behaviour is possible.

HORMONES OF THE ADRENAL GLAND
Corticosteroids

The published information about corticosteroid production and metabolism in pregnancy is generally unsatisfactory but the balance of evidence suggests increased secretion and there is firm evidence that metabolism is altered: concentrations in blood are raised with increased binding to plasma protein and a reduced rate of turnover. The earliest evidence was circumstantial: that rheumatoid arthritis improved during pregnancy in the same way as it was subsequently shown to improve when cortisone was given. Since the 1940s a considerable amount of information has accumulated, all pointing towards increased secretion. The estimation of corticosteroid hormones is somewhat confused by a wide variety of methods of assay.

The adrenal cortex obviously remains the primary source of

corticosteroid production in pregnancy but there is some evidence to suggest that the placenta and even the foetus also may contribute. The evidence is reviewed by Diczfalusy and Troen (1961). Evidence in favour of placental production is largely circumstantial and rests on the fact that a number of women with Addison's disease have shown some clinical improvement during pregnancy and corticosteroid excretion has risen in adrenal-deficient women during pregnancy. But such signs are not invariable and in one subject, adrenalectomized for Cushing's disease, who showed increasing corticosteroid excretion, it was suggested that pregnancy might have stimulated adrenal rests (Kreiger, Gabrilove and Soffer, 1960). Other experiments have so far failed to answer the question. Troen (1961b) perfused placentae for some hours and recovered slightly greater quantities of corticosteroids than could be found by analysis in a series of control placentae not perfused. He admitted that the findings were equivocal. Both Bayliss *et al.* (1955) and Salhanick (1960) reported the same concentration of 17-hydroxy-corticosteroids in uterine vein blood as in peripheral blood.

The foetus is undoubtedly equipped to make its own corticosteroids, and they probably can pass to the maternal circulation (Migeon, Bertrand and Gemzell, 1962) but the evidence from studies of adrenal-deficient women in pregnancy suggests that the foetus contributes only a negligible quantity. There is a considerable collection of evidence to show that corticosteroid in urine is raised during pregnancy, although the amount of increase is not clear and estimates are confused by variations in methods of assay. A substantial increase in the excretion of aldosterone seems undoubted (Jones *et al.* 1959; Martin and Mills, 1956) and there may be more 17-oxosteroids and 17-oxogenic steroids (previously 17-ketosteroids and 17-ketogenic steroids) in urine (Birke *et al.* 1958; Cope and Black, 1959; Steinbeck and Theile, 1962). Martin and Mills (1958) describe only a possible small and insignificant rise and say that the apparent excess of 17-oxosteroids is probably due to the fact that the Zimmermann reaction measures also 20-ketone metabolites of progesterone. There is no evidence of increased production of androgens during pregnancy.

The concentration in blood of corticosteroids, largely cortisol (hydrocortisone) rises progressively during pregnancy (Bayliss *et al.* 1955; Birke, *et al.* 1958; Martin and Mills, 1958; Bro-Rassmussen *et al.* 1962) and by the end of pregnancy is probably 2 or 3 times the non-pregnant. It is generally considered that the increase of plasma corticosteroids is due entirely, or almost entirely, to increased binding by plasma protein and that the pattern is similar to that after oestrogen administration to men and non-pregnant women (Peterson *et al.* 1960; Mills *et al.* 1960). But Doe *et al.* (1960) considered that the pattern of protein binding in pregnancy was not the same as that induced by oestrogen. When oestrogen is given all the added blood corticosteroid is protein-bound; in pregnancy some of the increase is not protein bound and that, Doe *et al.* claim, fits in with the clinical picture of 'mild adrenocortical hyperfunction' in pregnancy: striae in the skin, glycosuria, hypertension and increased fragility of cutaneous blood vessels. The same view is held also by Poidevin (1959). Doe's account of events would explain also why the increased protein binding in pregnancy is not accompanied by reduced excretion in urine, as happens when protein binding is increased by oestrogen administration. Whether or not this is so, increased protein binding greatly affects corticosteroid metabolism and slows the rate of disappearance of corticosteroids from the plasma.

The rate of secretion of corticosteroids has been measured in several laboratories by application of the dilution principle: hormone labelled with a radioactive isotope is given and the ratio of labelled to unlabelled metabolite is measured in the urine. Cope and Black (1959) compared eight women in late pregnancy with 8 non-pregnant women and found a two to three-fold increase in cortisol production; it averaged 25 mg per day with a range of 20 to 40 mg.

Jones *et al.* (1959) found aldosterone secretion in six women in late pregnancy to be between 248 and 1100 μg per 24 hours (normal non-pregnant mean, 192 μg) and Van de Wiele *et al.* (1960) found rates of 1040, 1210 and 2250 μg per day in three normal women in late pregnancy. It is not possible to explain the conspicuously wide variation but it can fairly be concluded that the rate of secretion in late pregnancy is much above normal.

Without much more information it is difficult to fit the changes we have described into a consistent pattern of changing physiology in pregnancy. There is little beyond the suggestion that progesterone tends to cause sodium loss by the kidney and that aldosterone secretion rises to combat it (Landau, Plotz and Lugibihl, 1960).

Catecholamines

Hormones of the adrenal medulla, adrenaline and noradrenaline, are difficult to measure and what little evidence there is for a changed excretion in pregnancy is not convincing. Stone *et al.* (1960) in a largely cross-sectional study, measured the changes in concentration of adrenaline and noradrenaline in blood. In comparison with non-pregnant controls they found in the second trimester a statistically significant increase in the level of adrenaline and a statistically significant decrease in the level of noradrenaline, a difference which occurred in 'more than 50 per cent' of subjects. We would like to see this somewhat curious pattern confirmed before either accepting it or commenting on it. Concentrations in blood were estimated also by Israel *et al.* (1959) because it was thought that those hormones might influence labour. Concentrations were not different from the normal in non-pregnant women and there was no relation to performance in labour.

THE THYROID GLAND

In pregnancy the thyroid gland enlarges in from 25 to 80 per cent of women (Freedberg, Hamolsky and Freedberg, 1957), but the results of published surveys are difficult to interpret; none has included a group of non-pregnant control women and the criteria of enlargement are seldom clear. In a recent Aberdeen study (Crooks *et al.* 1964) 70 per cent of 184 pregnant women were found to have a thyroid gland which was both visible and palpable compared to 37 per cent of 116 non-pregnant women of similar age. The phenomenon was discussed almost ninety years ago by Tait (1875) but it had been recognized much earlier; the ancient Egyptians made use of it as a test for pregnancy by tying the stem of a plant around a woman's neck; pregnancy caused the gland to swell and broke the stem. We have been told by Dr Aboul-Khair that there is a carved stone in the Museum of Antiquities in Cairo showing the marriage of a young queen of the second dynasty with a stem tied round her neck.

The significance of the thyroid swelling in pregnancy has been the subject of considerable debate and many in the past have believed the pregnant woman to be hyperthyroid. As confirmatory evidence they have pointed to other signs of hyperthyroidism which appear in pregnancy: the increased oxygen consumption, the increased pulse rate, the intolerance of heat and the raised levels of serum protein-bound iodine. We have discussed elsewhere the first three of these signs: we hold that the increased oxygen consumption can be accounted for by the oxygen consumption of the foetus and added maternal tissue and by the extra work of the heart and respiratory muscles. The increased pulse rate is associated with the necessary increase in cardiac output in pregnancy and the intolerance of heat shows that the peripheral vasodilatation and overbreathing are barely sufficient to dissipate the extra heat. The increase in serum protein-bound iodine is no more than an increase in the amount of thyroxine-binding globulin, to be discussed below. Positive evidence against the suggestion of hyperthyroidism is the anabolic nature of metabolism in pregnancy, the gain in body weight, and the increase in the level of serum cholesterol, when hyperthyroidism is invariably a catabolic state, and a marked rise of serum cholesterol is generally regarded as a sign of hypothyroidism. In short there is every reason to believe that the increase in size of the thyroid gland is not associated with an increase in the production of thyroid hormone; in fact a rise of maternal metabolic rate would be an additional embarrassment.

There have been remarkably few histological studies of the thyroid gland in pregnancy. Stoffer et al. (1957) could find only four series in the literature with a total of 28 glands; 22 of these had increased colloid and 24 hypertrophic epithelium. Tait (1875) who was not quoted had found a similar picture. Stoffer et al. themselves studied 65 thyroid glands removed at autopsy from women at all stages of pregnancy. The average gland was not much heavier than what they regarded as normal, but they confirmed the earlier findings that there was both an increase in the size of follicles with abundant colloid and some epithelial hypertrophy. They give no information about the relation of the stage of gestation to these changes.

An increase in circulating protein-bound iodine (PBI), now taken normally to be thyroxine iodine, is well established and the evidence is reviewed by Freedberg, Hamolsky and Freedberg (1957). The normal level of PBI in serum of non-pregnant women is about 5 μg per 100 ml; in pregnancy the mean values vary from about 8 to more than 10 μg per 100 ml. It is likely that the increase occurs within the first two months of pregnancy. Unbound thyroxine is no more than one part in a thousand of protein-bound thyroxine (Osorio and Myant, 1960). It is not known whether the concentration of free thyroxine changes in pregnancy; there is no evidence of a change. Increased levels of PBI are almost certainly due to increase of protein-binding globulin (Dowling, Freinkel and Ingbar, 1956; Robbins and Nelson, 1958) which is probably induced by oestrogen. Dowling, Freinkel and Ingbar (1960) showed that the administration of diethylstilboestrol or oestradiol benzoate to normal subjects raised the concentration of thyroxine-binding globulin. The peripheral turnover of labelled iodine was reduced to balance the large pool of hormone and give the same daily disappearance of hormonal iodine, a situation which seems likely to hold also in pregnancy.

Studies by Man and her colleagues (for example, Man *et al.* 1951) have shown that low PBI in early pregnancy is often associated with abortion, which accords with the theory that the increased protein binding is elicited by oestrogen, since a depressed secretion of oestrogen will doubtless be associated with failing pregnancy. That is, a lower than normal PBI is another manifestation of a failing pregnancy; it does not by itself 'predispose to first-trimester miscarriage' as Freedberg *et al.* (1957) suggest.

Until recently there have been few studies in pregnancy with radioactive iodine. Pochin (1952) measured the neck-thigh ratio of radioactivity, 4 hours after a dose of ^{131}I, as an index of the rate of clearance of iodine from the blood by the thyroid. The ratio was considerably higher in pregnancy than some weeks post-partum. Halnan (1958) confirmed this: he found neck-thigh ratios throughout pregnancy to be considerably above the ratios in the same women six weeks post-partum and in normal non-pregnant women.

The whole picture of thyroid behaviour in normal pregnancy has now been clarified by Aboul-Khair (to be published). In fifteen normal pregnant women studied serially from early pregnancy with the more acceptable isotope [132]I (half life 2.3 hours) he measured the clearance of iodine by thyroid and kidney, plasma inorganic iodine and the absolute iodine uptake by the thyroid gland. The results are shown in Table 6.1 and Figure 6.5. Renal clearance of iodine is considerably increased so that iodine is lost in the urine, another example of the curious waste of nutrients by the kidneys in pregnancy (see p. 124). As a result the inorganic iodine of plasma falls to half its normal concentration or less and the thyroid gland

TABLE 6.1. Renal Clearance of Iodine, Plasma Inorganic Iodine, Thyroid Clearance of Iodine and Absolute Iodine Uptake in 15 Normal Pregnant Women. (Unpublished data, Aboul-Khair)

Measurement	Weeks of pregnancy					Weeks post-partum			Non-pregnant control
	up to 12	16	24	32	36	2	6	12	
Renal clearance of iodine ml per min ± S.E. mean	48.1 ±4.4	57.9 ±2.4	61.9 ±4.1	63.2 ±3.1	56.1 ±3.3	45.3 ±5.9	32.7 ±2.6	34.3 ±1.4	31.1 ±3.7
Plasma inorganic iodine μg per 100 ml plasma ± S.E. mean	0.13 ±0.02	0.12 ±0.02	0.06 ±0.02	0.08 ±0.01	0.12 ±0.03	0.11 ±0.03	0.18 ±0.04	0.15 ±0.07	0.20 ±0.02
Thyroid clearance of iodine ml per minute ± S.E. mean	48.7 ±5.8	48.5 ±5.9	49.7 ±6.2	47.8 ±4.9	53.1 ±3.4	36.7 ±5.1	22.8 ±4.7	21.0 ±4.2	15.00 ±1.7
Absolute iodine uptake by gland μg per hour ± S.E. mean	3.42 ±0.6	3.42 ±0.5	1.63 ±0.2	2.10 ±0.2	3.82 ±0.9	2.53 ±0.4	2.07 ±0.4	1.65 ±0.3	1.73 ±0.2

must clear at least twice the normal volume of blood each minute to maintain a normal iodine uptake. Under standard conditions, absolute iodine uptake by the thyroid gland is within euthyroid limits throughout pregnancy, although nearer the levels shown in simple goitre than in average non-goitrous subjects.

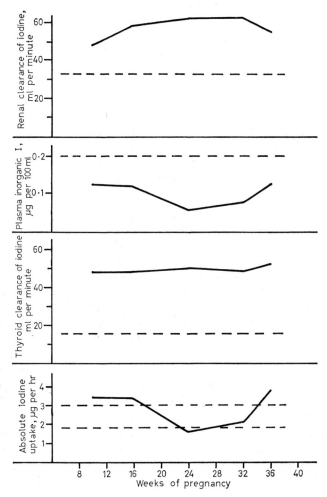

FIGURE 6.5. Iodine metabolism in pregnancy. The dotted lines show the usual non-pregnant levels; for absolute iodine uptake the upper dotted line is the average for simple goitre (From unpublished data supplied by Dr S. Aboul-Khair)

The goitre of pregnancy is therefore, at least in part, a goitre of iodine deficiency; not the usually recognized dietary lack, but a deficiency of iodine in the immediate environment of the gland. Tait in 1875 had the right answer when he described the swelling as 'a true hypertrophy, due probably to an increase of the amount of work the gland has to do'.

The relationship between the thyroid function of mother and foetus has been reviewed recently by Smith and Montalvo (1961). Most experimental studies have been made with laboratory animals and it is not possible to transfer the results to human pregnancy, but several points have been established. Thyroxine can cross the placenta from mother to foetus but does so extremely slowly; the passage of triidothyronine is a little more rapid (Grumbach and Werner, 1956). There is evidence that the foetus is manufacturing its own thyroxine by about 19 weeks of gestation but if it fails to do so the transfer of maternal thyroxine is not sufficient to compensate and normal foetal development may be impaired.

INSULIN

It is not possible to discuss insulin in pregnancy adequately without discussing changes in carbohydrate metabolism in general, so both are included in this section. Changes in hormonal control of carbohydrate metabolism in normal pregnancy have tended to be obscured by the overwhelming weight of studies of the effects of pregnancy on women with diabetes mellitus or 'prediabetes'.

A full discussion of diabetes in pregnancy is outside the scope of this book but we are unable to exclude it altogether because it is well known that a diabetic state can appear during pregnancy in an apparently normal woman, and the question arises whether normal pregnancy in a normal woman can provoke diabetes. There is little doubt that established diabetes is made worse by pregnancy; that diabetes may appear for the first time in pregnancy and then disappear after delivery; and that in some pregnant women who do not show signs of diabetes evidence of it can be provoked by the administration of cortisone (Jackson, 1961a, 1961b). Diabetes may become established many years after a pregnancy in which signs of it were apparent: for example, characteristically large infants are produced by diabetic and pre-diabetic mothers and in a series of 61 women examined 13 years after having a baby of $10\frac{1}{2}$ lb or more,

20 had definite or probable diabetes and it was considered likely that a number of others, who were obese, would become diabetic (Fitzgerald *et al.* 1961a). Jackson (1952) described similar statistics for a South African population.

The diabetic trait, which may never become overt, is probably more common in the population than attendance at diabetic clinics would imply and the possibility that many women may have it and therefore an abnormal response to pregnancy makes the study of normal pregnancy more difficult. Average figures from an unselected sample of apparently normal pregnant women may be influenced by a few who are in fact not normal.

Whether pregnancy is truly diabetogenic, in the sense that it causes diabetes which would otherwise not have arisen, is debatable. Jackson (1961b) claims that it is not, but two studies (Pyke, 1956; Fitzgerald *et al.* 1961b) have shown very persuasively that while males and nulliparous females have a similar incidence of diabetes at all ages, there is an increasing incidence of diabetes with increasing parity. Fitzgerald *et al.* for example, in an exceptionally well controlled study, showed that for diabetes diagnosed between the ages of 50 and 79 the incidence in women who had had 6 or more children was over 45 per cent. It has been argued that the excess could be explained by greater fertility among diabetics; in other words that the diabetic constitution conditioned the high fertility rather than the reverse. Such a proposition is difficult to disprove, but the fact that married nulliparae, who are presumably of low fertility, have the same incidence of diabetes as unmarried nulliparae whose fertility is likely to be average, is against it. One puzzling feature of the relation between parity and diabetes, shown by both Pyke and Fitzgerald *et al.*, is that the mean age of onset of diabetes is not affected by parity. That is, repeated pregnancy does seem to cause diabetes; it does not speed its appearance.

The cause of the particularly large babies of diabetic mothers has not been satisfactorily explained. It was once thought that their size was due to excess secretion of growth hormone by the mother, an explanation most unlikely to be correct; women with active acromegaly have babies of the usual size (Jackson, 1955) and it is in any case doubtful whether growth hormone can cross the placenta. The suggestion by Osler and his colleagues, for example Osler and Pedersen (1960), that these infants are no more than obese because they are subject to a high blood sugar throughout pregnancy does not fit the facts: big babies are born to 'prediabetics' who do not have a high blood sugar in pregnancy, and Cardell (1953), for example, has shown that babies of diabetic mothers are longer and have bigger organ weights than infants from non-diabetic mothers.

The most plausible explanation for the big babies of diabetic mothers has been put forward in a detailed review of recent evidence by Farquhar (1962). The main points are these: there is, even in normal subjects, an antagonist to insulin, and high levels of it are present in the diabetic and 'prediabetic' (Vallance-Owen and Lilley, 1961). The antagonist appears to be a polypeptide, dialysable and almost certainly capable of crossing the placenta; it opposes the activity of insulin in glycogen formation in muscle, but not in lipogenesis. The over development of pancreatic islet tissue in the baby, which has been shown by many workers, could therefore be explained as a compensatory reaction, and would in turn explain the greatly increased tolerance of glucose injected intravenously which is shown by newborn infants of diabetic mothers (Baird and Farquhar, 1962). Thus the foetus of the diabetic mother is subject to high levels of blood sugar because of hyper-glycaemia in the mother and has an increased output of insulin whose action in muscle is probably opposed by insulin antagonist from the mother. But lipogenesis, and probably the effect of insulin on skeletal growth are unaffected so that the baby grows more quickly and becomes fat.

Burt (1960) has recently reviewed the subject of carbohydrate metabolism in pregnancy, a field to which he has himself con-tributed extensively. Evidence was presented earlier (Burt, 1954) to show that the oral but not the intravenous glucose tolerance test is often abnormal. A lag type of curve is commonly found. Burt suggests a change in gastro-intestinal absorption of carbohydrate, not in metabolism, which is unlikely (see Chapter 13).

There is ample evidence of loss of insulin sensitivity particularly in late pregnancy; a standard dose of insulin causes a smaller fall in blood glucose, blood inorganic phosphate and blood amino acids and a smaller rise in blood lactate. The nature of the insulin 'resistance' is not known. Burt speaks of insulin antagonism and considers that increased adrenocortical activity in late pregnancy (see p. 170) may be, at least in part, responsible. Little is known of the biochemical mechanism; but one suggestion is that a block may occur between glucose and pyruvate in the glycolytic cycle, possibly between glucose and glucose 6-phosphate (Burt and Pulliam, 1959). Another influence may be an increased rate of destruction of insulin. Freinkel and Goodner (1960) have demonstrated in the human placenta a proteolytic enzyme system capable of inactivating insulin, similar to the liver 'insulinase' prepared from animals.

Sugar is commonly found in urine from pregnant women. In a large serial study of 245 pregnant women, and using sensitive laboratory methods including chromatographic identification, Flynn, Harper and de Mayo (1953) found a positive Benedict's test in 72.9 per cent. After mid-pregnancy lactosuria was more common than glycosuria and occurred in about half the women; the incidence of glycosuria, with levels usually less than 67 mg per 100 ml of urine, rose rapidly after the 3rd month to fluctuate between 20 and 30 per cent.

We have pointed out in Chapter 4, that the greatly raised glomerular filtration rate in pregnancy presents much more glucose than normal to the tubules for reabsorption, and if the blood sugar is raised by quite modest amounts there may be more than the tubules are capable of reabsorbing. There is no evidence of a reduction of the renal threshold in the sense that the capacity of the tubules to reabsorb glucose is reduced.

Altogether the evidence of loss of sensitivity to insulin with prolonged circulation in the blood of glucose, amino acids and inorganic phosphorus suggests to us a device to retard storage in maternal tissues and give the foetus additional opportunity to acquire those nutrients. The device must greatly facilitate pickup by the placenta, and even if it means some loss in urine, the probability is that what is lost in urine is more than offset by gain to the foetus.

GLUCAGON

In one study of 12 women at 3, 6 and 9 months of pregnancy, Cassano and Tarantino (1959) found that an injection of 0.007 mg glucagon per kg body weight had a smaller effect at 6 months of pregnancy than at 3 and 9 months, or in the non-pregnant subject. Compared to a non-pregnant increase in blood glucose of 45 mg per 100 ml reached after 20 minutes, the woman 6 months pregnant had a rise of only 24 mg per 100 ml reached after 30 minutes.

CHAPTER 7

Preparations for Breast Feeding

Throughout pregnancy preparations are made for the nutrition of the foetus after birth. Nutrients are stored by the mother for use during lactation; the glandular tissue of the breasts develops and begins, even in early pregnancy, the manufacture of milk; and the nipples become larger and more mobile.

CHANGES IN THE BREASTS

Tenderness of the breasts, a tingling sensation or 'heaviness' and even obvious enlargement are early indications of pregnancy. The initial rapid enlargement during the first two months of pregnancy is probably little more than a vascular engorgement. When breast volume is measured before 10 weeks of pregnancy, and again at 12 to 14 weeks, there has often been a reduction between the measurements (Hytten, unpublished data). Thereafter, the breast enlarges progressively throughout pregnancy for the most part by growth of the gland. Some of the breast enlargement may be due to increase in subcutaneous fat, but there is no evidence, and our impression is that fat in this site does not usually increase.

The stimulus to growth of the mammary gland is presumed to be hormonal, but whether oestrogen and progesterone are both necessary in man is not known (Chapter 6).

Variation in breast enlargement

There is a striking individual variation in growth of the breasts in pregnancy, variation on a scale which is probably unknown outside the human species. In 143 primigravidae whose left breasts were measured by a displacement method at the end of the first trimester of pregnancy and again at term, the increase for a single breast ranged from zero or even a small loss of volume to as much as 880 ml with a mean value of about 200 ml. Measurements in 73 multigravidae showed a smaller range about a similar mean value. (Unpublished data, Hytten 1954b).

The increase in breast size in primigravidae declined with age from a mean of 234 ml for 14 women under 20 to 79 ml for 15 women over 30. The difference is obvious clinically: the young primigravida of 18 is often embarrassed by her rapid breast enlargement as early as the 2nd or 3rd month of pregnancy and her breasts are often tense and tender. The primigravida of 30 is more often unaware of any breast change. The effect of age on breast enlargement in multigravidae is less striking.

As might be expected, the performance in lactation is related to the growth in size of the breast. In 77 primigravidae where sufficient data were available, the correlation coefficient of breast enlargement and 7th day milk yield was 0.46, and the coefficient rose to 0.53, when the effect of age was eliminated. The small difference is not significant statistically, but suggests that for a given breast enlargement, the younger primipara produces more milk than the older; that is, she may be more physiologically efficient. Further evidence of decreased efficiency of the mammary gland with increasing age is the steady decline in fat content of 7th day milk from a mean of 3.25 per cent in primiparae under 20 to 2.83 per

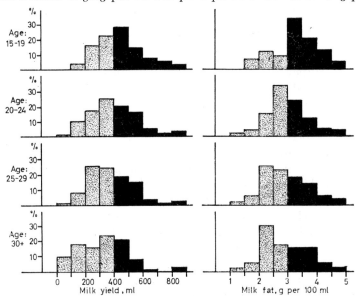

FIGURE 7.1. The effect of maternal age on the yield and fat content of 7th day milk. 509 Aberdeen primiparae. Arbitory divisions at 400 ml and 3.0 g/100 ml have been made to emphasize the difference between groups.

cent in primiparae of 30 and over (Baird, Hytten and Thomson, 1958). (Figure 7.1).

We can only speculate on the changes that may occur in breasts which do not function for many years after sexual maturity, but it is tempting to attribute the reduced efficiency of lactation in older primiparae to a process analogous to disuse atrophy. Apparently, the changes in the breast which are said to occur during the menstrual cycle (Ingleby, 1949) are not enough to prevent this 'atrophic' effect.

Age is not the only, or even the major influence, on individual variation in breast enlargement; genetic differences may be more important. There has been little or no natural selection for lactational ability in man because, in contrast to all other mammals, the ability of a mother to lactate has probably never been a necessity for the survival of her child; substitute mothers or substitute milks have always been available for the human infant. Anatomical confirmation of these individual differences has been provided by Engel (1941, 1947) who examined, at autopsy, the breasts of 80 women who had died soon after delivery. Only 20 to 30 per cent of the breasts 'contained glandular tissue in the same abundance as animals such as cows, dogs, guinea-pigs and others which were examined for comparison'. Another 30 to 40 per cent were grossly deficient; they consisted largely of fibrous tissue and fat.

The overall size of the breast, as distinct from its increase in size during pregnancy, is poorly related to function and is less variable than its ability to produce milk. This suggests that, in man, the breast has become more important as a sex symbol than as an organ of infant nutrition.

The early enlargement of the breast in pregnancy may have a functional importance. There is no doubt that it is capable of some function during the first trimester; lactose may appear in the blood and urine (Flynn, Harper and de Mayo, 1953) and secretion can sometimes be expressed from the nipple. Galactose is a vitally important structural sugar needed for such substances as chorionic gonadotrophin, and for mucopolysaccharides and cerebrosides necessary for foetal growth. It would be dangerous for the foetus to depend on galactose in his mother's diet and it may be that the supply of galactose comes from the mammary glands. In theory, the reaction by which many tissues convert galactose to glucose is reversible, but there is no evidence that the reverse conversion actually occurs except in the mammary gland and it would be of great interest to know whether normal foetal growth would be possible after bilateral mastectomy if galactose were excluded from the diet.

CHANGES IN THE NIPPLES

During pregnancy the nipples enlarge and become more mobile. The areolae also enlarge and, at least during the first pregnancy, become more deeply pigmented. Montgomery's tubercles increase in prominence, probably because, as histochemical studies suggest, they may be rudimentary mammary glands (Giacometti and Montagna, 1962).

Some of these changes were measured in an investigation reported by Hytten and Baird (1958). Three measurements were made serially from early pregnancy in 170 primigravidae and 104 multigravidae: the diameter of the areola, the diameter of the nipple, and the 'bite'—the minimal thickness of tissue behind the nipple. The last was estimated by compressing the areola immediately behind the nipple in the position where the baby makes its grip for sucking, with $\frac{1}{4}$ inch diameter ball-ended callipers. It is an index of the mobility of the nipple, its ability to be pulled out and therefore effectively grasped by the sucking infant. If the nipple will not pull forward, the calliper ends cannot be approximated and will therefore register a large bite; conversely, the nipple which is easily mobile has loose, readily-compressed tissue behind it and therefore a small bite.

Diameter of the areola

The diameter of the areola increased progressively throughout pregnancy. For primigravidae the mean increase was from 34 mm in early pregnancy to 50 mm in the early puerperium; for multigravidae there was a similar increase from 36 to 52 mm. In primigravidae, but not multigravidae the increase in areola diameter was less as maternal age increased (Table 7.1).

Diameter of the nipple

The nipple itself was difficult to measure; its size varied with its degree of erection which could not easily be controlled. There was no doubt however that the diameter increased during pregnancy

TABLE 7.1. The Effect of Age in Primigravidae on Increase
of Areolar Diameter during Pregnancy

Maternal age	Number of Subjects	Mean diameter of areola, mm		Increase per cent
		Early pregnancy	Early puerperium	
15–19	14	35.8	58.4	63
20–24	90	34.0	51.6	52
25–29	48	34.0	48.5	43
30 and over	18	33.0	44.2	34

from about 9.5 mm to 11.5 mm in primigravidae, and from 10 to
12.5 mm in multigravidae. There was no obvious age difference.

Mobility of the nipple

There was an improvement in the mobility of the nipple during
pregnancy with a reduction in the 'bite'. A 'bite' of 4 mm or less
indicates a nipple whose protractility would be considered satisfactory by any clinical criterion; at 6 mm many nipples appear
clinically unsatisfactory and above 6 mm almost all nipples would
be regarded as defective. In early pregnancy, only 40 per cent of
primigravidae had measurements of 4 mm or less, but the proportion had risen to almost 80 per cent by the puerperium. As a
prediction of function these measurements proved sound. Of 144
primigravidae whose 'bite' post-partum was less than 6 mm, only 4
had difficulty with the baby fixing; of the other 26 whose measurement was 6 mm or more, 9 had difficulty.

In multigravidae the mean 'bite' was initially much smaller than
in primigravidae, and the improvement during pregnancy was less
striking.

Maternal age had no apparent effect on the measurement of the
'bite', possibly because the processes responsible, unlike growth,
are less influenced by age. We have discussed the possible
mechanism for the increased mobility of the nipple in the Chapter
on hormones. Both oestrogens and relaxin may play a part in the
altered physical properties of connective tissue.

Clinical implications

It is widely believed that many women have nipples which require treatment during pregnancy to make them suitable for breast feeding. The opinion was first made popular by Waller (1939) who subsequently described a test for the detection of defective nipples: 'In imitation of the action of the baby's jaws the areola is pinched [by the thumb and forefinger] just beyond the nipple's base': if the nipple projects when this is done it is considered to be 'protractile' and therefore satisfactory (Waller, 1946). Of 200 primigravidae examined by Waller, 56 had 'poor protraction' and only 49 'good protraction'. On a similar basis Blaikley et al. (1953) thought that 52 of 234 primigravidae had nipples which required antenatal treatment because they were 'poorly protractile', and Naish (1948) stated that 'retracted nipples and nipples poorly formed are a common abnormality' requiring treatment in early pregnancy. Manual expression of colostrum, manipulation of the nipple, and the wearing of nipple shields during the last three months of pregnancy were claimed by both Waller and Blaikley et al. to give excellent results.

Antenatal treatment of the nipple by some form of manipulation has not been universally approved. The Ministry of Health (1944) for example, discussing the problem of why some women dislike breast feeding said: 'In some cases this distaste may have been engendered by an unnecessarily elaborate routine prescribed during the antenatal period. . . . It is, we fear, bordering on the paradoxical to impress upon the ordinary expectant mother that breast feeding is a normal, easy and natural process, if at the same time the advice she receives as a routine imposes on her the need for an elaborate daily ritual of preparation. We think it possible that with an anxious type of woman too much insistence on preparation of the breasts may alarm and discourage her to such an extent that she will refuse to initiate breast feeding'. In the only published controlled trial of breast preparation in pregnancy, Ingelman-Sundberg (1958) concluded that it was of no value.

The changes we have described suggest that what is claimed for antenatal treatment of the nipple can be attributed to normal physiological changes. The same can be said of claims that failure to breast feed a first baby because of defective nipples can be changed to success with the second baby after treatment during the second pregnancy (Naish, 1948). Improvement between first and second pregnancies is to be expected in more than half such women without treatment. Whether the small group of women whose nipples do not undergo the usual physiological changes would benefit from the local treatment usually advocated is doubtful, and the efficacy of treatment could be assessed only by a closely controlled trial on a sufficient scale.

STORAGE OF NUTRIENTS FOR LACTATION

We discuss at length in Chapter 12, the phenomenon of fat storage in pregnancy. The estimated average increase in body fat of about 4 kg or about 9 lb may represent an energy store of some 35,000 kcal, enough to subsidize lactation for 4 months at the rate of nearly 300 kcal daily. Evidence from farm animals shows that calcium is stored in pregnancy and mobilized for milk secretion. It seems likely that, if the supply is adequate, women also will store calcium; we have no information. It is unlikely that any other nutrient is stored in important quantities; in particular there is no good evidence that women store protein in pregnancy which they could mobilize for lactation. Indeed the low protein content of human milk, about 1 per cent (Hytten, 1954a), is so easily found in a diet which supplies sufficient energy, that storage for this purpose would be unnecessary.

CHAPTER 8

Respiratory Exchange and Supply of Nutrients to the Foetus

GENERAL CONSIDERATIONS
Morphology of the placenta

The origin and growth of the placenta is discussed elsewhere (p 262). Here we are concerned with the placenta not only as an 'extra-corporeal extension of the foetal capillary bed' but also as an organ with respiratory, hepatic and renal functions. We are not primarily concerned with how the placenta functions or with the requirements of the foetus, but only with how much the mother must provide so that the needs of the foetus may be met; and the efficiency of transfer by the placenta may have some effect on the total to be provided.

Growth of the placenta continues throughout gestation and is at first ahead of growth of the foetus (Hamilton and Boyd, 1951; Crawford, 1959, 1962). Crawford estimates that the placenta has its full number of cotyledons by the end of 12 weeks and further growth is by increase in number, branching and length of the villi. The placenta weighs about 200 g at 12 weeks and 650 g at term.

Surface area, as measured by counting nuclei per unit of chorion surface, is 6.4 ±0.3 m² (Bartels, Moll and Metcalfe, 1962), or, as estimated from planimetric measurement of prepared sections, from 10.29 to 14.5 m² (Wilkin, 1957; Clavero and Botella Llusiá, 1963). The electron microscope has revealed an enormous additional surface of microvilli, but it is not clear whether they have an absorbing surface in the ordinary physico-chemical sense or are adapted to engulf particles, too large for absorption through the cell surface, by the process called pinocytosis. Microvilli occur also on the surface of gland cells whose function is secretion (Amoroso, 1961).

The foetal capillaries in the placenta are covered with a layer of cytotrophoblast and one of syncytiotrophoblast, and the two, no matter how thin they become, are always demonstrable in the chorionic villi (Amoroso, 1961). The distance across which transfer must occur is given by Bartels, Moll and Metcalfe (1962) as 5.5 μm of tissue and 1 μm of plasma. The tissue barrier is therefore between 5 and 10 times as thick as that across which transfer of gases takes place in the lung.

Transfer

At one time the two-layer barrier between maternal and foetal blood was regarded as a semi-permeable membrane and what the foetus acquired as an ultrafiltrate of maternal plasma. When that simple hypothesis was shown to be inadequate to describe transfer from mother to foetus, a much more elaborate scheme was adopted involving 'diffusion', 'facilitated diffusion', 'active transport' and finally pinocytosis. How many of the concepts defined by Danielli and described recently by Widdas (1961), are required to explain transfer across the placenta is difficult to judge. It seems reasonable to suppose, and is conceded by Barron (1960), that simple diffusion suffices to explain passage of gases and water. The main stumbling block to acceptance of simple diffusion as the mode of transfer of other substances is that so many are found in higher concentration in foetal than in maternal blood. But the gradient is not directly from maternal blood to foetal blood, but first from maternal blood to syncytiotrophoblast where all sorts of complexes, proteins, enzymes, nucleic acids, high energy phosphates and hormones, are built up. The surplus, or perhaps on occasion an augmented supply, then goes to cytotrophoblast where further syntheses and conversions go on. We do not, in fact, know what the gradients in simple diffusible substances may be between those layers or between cytotrophoblast and foetal blood. It should be remembered that Christensen and his colleagues demonstrated that active growing and metabolizing animal tissues, including the uterus, concentrate free amino acids in intracellular water (Christensen and Streicher, 1948; Noall et al. 1957). Possibly the final transfer is from a high concentration of free metabolites in cytotrophoblast to foetal blood.

Pinocytosis has now been described in intestinal epithelium, the placenta (Brambell and Hemmings, 1960) and the secretory epithelium of some glands; all of those surfaces are liberally supplied with microvilli. It is not clear whether the microvilli of intestine and placenta are receptor devices tuned to accept large molecules of one specific structure only, or whether they are used to engulf a wide range of large molecules. We know that maternal plasma proteins are not identical with foetal plasma proteins of the same electrophoretic group. But amino acids pass the placenta easily, with some structural selection, but still freely. There is no reason to suppose that maternal proteins are needed or would be of help to the foetus if they were transferred intact. The same holds for lipids in general. Acetyl coenzyme A passes and can act as precursor of fatty acids and lipids. Sugars pass freely, if with some differences in rate of transfer, and probably all the other components of nucleic acids and blood group polysaccharides, or their simpler precursors. There is no definite evidence that proteins, lipids and nucleic acids are transferred intact by pinocytosis or otherwise. Whatever doubt there may be about the origin of those large molecules, there can be none that the foetus synthesises its own blood group antigens. On the whole it seems probable that the foetus synthesises its own large molecules, with the exception of γ-globulin.

The foetus at birth has only maternal γ-globulin and 'nearly a full complement' of maternal antibodies (Engle and Woods, 1960). It has been thought that the failure of the foetus to provide itself with γ-globulin might be due to the late, post-natal appearance of plasma cells, but Silverstein and Lukes (1962) have shown that the foetus can produce plasma cells in response to intrauterine infection and the premature infant is well able to form antibody of its own (Uhr et al. 1962). Silverstein et al. (1963) demonstrated that the foetal lamb is capable of forming specific antibody to bacteriophage as early as the 66th day of a 150 day gestation and to other antigens at different times later in pregnancy. The earliest, anti-phage, antibody was a macroglobulin and only in the older foetuses were appreciable amounts of γ-globulin formed.

That the human foetus relies on maternal γ-globulin to provide its antibodies for the immediate post-natal period and refrains, or is restrained, from making its own, may bear on the immunological puzzle of placentation.

The immunological puzzle

At first sight placentation would seem to be impossible. The trophoblast is foetal tissue, genetically foreign to the mother, and should be destroyed by an immunological reaction. Although

transplantation immunity is an important field of research, attention has been directed to placentation only recently and little is
known about why the placenta survives.

Medawar (1953) suggested that the privileged position of the
product of conception might be due to any or all of three things:
lack of antigenicity of the placenta, anatomical isolation of the
foetus from the mother, and immunological inertia of the pregnant
woman.

For both man and animals there is ample evidence that the
pregnant mammal is not immunologically inert. For example,
Bardawil *et al.* (1962) have shown that skin homografts are rejected
normally by pregnant women, and the mother may, when chal-
lenged, show a normal immunological response to foetal antigens
such as red cell antigens of the ABO and Rh series, and also antigens
associated with leucocytes and platelets (Van Rood, Van Leeuwen
and Eernisse, 1959).

That some tolerance of the foetal tissues may be induced in the
mother is suggested by experiments described by Breyere and
Barrett (1960). When female mice of an inbred strain were mated
with males of another inbred strain, skin grafts from the male strain
to the females survived progressively longer with increasing parity
from about 14 days in the virgin mouse to about 24 days after 4 or
more cross-bred litters had been born. That there was no effect of
parity *per se*, was shown by the rejection of skin grafts from males to
which the females were not bred.

Woodruff (1957) has favoured the possibility of anatomical
isolation. He showed in rats and rabbits that when females were
sensitized to their mates by skin grafts, a succeeding pregnancy
went successfully to term even though limbs from the unborn
foetuses grafted on to the mother were rejected.

There can be no question of anatomical isolation of the placenta
in man. It is accepted as a homograft even when, in abdominal
pregnancy, it implants in the ovary or peritoneum and Douglas *et
al.* (1959) have presented convincing evidence that trophoblast is
often broken off from the villi and swept into the maternal circulation.

That placental tissue, genetically foetal, is in direct contact with
maternal tissue and that the mother is capable, perhaps with some
modification of forming antibody to foetal antigen, leaves us only
with Medawar's third possibility to explain the success of this

unique homograft: the placenta must be non-antigenic. But it is not. Hulka, Hsu and Beiser (1961) showed that blood-free human trophoblast does have antigens. They were unable to demonstrate circulating antibody to trophoblast during pregnancy, but they showed quite clearly, by fluorescence technique, that five women studied had circulating antibody, each to her own placenta, a few days *post-partum*. Their explanation was that the large surface of trophoblast absorbs the circulating antibody, and consequently it becomes apparent only when the absorbing surface is removed. An alternative explanation could be that there is some central inhibition of the formation of antibody to trophoblast during pregnancy.

In mice, Dancis, Samuels and Douglas (1962) showed that the placenta not only was antigenic but also contained immunologically competent cells capable of making antibody to host tissues. As they conclude 'this makes even more remarkable the success of the placenta as a homograft'; and the puzzle remains.

Brown (1963) found foetal red cells in the circulation of 83 of 165 women after normal labour. We do not know whether leakage occurs as often before labour but if it does, then the fact that only a small proportion of women form antibodies to incompatible foetal cells suggests again that a mechanism of tolerance may be operating. But incompatibility associated with blood group differences is apparent in human pregnancy. Matsunaga and Itoh (1957–58) demonstrated in two Japanese villages that ABO blood group incompatibility of husband and wife resulted in a considerable excess of abortions: there was 1 abortion in 6.5 pregnancies in incompatible matings compared with 1 in 10 pregnancies where the blood groups of husband and wife were compatible.

Waterhouse and Hogben (1947) in a study of 1239 families described a highly significant shortage of group A offspring in the mating class Father A × Mother O as compared with the reciprocal class Father O × Mother A and a shortage of group B offspring in the mating class Father O × Mother B compared with the reciprocal class Father B × Mother O. This has been interpreted as indicating losses due to blood group incompatibility but detailed examination of the data (Allan, 1953) suggests that the differences are more likely to be due to differences of fertility, fathers of group A and mothers of group B being the least fertile. The association of blood groups with differences of sex ratio is discussed on p. 385.

TRANSFER OF GASES

Oxygen

The supply of oxygen to the foetus has two main points of interest: it must be sufficient in quantity to cover the energy expenditure of the foetus, and the necessary amount must be delivered at such a tension that it can penetrate into the tissues. The second consideration, vital to tissue respiration, has received relatively little study.

We will examine first information relating to the transfer of oxygen, and then attempt to picture the whole situation from the foetal point of view. We will do that in spite of having said we are not concerned with foetal physiology because the needs of the foetus dictate the maternal adjustments to be made.

ADULT AND FOETAL HAEMOGLOBIN

Oxygen is transported in blood in solution in the plasma and in combination with haemoglobin in the red cell. Dissolved oxygen is quantitatively of little importance, about 0.25 ml per 100 ml blood, and only haemoglobin oxygen need be considered. When exhaustively dialysed, adult and foetal haemoglobins have the same dissociation curve but they carry different associated substances and move in different environments in the red cell and plasma (Allen, Wyman and Smith, 1953). The affinity of blood for oxygen and the speed with which it will liberate oxygen depend on the tensions of oxygen and carbon dioxide and the pH of the blood, and, of course, on the concentration of haemoglobin in the blood. A gram of haemoglobin combines with 1.34 ml oxygen. Adult blood in pregnancy carries an average of 11 or 12 g haemoglobin, 15 or 16 ml oxygen per 100 ml when saturated. Foetal blood, with 16 or 17 g haemoglobin can carry up to 23 ml oxygen per 100 ml.

In the early stages of growth, up to the end of the first month when a primitive circulation is established, respiration in the embryo is by the direct oxidation and reduction of the many compounds later active in tissue cell metabolism. When the structure of the embryo becomes too complicated and distances too great for direct oxidation, the blood takes over as intermediary. The composition of foetal blood is such that its affinity for oxygen at such tensions of oxygen and carbon dioxide as prevail in the placental circulation is higher than that of the mother, and at low oxygen tensions and high concentrations of carbon dioxide its affinity for oxygen is less than that of the mother. In consequence haemoglobin in foetal blood extracts more oxygen from the supply in the inter-villous space than it would if it were in maternal blood, and as it traverses the body, foetal haemoglobin continues to liberate oxygen when haemoglobin in maternal blood would not. Van Slyke (1959) said, if maternal blood at 30 mm Hg oxygen tension and 60 per cent saturation equilibrates with foetal blood in the intervillous space, the foetal blood will be 70 per cent saturated.

OXYGEN TRANSFER: BASIC MEASUREMENTS

Many detailed studies have been made of oxygen transfer from mother to foetus in the sheep and rabbit by Barcroft and his disciples. It is not possible to make similar studies in women. Indeed the number of measurements that can be made is small, most of them are made at caesarean section and it is inevitable that they should be eked out with assumptions. The measurements that can be made in late pregnancy are of oxygen capacity and saturation in maternal and foetal blood, and of blood flow, by indirect measure-ment with nitrous oxide or a radioactive element injected into the circulation. Several workers have measured oxygen saturation but only three studies in which blood flow was measured have been found.

Blood flow in the uterus. The techniques used and the possible validity of the results of those three studies have been discussed in Chapter 2. They are the basis of all subsequent estimates of the oxygen consumption of the foetus: alternatively, the estimates of blood saturation are used with assumed values for the oxygen con-sumption of the foetus to estimate blood flow. Before we summarize the results, it should be said that a single estimate of oxygen tension and saturation describes only the conditions at the moment of sampling and is not necessarily a measure of requirement. The amount of oxygen removed from maternal blood during transit through the intervillous space, or from umbilical vein blood during transit to umbilical artery, represents foetal requirement only if the whole system is functioning fully and freely, without let or hind-rance. Barron (1960) said, 'To date no one has measured the rate of oxygen consumption of a fetus *in utero* in circumstances in which it was known that the fetus was meeting all its metabolic require-ments by oxygen derived from the fetal blood and not developing an oxygen debt'.

Assali and his associates made two series of measurements. The later, on women between the 9th and 28th weeks of pregnancy, is of interest chiefly for the comparison of a flowmeter with the nitrous oxide method of estimating blood flow (cf. Chapter 2) and for the suggestion that, per unit weight of the pregnant uterus, blood flow and oxygen consumption are constant during the interval studied (Assali, Rauramo and Peltonen 1960). The first series deals with blood flow in late pregnancy (Assali *et al.* 1953b). Measurements were made on 7 women between 37 and 40 weeks of pregnancy. In terms of cc oxygen per 100 cc blood per minute the range was from 12.2 to 18.5, with an average of 15.1. Weights of foetuses were not given. Instead, the report says: '. . . if we accept Chesley's figures of 5 kilograms as being the approximate weight of the uterus, fetus, and amniotic fluid at the end of gestation, the blood flow for the entire uterus would be close to 750 cc per minute'. What Chesley really included in the weight of 5 kg was the product of conception, 'baby + afterbirth + amniotic fluid'.

The reports of the Boston group (Romney *et al.* 1955; Metcalfe *et al.* 1955) show minor differences in detail. In the first publication, the average blood flow in the uterus was estimated to be 518 cc per minute, with a range from 255 to 840 cc.

Those two estimates, the one of a uterine blood flow of 750 and the other of 518 cc per minute, are usually quoted, not as two independent averages, but as if they represented the range of one, or a number of homogeneous series. The total range in the two series taken together was from 255 to 925 ml per minute. In their latest review Bartels, Moll and Metcalfe (1962) give the rate of blood flow as 'between 500 and 750 ml per minute' and add: 'If one assumes that approximately 25 per cent of this blood does not enter into gas exchange with the fetal blood, a figure for the blood flow through the intervillous space of 375 to 560 ml per minute is reached'.

Browne's (1959) estimate of blood flow with radioactive sodium and an assumed value for the oxygen consumption of the foetus, was 600 ml per minute in normal women and only 200 ml in the hypertensive.

Blood flow in the cord. Metcalfe (1959) summarized the evidence from analyses of cord blood as giving an arterio-venous difference of between 4.5 and 7.2 volumes per cent. Estimates of the oxygen consumption of the foetus, he said, range between 4 and 7.5 ml per kg per minute. From those figures, assuming a foetal weight of 3.3 kg, cord blood flow ranged from 200 to 550 ml per min. Bartels (1959) reported the oxygen content of umbilical vein blood as 10.6 and of umbilical artery as 2.9, with, on his figures, a mean difference of 7.2 volumes per cent. With an assumed value for the oxygen uptake of the foetus of 6 ml per kg per minute and an assumed weight of 3.3 kg, cord blood flow was computed to be 360 ml per minute. Later, Bartels, Moll and Metcalfe (1962) scaled down the arterio-venous difference in cord blood to 6.7 volumes per cent, the oxygen uptake of the foetus to 5 ml per kg per minute and only foetal weight remained the same. The reassessment of the arterio-venous difference came from a collection of averages with a range from 5.00 to 9.60 and an unweighted general average of 6.9 volumes per cent. On the new basis the estimate of cord blood flow was 250 ml, with a range from 165 to 330 ml per minute.

Oxygen in blood in the intervillous space and umbilical cord. Recorded data for oxygen in the intervillous space and umbilical vessels are unsatisfactory. The range is so wide, where the infant is described as normal as well as where it is said to be anoxic, that means derived from such ranges are valueless.

On the subject of sampling the blood in the umbilical vessels Barcroft (1946) said:

'Nothing is easier than, armed with a syringe, to open the abdomen of a pregnant animal, open the uterus, expose the cord, and after the vessels have eluded the point of the syringe a time or two (which they are very likely to do) obtain two samples of blood for analysis, and when that has been done to say the umbilical artery and vein of the foetus contain respectively such and such quantities of oxygen. Such results are frankly worthless—some guarantee must be given that the blood in these vessels, so sensitive to any kind of manipulation, is coursing at the normal rate; some guarantee must be given that the foetus is in a normal state; some guarantee must be given, and this is often overlooked, that the circulation in the mother is also normal: and lastly when the worker has satisfied his readers and, what is probably more difficult, himself, that the data are as nearly correct as may be, there remains the question—to what stage of pregnancy do they refer?'

The position is no better when blood in the intervillous space is sampled. It receives blood at arterial oxygen tension and discharges venous blood, so that it must contain a non-homogeneous mixture

TABLE 8.1. Tension of Oxygen and Oxygen Saturation of Umbilical Cord Blood at Term

Authors	Subjects	Oxygen Saturation, per cent		pO₂, mm Hg	
		Umbilical vein	Umbilical artery	Umbilical vein	Umbilical artery
Walker (1954a)	10 subjects; normal spontaneous delivery	48.3 (13.4 to 60)	19.6 (0.9 to 28.8)	21.5	12.0
	8 subjects; difficult labour, no foetal distress	45.5 (27.6 to 57.3)	16.8 (4.0 to 30.0)	20.5	11.0
	11 subjects; recent foetal distress	23.2 (8.0 to 32.1)	4.8 (0.0 to 11.9)	13.0	5.0
McKay (1957)	Uncomplicated vertex deliveries				
	26 subjects at 35–38 weeks	72.7 ± 4.62	38.2 ± 4.29	31	18
	60 subjects at 39–41 weeks	64.4 ± 4.53	31.2 ± 4.53	27	16
	26 subjects at 42–43 weeks	53.9 ± 5.63	20.2 ± 6.13	24	12
Turnbull and Baird (1957)	Uncomplicated deliveries. Calculated from equation for primigravidae aged 25				
	38 weeks	55	28	24	15
	40 weeks	48	21	21	13
	42 weeks	41	14	19	10

TABLE 8.1. (continued)

Authors	Subjects	Oxygen Saturation, per cent		pO₂, mm Hg	
		Umbilical vein	Umbilical artery	Umbilical vein	Umbilical artery
James et al. (1958)	55 vigorous infants at birth	49	22	22	13
Prystowsky, Hellegers and Bruns (1960)	3 normal women at elective caesarean section at term	71.0; 66.1; 52.3	26.7; 30.6; 34.2	31; 30; 24	15; 16; 18
Sjöstedt, Rooth and Caligara (1960)	69 uncomplicated vaginal deliveries	60.1	23.7	28.9	16.9
Vasicka et al. (1960)	19 normal vaginal deliveries and 12 caesarean sections at term	No data	No data	20.73	10.2
Dunphy (1962)	95 women with spontaneous or low forceps deliveries; duration of pregnancy less than 43 weeks	56.8 (23.1 to 88.5)	29.0 (2.7 to 64.6)	24 (13 to 46)	15 (2 to 27)

which a single sample cannot possibly describe. Fuchs, Spackman and Assali (1963) have demonstrated the lack of homogeneity in a recent study. In one subject at ceasarean section the pO_2 of arterial blood was 101 and of blood from the uterine vein 50 mm Hg. Two samples ostensibly from the intervillous space gave oxygen tensions of 90 and 52 mm Hg but the workers themselves say the intervillous space is so closely packed with villi that it is impossible to know when a needle is in it. The samples taken may have been from blood vessels.

In Table 8.1 we have collected illustrative studies. Oxygen tension is not usually measured in such studies and the figures in Table 8.1 for pO_2, with the exception of those of Prystowsky, Hellegers and Bruns; Sjöstedt, Rooth and Caligara, and Vasicka et al., are derived from data for oxygen saturation, the corresponding tensions being read from the oxygen dissociation curve of foetal blood in Figure 8.1 (Darling et al. 1941).

It is obvious that vaginal delivery is attended by episodes of oxygen deprivation which if continued for any length of time would be incompatible with survival of the foetus and cannot be taken as representing conditions in utero. We are supported in this view by those studies in which saturation and oxygen tension were measured together. It will be seen that the points all lie slightly to the right of the dissociation curve, suggesting some accumulation of carbon dioxide, even in those that appear to offer a reasonable approximation to normality. Some of the wide scatter of results is probably due to the technical difficulties described by Barcroft; some may be due to acute deprivation of oxygen associated with delivery. James and Burnard (1961) found the oxygen saturation of umbilical arterial blood in 55 babies in excellent condition at birth (Apgar scores 9 and 10) to range from 0 to nearly 70 per cent. There is no need for further comment on such data as criteria of normality.

Nevertheless, there is a clear trend to lower oxygen saturations with postmaturity (McKay; Turnbull and Baird), associated with clinical signs of hypoxia. For that reason we have to consider what are the safe physiological limits of oxygen tension and possible protective devices against deprivation.

EMERGENCY MEASURES

The foetus may make use of any of four protective devices to help to

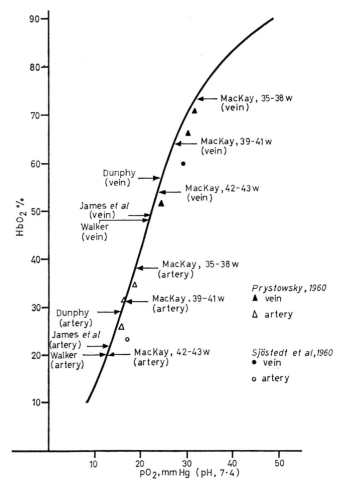

FIGURE 8.1. Published estimates of oxygen saturation and tension in foetal blood referred to the dissociation curve of foetal blood

assure adequate oxygen supply. The first is a mechanism built into the placenta and is presumably ready at any time to meet sudden deprivation. It is, in a sense, a reversion to an earlier method of respiration as in the embryo before establishment of the circulation and is well known in the metabolism of cells and tissues, for instance in the anaerobic respiration of intense muscular effort, as in sprinting. It has been demonstrated by Huckabee *et al.* (1962) in the foetal goat. When the supply of oxygen to the mother is artificially reduced so that oxidation in foetal tissues is incomplete and lactic acid accumulates, the excess is arrested in the placenta and is presumed to be oxidized there by oxygen from highly oxidized phosphorus-containing nucleotides. As long as such oxidation continues the foetus is respiring in part anaerobically, but the combined metabolism of foetus and placenta is not anaerobic. The condition for such respiration is that there should be enough oxygen to penetrate the cells of the placenta but not enough to traverse it to reach the foetal blood in adequate amounts. There is no doubt, under marginal conditions, the device may be life saving in the ungulate; it does not follow that it would have the same significance for the human foetus, first because the human placenta is in so much more intimate contact with maternal blood, and second, because possibly the human foetus may be more sensitive to partial anoxia.

Second, there is the reaction by which excess of oxygen contracts and excess of carbon dioxide dilates the placental vessels so adapting blood flow to oxygen demand (Panigel, 1962).

The other two methods of protection are designed to deal, not with sudden emergency, but with chronic shortage. The first of these can operate only if the shortage is established early in pregnancy. If, for example, the mother is living in an atmosphere where oxygen tension is low, as at high altitudes, the placenta is bigger in size and weight than at low altitudes (Prystowsky, 1960). Such compensatory growth is not possible after the first few weeks of pregnancy.

The second protective mechanism is polycythaemia which increases the oxygen carrying capacity. It occurs in both mother and foetus at high altitudes, of greater degree in the foetus, as might be expected since it gets its oxygen at second hand. This is what Barcroft called the 'Everest reaction', though it was first seen in the Andes.

That the conditions in which the human foetus respires in late pregnancy may elicit the Everest reaction was first shown by Walker and Turnbull (1953) and Walker (1954a). In a study of oxygen capacity and saturation in cord blood at delivery they found that a number of infants showed progressively lower oxygen saturation and higher haemoglobin concentration with the duration of pregnancy after term and they suggested that the reduced 'margin of safety' might account for the more frequent occurrence of intrauterine death, associated with asphyxial changes, when pregnancy continued after term. The hypothesis was applied with success by Baird (Turnbull and Baird, 1957; Baird, 1960, 1963) to reduce the incidence of perinatal infant death, especially the infants of elderly primiparae, by induction of labour at or shortly after term, or by caesarean section if there was evidence of foetal distress.

That the foetus may be subjected to oxygen deprivation if pregnancy continues past term seems established by both the epidemiological evidence of a reduced foetal death rate with asphyxia *in utero* when labour is induced at term, and the fact that the protective device of polycythaemia in the foetus comes into action.

Just where the block to oxygen supply occurs is not known. It is unlikely to be caused by failure of the mother to deliver sufficient oxygen to the intervillous space; perhaps the placenta itself is at fault or is impaired in function by deposition of fibrin on its outer surface. The *amount* of oxygen reaching the foetus may not be greatly reduced and indeed the danger of anoxia is not apparent from the figures which are claimed to show it. In the data of Turnbull and Baird (1957) for example, the oxygen saturation in umbilical vein declined as pregnancy progressed beyond term, but the oxygen saturation in the artery declined in parallel so that the available oxygen per unit volume of blood was apparently unaltered. The importance of the low saturations lies in the low partial pressures of oxygen from which they arise. From the data plotted in Figure 8.1 with the dissociation curve of foetal blood it seems highly probable that the oxygen supply to the foetal tissues will be prejudiced if the partial pressure falls below 15 mm Hg, giving oxygen saturations of 30 per cent or less. The distressed infants of Walker's study and the postmature infants described by McKay and Turnbull and Baird were anoxic because of insufficient *pressure* of oxygen.

SUBSIDIARY OBSERVATIONS

In a discussion of the effect of giving oxygen to the mother on the oxygen supply to the foetus Prystowsky (1959) said that the pO_2 in the intervillous space rose from 40 to 60 mm Hg and the percentage saturation of the blood from 66 to 92. In agreement with Prystowsky, McClure and James (1960) record that when mothers were given oxygen for 10 minutes or less, for 11 to 15 minutes, or for more than 15 minutes before delivery, the pO_2 of umbilical blood was 31.0, 34.4 or 40 mm Hg. Barron (1959), nevertheless, doubted that raising the tension on the maternal side of the placenta would necessarily raise that on the foetal side. 'There is evidence' he said 'in two species, that in those circumstances the foetus apparently decreases the size of his capillary bed or modifies his circulation rate so that he gets his oxygen in the amount and at the tension he wants it'. Panigel (1962) also suggests the possibility of control by the foetus when he says that raising the oxygen tension in a placental perfusate contracts the capillaries and raising the carbon dioxide dilates them. The obvious contradiction may be resolved by the difference between the observers; Prystowsky and McClure and James were speaking of administration of oxygen at delivery; Barron probably of normal control *in utero*. We have just seen reason to believe that the power of control fails at low oxygen tensions.

THE FOETAL OXYGEN SUPPLY: ESTIMATES FROM
BASIC MEASUREMENTS

The data just described have been used in various combinations to estimate oxygen supply to, or consumption by, the foetus. With such wide ranges of variation it is difficult to judge what should be taken to represent the 'normal'. Perhaps, allowing for the accumulation of disturbances at delivery, it would be correct to choose the higher oxygen contents as representing normal pre-labour levels, but the custom has been to use averages or ranges.

Assali *et al.* (1953) assessed the oxygen consumption of the uterus as between 0.54 and 1.45 ml per 100 g per minute. Applied to an assumed weight of uterus and contents at term of 5 kg, total consumption becomes 27 to 72.5 ml oxygen per minute. The higher estimate is equivalent to 104 litres per day, or about 140 kcal per kg per day. The basal metabolic rate of a 56 kg non-pregnant woman is about 1400 kcal daily, or 25 kcal per kg, so that the higher estimate is obviously absurd. Even the lower limit of 27 ml per minute for the 5 kg uterus means 39 kcal per kg per day and is 50 per cent above the non-pregnant rate adopted for comparison, and therefore improbably high. From the oxygen contents of umbilical vein and artery Assali *et al.* estimated the oxygen consumption of the foetus (meaning probably foetus plus placenta) at only 16 ml per minute, equivalent to 29 kcal per kg, in better agreement with, but still above the putative maternal non-pregnant basal metabolic rate.

In Table 8.2 is reproduced part of the table in which Romney, Metcalfe and their associates (1955) presented data for 12 women showing an average oxygen consumption of 23.8 ml per minute or 36 kcal per kg, which is nearly 40 per cent above maternal non-pregnant basal rate. If we omit the three highest values, which are

TABLE 8.2. Uterine Arterial and Venous Oxygen Content, Blood
Flow and Oxygen Consumption (Romney *et al.* 1955)

Foetus kg	A-V oxygen difference cc per 100 cc	Blood flow cc per min	Oxygen consumption cc per min
3.5	3.0	590	17.7
3.1	3.4	535	18.2
3.0	5.0	330	16.4
3.2	3.8	560	21.3
3.1	3.4	480	16.4
3.7	4.7	315	14.8
3.7	2.7	840	22.7
2.9	5.1	255	13.0
2.9	6.5	335	21.8
3.6	6.1	510	31.0
3.2	6.3	770	48.5 (57.0)*
3.5	6.3	700	44.0
3.3	4.7	518	23.8

* The figure 57.0 is given for this case in the paper by Metcalfe *et al.* (1955) who report the same data.

so far out of line as to suggest a technical error, the averages become: foetal weight 3.2 kg, arteriovenous oxygen difference 4.2 ml per 100 ml blood, blood flow 470 ml and oxygen consumption 18 ml per minute. That gives approximately 26 kcal per kg per day, in agreement with maternal basal rate.

It seems fair to conclude that the nitrous oxide method over-estimates blood flow, sometimes seriously. Arterio-venous oxygen difference may also be overestimated.

To estimate what flow of blood would be required to meet the needs of the foetus, Browne (1959) assumed a requirement of 25 ml per minute, attributing the estimate to Villee who had suggested that, according to the literature, the foetus at term uses 24 ml per minute or 35 litres a day. Browne next assumed a difference of oxygen content between the uterine artery and vein of 7 volumes per cent. On those chosen assumptions he argued that a flow of 350 ml per minute is sufficient to supply the needs of the foetus. The needs of the placenta and the uterus were not considered.

ENERGY EXPENDITURE OF THE FOETUS

The energy expenditure of the human foetus is usually estimated on the assumption that it can be expressed in kcal as a constant multiplied by a power of body weight less than unity, like that of an adult, or, what amounts to the same thing in theory, as the measured expenditure of the child soon after birth. Carpenter and Murlin (1911), who found that the energy output of a pregnant woman was the same as that of the same woman *post-partum* plus her baby, concluded that the baby's metabolism *in utero* was related to its surface area and therefore, per unit weight, considerably above that of its mother. But experiments on animals have shown that the foetus 'does not behave metabolically as a small homeotherm' (Kleiber, 1961). Much earlier than Kleiber, Barcroft (1936) said: 'The embryo has no surface, if the word surface is used in the physiological sense, intended to convey to the reader the idea of an area from which heat is dissipated'. Of his experiments on goats and sheep he wrote: 'For the low figures obtained for the foetus there appears to be a reason; the foetus has no cooling surface and is under no necessity to keep up its own body temperature. The heat which it produces must ultimately be dissipated by the mother and the greater the heat produced the greater the burden thrown upon the parent'. He explained part at least of the difference between the metabolic rate of his experimental animals *in utero* and after birth as due to the acquisition of muscle tone. The foetus, he said, is flaccid, and the effect of exposure was demonstrated by alternately lifting sheep foetuses out of, and replacing them in a warm bath.

There are other reasons why we cannot accept surface area, or the estimates of Carpenter and Murlin, as giving true estimates of foetal metabolism. Carpenter and Murlin computed the metabolic rate of the foetus on the assumption that the pregnant woman was equivalent in energy output to herself when non-pregnant, *plus* her foetus. But, apart from the foetus, the pregnant woman has many extra expenditures. We have already shown that a part of the rise in basal metabolic rate is due, not to the foetus, but to the extra work of respiration and the heart (p. 99, Chapter 3). If the mother's non-pregnant expenditure be taken as 1400 kcal daily, equivalent to about 200 ml oxygen per minute, and the pregnancy increase be taken as 14 per cent, her extra oxygen requirement per minute would be about 28 ml. If the oxygen consumption of the foetus were that most often assumed, about 25 ml for a weight of 3 kg, the total for foetus, placenta and uterus, 5 kg in all, would account for more than the whole increase.

A NEW ESTIMATE

The problem must therefore be formulated anew. If we consider the foetus as behaving metabolically as part of the mother's body, we still have no agreed basis on which to make our calculations. They should possibly be made in terms of metabolically active tissue and it might be argued that, weight for weight, the growing foetus would have more, and more active, tissue than the mother. On the other hand, the water content of the foetus is higher and the balance of probability, taking the excellent evidence from animal work into account, is that the metabolic rate of the foetus is, weight for weight, not greater than that of the resting, fasting, non-pregnant woman.

If equivalence per unit weight is assumed, it seems likely that an estimate of foetal metabolism will be too high, rather than too low.

On that assumption, calculations for the hypothetical standard healthy woman described in Chapter 13 would be as follows, to the nearest 100 g:

Weight of mother, non-pregnant: 56 kg
Basal metabolic rate: 1400 kcal daily or 200 ml oxygen per minute
Weight of term foetus: 3.3 kg
Weight of foetus and placenta: 4 kg
Weight of blood-free increment of myometrium: 0.9 kg
Weight of uterus, foetus and placenta: 4.9 kg

On that basis, the oxygen requirement of the foetus would be not more than 200 × 3.3/56, about 12 ml oxygen per minute; of foetus and placenta 14, and of uterus, foetus and placenta approximately 18 ml per minute, which is the same as our revised interpretation of the data of Romney et al. (1955) (Table 8.2 and related text).

The calculation may be checked in part by substituting estimates of the metabolism *in vitro* of placenta and myometrium. The substitution, according to Kleiber (1961) may legitimately be made because 'The effect of the metabolic regulators . . . appears to persist in the tissues after removal from the animal and to affect the respiration rate *in vitro*'. Friedman, Little and Sachtleben (1962) give the oxygen consumption of the gravid myometrium as between 3.3 and 4.2 ml per kg per minute, from which we may assume a possible average of 3.7. They report the oxygen consumption of term placentae to average 2.04 μl per mg dry matter per hour (range 1.13 to 2.58), which, for a 650 g placenta, dry weight 110 g, is 3.7 ml per minute. Villee's (1953) estimate for term placentae was similar, 1.9 μl per mg per hour, or 3.48 ml per minute for our standard placenta.

With those substitutions the total expenditure becomes: foetus, as before, 12 ml; placenta 3.7 and uterus 3.3 ml per minute; total 19, a little higher than when the whole is taken in proportion to maternal basal metabolism, but in sensible agreement with it.

If we accept the second synthetic estimate of 15.7 ml oxygen per minute as the probable requirement of foetus and placenta, and the difference in oxygen content between umbilical vein and artery as 4.5 or 5 volumes per cent, a blood flow in those vessels of 310 to 360 ml per minute would supply foetus and placenta. To supply 19 ml per minute for uterus, foetus and placenta at about the same oxygen difference, 380 or 420 ml would be required or, if the oxygen difference were as high as 7 volumes per cent, which seems to be as much as is likely to occur under normal conditions, 270 ml would suffice. These quantities are less than most of the estimates, and are probably well within the attainment of normal women.

Carbon dioxide

There is no question of difficulty in the transfer of carbon dioxide across the placenta in either direction. It diffuses through a wet membrane 20 or 30 times as fast as oxygen, and no doubt something similar would hold for a cellular barrier if the only problem was to get rid of carbon dioxide. The position is not quite that. In the first place, the carbon dioxide carried in solution in blood is only a small part of the whole. Most of it is carried as carbonate or bicarbonate, a small fraction in combination with haemoglobin. The equilibrium between the carbonates plays a major part in hydrogen ion regulation; the surplus over that required as carbonate is removed in respiration.

Only one study during pregnancy of carbon dioxide in blood and the relation between concentrations in maternal and foetal plasma has been found, that of Prystowsky, Hellegers and Bruns (1961). During repeat caesarean section in six healthy women plasma carbon dioxide, plasma bicarbonate, pCO_2, pH and physically dissolved CO_2 were measured in blood from intervillous space, umbilical vein and umbilical artery. In four of the six, cord blood was sampled less than a minute after maternal blood; in the other two there was a delay of 4 or 5 minutes before cord blood was sampled. In all cases, foetal carbon dioxide exceeded maternal by from 4.5 to 8.4 mm Hg when there was no delay, and by 17.5 and 20.5 mm Hg in two subjects where there was delay. Delay in sampling raised carbon dioxide tension in the foetus and slightly reduced it in the intervillous space. It is always difficult to be sure that conditions at term, or during caesarean section, are strictly comparable with those during uninterrupted pregnancy.

Maternal overbreathing, as described in Chapter 3, would reduce carbon dioxide tension in maternal blood and increase the gradient for transfer from the foetus.

Carbon monoxide

We have already seen in Chapter 1 that free carbon monoxide readily crosses the placenta. When it is used as Sjöstedt used it as a tracer for the estimation of blood volume, it overestimates maternal volume.

When it is given chronically in small doses there is time for equilibration with haemoglobin and a varying proportion of carboxyhaemoglobin results, reducing the carrying capacity of the blood. For that reason it might be expected that carbon monoxide poisoning during pregnancy would be teratogenic, like acute deprivation of oxygen by other means, and Haddon, Nesbitt and Garcia (1961) cite evidence that it is so.

In their study, Haddon et al. measured carbon monoxide concentration in the blood of 50 pregnant women who smoked cigarettes and 50 who did not. They found a significantly higher concentration in the smokers and a significantly high correlation between the concentrations in maternal and umbilical vein blood.

On the other hand acute poisoning causes death before any

appreciable amount of the gas is transferred to the foetus (Martland and Martland, 1950).

TRANSFER OF NUTRIENTS

Very many studies have been made to compare the composition of maternal blood with that of foetal blood. They do not contribute to our knowledge of transfer and no attempt is made to list them.

It is often stated that the rate of transfer of nutrients across the placenta become progressively faster from about the 12th week to term, or about term. The statement is imprecise because it is not made clear whether the increase is envisaged in absolute terms or in relation to foetal weight. On the foetal side, there will be a steady increase of total blood volume, but there is no evidence to show whether the amount passing through the placenta in unit time rises in proportion to total volume or not. According to Assali *et al.* (1960) maternal blood flow increases in proportion to foetal weight.

Improvement in rate of transfer is attributed also to greater 'permeability' of the placenta associated with thinning of the cellular barriers. It is difficult to see how that should be important unless the size of the molecules presented to the placenta is of primary importance. There is evidence for and against that view. According to Moya and Thorndike (1962), drugs of molecular weight less than 600 pass freely; those of molecular weight over 1000 do not pass at all, and those of intermediate weight have not been investigated. But size is certainly not the only determinant. Of plasma proteins as classified by electrophoresis and ultra-centrifuge, some of the 7S (Svedberg units) group pass so freely as to be in equilibrium on both sides of the placenta. But not all those in the 7S sedimentation group can pass. The $\beta_2 A$ moiety to which siderophilin (transferrin) belongs, is rejected. Freda (1962) says all the immune globulins belong to the 7S group but passage is decided, not by the size of the molecule, but by its structure as a γ_2-globulin. Morris (1963) writing of the transmission of homologous antibodies says '. . . it is conceivable that the receptor would be better adapted to receive the 'species-specific' part common to all the antibody molecules than the residual or antibody reactive parts whose structure must depend to some extent on the antigens which stimulated their production'.

Evidence in the same direction comes from the preferential

transfer of L-amino acids, and of D-xylose which is transferred at a rate four to five times that of L-xylose.

Derrington and Soothill (1961) have an interesting postscript to the question of molecular size. They planned to compare the concentrations in maternal and foetal sera and amniotic fluid of pairs of proteins of comparable size: albumin with siderophilin, 7S γ-globulin with coeruloplasmin, and α_2-glycoprotein with 19S γ-globulin. The third comparison could not be made because 19S γ-globulin was not found in amniotic fluid. The ratio of siderophilin to albumin in 14 comparisons, and of coeruloplasmin to 7S γ-globulin in 5 comparisons did not differ significantly between maternal serum and amniotic fluid, but there were significant differences for foetal serum. It would appear therefore that amniotic fluid protein is an ultrafiltrate of maternal, not foetal, serum.

Quantitative measurements

Many studies of transfer have now been made by injection of substances labelled with radioactive isotopes, or tracer amounts of the element to be measured, into the maternal circulation and estimation of radioactivity in foetal blood. The technique, in essence, is simple, but the attendant circumstances are complicated and liable to produce errors of interpretation.

In the first place any manipulation that is liable to change flow or hydrostatic pressure in the intervillous space will be liable to affect transfer. Dancis, Brenner and Money (1962) enter a caveat about experiments in which osmotic pressure is altered because shift of fluid may simulate a change in rate of transfer of solutes.

Second, it is the transfer of radioactivity that is measured and, strictly speaking, it is not always certain that, when it reaches the foetal circulation, the label is still attached to, and only to, the substance originally labelled. If it is, the label itself may alter the structure of the molecule to which it is attached and so effect transfer (Sternberg, 1962).

It would therefore serve no good purpose to summarize and discuss all those studies. Some of the results, all the same, deserve mention. The work of Flexner and his colleagues (1948) on transfer of sodium, measured with ^{24}Na in the blood of 16 women and in foetal plasma, was computed to be at the twelfth week 160 times and in the fortieth week 1100 times the amount incorporated in foetal tissues.

Fuchs (1957) provides evidence in the same direction for transfer of phosphorus, in the guinea-pig it is true, but of special interest because the technique is unusual. He measured maternal phosphate clearance and calculated that 'at term each foetus retains per hour as much P as is present in the form of inorganic P in the total maternal plasma volume'. Two points should be remembered. The massive retention includes phosphorus arrested in the placenta and that transferred to foetal bone and soft tissues; and the guinea-pig at birth is much more highly developed than the human child. A study of phosphate clearance in women might be enlightening.

With regard to quantitative estimates of net transfer to the foetus we can say nothing more informative than what is contained in the simple analysis of the foetus. The more important components are described in Chapter 12. A component not included there about which we have some information is fluorine, and that more on account of its present controversial public health interest than because of its importance in nutrition. According to American investigators (Gardner *et al.* 1952; Hodge and Smith, 1954) in areas where drinking water had fluoride added to the total concentration of 1 part per million, the placenta contained more fluorine than in areas of low fluorine supply. Placentae from Newburgh for instance had three times as much fluorine as those from Rochester. Also, the concentration of fluorine in placenta was many times that in circulating blood. Hodge and Smith say: 'How the fluoride is held in these organs is not known and whether the placenta really constitutes a barrier between the mother's blood and the foetus has not been established. The high concentration of fluoride suggests a protective role.' The behaviour of fluorine in relation to bone and teeth might suggest that accumulation of fluorine in the placenta would occur only where there was already deposition of calcium salts, in which case it is probably a late occurrence. The only information about fluorine in human foetal bone we have found is the work of Brzezinski, Bercovici and Gedalia (1960), who said that the bone of infants of mothers in Jerusalem, drinking water with 0.55 part per million of fluorine, had as much fluorine at the 9th month as was found in a new born infant in West Hartlepool where the water contains 1.5 ppm.

Problems of the production and transfer of hormones are discussed in Chapter 6.

TRANSFER OF HARMFUL AGENTS

We have discussed above the transfer of carbon monoxide, with special reference to cigarette smoking. The harmful agents most in mind at the present moment are probably radioactive elements in 'fall out' from the test explosion of atomic bombs. Sternberg (1962) classes the elements concerned as long-lived fission products, ^{90}strontium and ^{137}caesium, and those in which radioactivity is induced, which include many natural metabolites and one or two that we do not generally consider as natural. The natural metabolites, for instance iodine, cobalt, copper, zinc, carbon and hydrogen, are transferred in the same way as their stable isotopes. Radioactive strontium behaves like the stable isotope also, being discriminated against in favour of calcium. The menace *in utero* is probably negligible; a more real danger to infants is from milk after birth. Caesium behaves like potassium. The rare earths, like cerium and lanthanum, behave like colloids and are withdrawn from circulation by the mother, without danger to the foetus.

Microorganisms

We have seen that the transfer of antibodies from mother to foetus ensures protection of the child against common infections to which the mother is immune. Such protection lasts for from 2 or 3 to 9 months after birth, by which time the child is competent to meet infection with its own antibodies. But there are infections which damage the placenta and microorganisms can then spread to the foetus. Examples are tuberculosis and syphilis.

More difficult is the question of virus infections, of which the best known is rubella. Saxen (1962) gives a clear account of the epidemiology of virus infections in pregnancy. All of them have, at some time, been reported as teratogenic but much error and misinterpretation is due to poor reporting. Saxen and his colleagues made a careful study of an epidemic of ECHO-9 virus infection and showed that it is not teratogenic. After an epidemic of 'Asian' influenza there were more congenital malformations than normal, but the causation is not necessarily the same as with rubella. Leck (1963) in his study in Birmingham found more than double the incidence of oesophageal atresia, cleft lip, anal atresia and exomphalos following the 1961 influenza epidemic. There is a good deal of evidence from the induction of congenital malformations in animals by dietary deficiency of the mother, that the effect may be due, whatever the deficiency, to deprivation of oxygen, which implies interference with the respiratory enzymes of early foetal life, before an effective circulation provides a sufficient, more direct, supply of oxygen. Saxen suggests that some of the effects associated with virus infection may be due to high fever, or the drugs used in treatment, about whose possible teratogenic effects little or nothing is known.

Drugs

All inhalation anaesthetics resemble the gases in passing the placenta freely and exercising their effects on the foetus. The barbiturate anaesthetics also pass. Pentothal for instance reaches equilibrium on both sides of the placenta in about 3 minutes.

Tranquillizers like chlorpromazine cross the placenta but less rapidly, as do also hypnotics and sedatives like chloral hydrate, alcohol, paraldehyde. Some of these may be harmless enough but others like thalidomide are teratogenic. Robertson's (1962) study of the effect of thalidomide on male patients in a mental hospital, of whom a fourth developed glossitis and some fissuring of the mouth, cured by giving B vitamins, suggests that thalidomide, like rubella virus may interfere with enzymes in the foetus. On the whole drugs should be used with the greatest caution in pregnancy. That must also be true for narcotics, even if antagonists to the depressant effects have recently been shown to cross the placenta. Muscle relaxants have not been found in foetal blood.

All the antibiotics investigated so far have been transferred with ease to foetal blood.

Moya and Thorndike, to whose review (1962) we are indebted for a condensed account of the present position, sum up by saying that the majority of drugs in current use pass at a greater or less rate. They are of the opinion that transfer is linked to lipid solubility, as well as molecular size.

SUMMARY

To sum up what we know about transfer to the foetus we may say with Barcroft (1944) that 'it is obvious that everything necessary for the development gets through'. We have calculated that it is well within the circulatory capacity of the normal pregnant woman to supply the oxygen required by the foetus at its maximum about term. Possible limitations to that statement have been discussed with special reference to postmaturity. We have seen that the uterus and the growing cells of the foetus accumulate free amino acids and free inorganic nutrients; that sugar and the precursors of lipids and other large molecules pass freely. It seems most likely that, under normal conditions, many or most nutrients pass through the foetus in quantities much larger than are retained.

P

CHAPTER 9

Weight Gain in Pregnancy

The range of weight change in pregnancy is wide, from loss to a gain of 60 lb or more. A normal outcome may be found anywhere in the range and it is difficult to define either a normal or an optimum gain. For the present we must be content with a general picture and an estimate of what, on the average, a healthy woman gains.

Such an average estimate is needed as a framework for many calculations that will be made in this book, and, for reasons that will be explained below, it is important that the average healthy woman to be measured should not be arbitrarily restricted in what she may eat and how much of it. To procure an array of measurements from which to derive such an average gain would not, at first sight, appear to involve any special difficulty and indeed body weight has probably been recorded in a haphazard sort of way more often than any other measurement made during pregnancy. Nevertheless there is very little useful information in the literature about the optimum, or even the average weight gain. Much of the recorded information is unacceptable for one or more of three main reasons: (i) weight gain has been manipulated by restriction of diet, (ii) abnormal pregnancies have not been excluded; and (iii) an estimate is made for the whole of pregnancy without any statement of how the gain in early pregnancy was measured or estimated. For our present purpose corresponding criteria of acceptability of records are: (i) absence of manipulation of diet; (ii) information about the health of subjects so that the abnormal may be omitted, and (iii) measurements must be recorded for at least the last two-thirds of pregnancy. Reasons for these stipulations are set out below.

PUBLISHED RECORDS OF WEIGHT GAIN
Manipulation of weight gain

In a study of physiological adaptations in pregnancy it seems to us that the correct starting point is the healthy young woman who eats to appetite, even though, in a sophisticated society, appetite is not the only determinant of food intake. Unfortunately it is difficult to find records for such women because, even before reports of systematic weighing were published, obstetricians were using restricted diets with a view to reduction of weight gain. Prochownick (1889, 1901) is usually credited with the idea of restriction to procure easier delivery, and his work will be discussed in Appendix A, but there is good evidence that restriction of diet was practised long before the end of the century. According to Mussey's (1949) review, Cazeaux (1850) in his Treatise of Obstetrics disapproved of the practice and Prochownick himself cites earlier and contemporary observations and opinions.

Prochownick's main aim, as set out in Appendix A, was to get live babies from women with contracted pelves. It is true that the weight of the baby is related, at least statistically, to the weight gain of the mother and control of diet with a view to easier labour, had there been no other motive for restriction, might have disappeared with rachitic pelves. But Prochownick was concerned also to limit the weight gain of obese women who had already had difficult labours and, probably quite independently of Prochownick, there arose in America the now world-wide idea that for women a slim figure is the ideal and that a slim figure must be restored after pregnancy. In the 1920s some attempts were made to analyse maternal weight gain in terms of its components. Hannah (1925) and Slemons and Fagan (1927) computed the average desirable gain to be 15 lb, about 10 lb for the foetus, placenta and liquor, and the remaining 5 to cover the enlargement of the uterus and breasts and the increase of blood volume. Any gain above 15 lb was assumed to be fat. Slemons and Fagan sum up the implications by saying that this 'places in the hands of the obstetrician a potent argument which will influence his client to avoid gaining weight unnecessarily.'

Apart from contracted pelvis and the avoidance of obesity or preservation of the figure, a third inducement to restriction of diet appeared about 1920 in the observation that pre-eclampsia occurs more often in women who have made large gains of weight, regardless of the weight of the baby. It is not certain when the validity of that observation was first recognized. It was mentioned by Davis in 1923 and with increasing frequency towards the end of that decade. Chesley in 1944 reviewed in detail most of the published records of weight gain up to that time, and found almost complete agreement that women who developed pre-eclamptic toxaemia in general put on more weight than the average. The finding has been widely confirmed since. The analysis made by Thomson and Billewicz (1957) will be discussed later.

At least one generation of American women, even without specific instructions from their doctors, will have been influenced by one or other of these desires, to have an easier delivery or to preserve their figures; and they will have had the encouragement of obstetricians to avoid pre-eclamptic toxaemia. The more recent menace of obesity and cardiovascular disease cannot be ignored as a possible further inducement to dieting. As a result the average recorded weight gains of American women are usually less than those of European women. Probably some at least of them were recorded as a check on, and evidence of, the success of restriction of diet, and certainly they cannot be taken to show what women, eating to appetite, will gain. The loss of the American data for our purpose is the more unfortunate in that most of the American series relate to private patients from the upper income groups and might be taken to represent healthy, well-nourished women. Not only so, but as British and other obstetricians are converted to the current theory that pre-eclampsia can be controlled by limiting diet, records for unrestricted women will become increasingly scarce.

Health of the subjects

Some papers give no information at all about the health of the women measured and some do not even record parity. Obstetric medicine, like medicine in general, is concerned much more with the abnormal than with the normal. Further, the judgement of normality can be made only in retrospect, and the idea of assembling records so that, at the end of pregnancy, the normal may be singled out, is new and as yet unfamiliar. It is not surprising that all published arrays are a mixture of the pathological and the non-pathological; a statistically random sample of a population of pregnant women, perhaps, but not what we require to establish a normal standard.

Estimation of early weight gain

In published records it is not always clear when subjects were first weighed, or whether the 'total' weight gain recorded was that measured, usually from the third or fourth month, or included an estimate of weight gained during the earlier months to give an estimate for the whole of pregnancy. When such an estimate is made for the whole of pregnancy, it is usually based on what a woman said she weighed before she became pregnant. There is no series available of women accurately weighed from before pregnancy.

The published records

We have found in all 32 papers with information about weight gain in the last two-thirds of pregnancy. The data are presented in Table 9.1. When we have amassed that body of information, little of it meets the other criteria of acceptability for the establishment of normality. In many of the studies diet was deliberately restricted and in others from the United States, even when nothing is said about diet, restriction must be suspected because of the general attitude of American obstetricians and women alike to the question of diet and obesity. Still, some preliminary analyses may be made.

MODIFYING CHARACTERISTICS
OF THE WOMEN
Effect of age and parity

No study so far has attempted by statistical analysis to separate the effects of age and parity. In his survey of published work Chesley (1944) found almost complete agreement that, disregarding parity, younger women put on more weight than older. In primigravidae Thomson and Billewicz (1957) found that the younger gained more than the older, but the differences were small.

There is no agreement about the effect of parity, even disregarding age. A majority of records where parities are distinguished show multigravidae to gain less than primigravidae, and in about half of these records the difference is about 2 lb. For example Humphreys (1954) gives the weight gain of primigravidae as 25.77 lb and of multigravidae as 23.5 lb. But there is no evidence to show whether the smaller average gain of multigravidae, if a smaller gain be finally established, is due to higher average number of pregnancy, or age itself, or a combined effect of the two variables.

Effect of antecedent body weight

Those who were the first to study body weight in pregnancy, most

Author	Year	Place	Subjects	Parity	Numb
Davis	1923	U.S.A.	Private patients. No further description	Primigravidae Multigravidae	111 } 39
Hannah	1925	U.S.A.	Unspecified. Included a number of obstetric and medical abnormalities. Toxaemia not mentioned	Primigravidae Multigravidae	119 117
Randall	1925	U.S.A.	'Unselected' normal pregnancy	Primigravidae Multigravidae	200 100
Kerwin	1926	U.S.A.	No information except mostly from 'labouring class'	Not stated	147
Slemons and Fagan	1927	U.S.A.	Unspecified but implication that toxaemia excluded	Not stated	500
Trillat	1928	France	Healthy hospital and private patients	Primigravidae Multigravidae	172 80
Plass and Yoakam	1929	U.S.A.	Private patients normal pregnancy	Mostly Primigravidae	48
Bingham	1932	U.S.A.	No toxaemia, otherwise unspecified	Primigravidae Multigravidae	599 689
Cummings	1934	U.S.A.	Normal private patients	Primigravidae Multigravidae	656 344
Lawson	1934	U.S.A.	Normal private patients in 'comfortable circumstances'.	Not stated	220
Pugliatti	1937	Italy	Abnormalities excluded.	Not stated	200

ht Gain in Pregnancy

ipulation of diet	Weight gain calculated from:	First weighed	Total Gain	Range	Net Gain post-partum
			lb	lb	lb
icted: tail	Not stated	Not stated	21	Not stated	Not stated
iction of 'fats and hydrates' to nt 'abnormal gain' should not exceed	Not stated	Not stated	14.19 12.19	−20 to +41 −25 to +35	Not stated
icted to avoid ssive gain'	'Onset of pregnancy'	Not stated	23.2 21.0	Not stated	Not stated
icted: no detail	12th week	12th week	16.5	+6 to +38	At 6 weeks, −0.17
ted to 'about 2000	Not stated	Not stated	16.5	Not stated	Not stated
nformation	'Habitual weight'	Only a few before the 3rd month.	20.6 21.8	+2.7 to +47.0	Not stated
nformation	Not stated	3rd month	37.4	Not stated	At 2 weeks, +17.6
ohydrate restricted exercise prescribed	Stated 'normal weight' before pregnancy	Not stated	19.9	Not stated	Not stated
ral advice. No npt to influence nt gain	Stated 'normal weight' before pregnancy	Not stated	24.12 24.02	Not stated	Not stated
120 gained average lb. Next 100 were to this if possible, consequent much er variation	'Definitely known' weight before pregnancy	Very early in pregnancy	24.0	−12 to +44	Not stated
nformation	1st month	1st month	22.8	Not stated	Not stated

TABLE

Author	Year	Place	Subjects	Parity	Num
Bray	1938	U.S.A.	Healthy women Toxaemia excluded	Primigravidae ⎱ Multigravidae ⎰	69
Mauks	1939	Hungary	Healthy women from clinic and domiciliary practice	Unstated ⎱ mixture ⎰	376
Arnold	1940	U.S.A.	No description except toxaemia excluded	Not stated	116
Stander and Pastore	1940	U.S.A.	Normal healthy pregnancies	Primigravidae Multigravidae	1227 1097
Beardsley	1941	U.S.A.	Private patients of 'average initial weight' 2 'toxaemias' included. No other pathology mentioned	Primigravidae Multigravidae	119 81
Granger	1941	U.S.A.	Consecutive private patients, 6 with mild pre-eclamptic toxaemia and 4 with essential hypertension included	Not stated	100
Kuo	1941	China	200 normal women selected from 4175 deliveries for completeness of records, health, etc	Primigravidae Multigravidae	101 99
Waters	1942	U.S.A.	Hospital subjects Abnormalities included	Not stated	3230
Kerr	1943	U.S.A.	Healthy normal Pre-eclampsia, vomiting and *those who lost weight* excluded	Primigravidae	500
Robinson *et al.*	1943	U.S.A.	Normal private patients 'well situated economically'	62% Primigravidae	484

ued)

pulation of diet	Weight gain calculated from:	First weighed	Total Gain	Range	Net Gain post-partum
			lb	lb	lb
formation	Stated pre-pregnancy weight	Not stated	24.35 23.36	Not stated	Not stated
icted to avoid ssive' weight gain	Stated pre-pregnancy weight	Not stated	22.0	+6.6 to +39.5	2nd week, +4.4
, but 3–6 grains id daily for at 6 months	Not stated	Not stated	18.2	Not stated	Not stated
formation	Not stated	6 weeks (from graph)	28.3	Not stated	6 weeks +9.8
'weight manage- ' Aimed at 25 lb e 'normal' weight	Not stated	Before 4th month	25.9 23.18	Not stated	Not stated
i to limit gain to first trimester; a week in second ester; 1 lb a week ird trimester	Not stated	Not stated	23.3	Not stated	Not stated
e	'Non-pregnant weight'	During first 3 months	23.39 21.29	Not stated	Not stated
tioned to limit ht gain . . . to 5 lb'	'Usual weight'	2nd–6th month	23.2	−5 to 55 or more	Not stated
nformation	3rd month	3rd month	22.9	Not stated	Not stated
rweight subjects icted. Underweight ects encouraged to	'Usual weight'	3–4 months	24.3	No data	6 weeks, +2.0

TABL

Author	Year	Place	Subjects	Parity	Num
Beilly and Kurland	1945	U.S.A.	Normal private patients pre-eclampsia excluded	Not stated	979
Scott and Benjamin	1948	U.K.	Unselected patients at a London ante-natal clinic	Not stated	360
King	1949	U.S.A.	'Consecutive, un-selected private patients'. Pre-eclampsia excluded	Not stated	226
Tompkins and Wiehl	1951	U.S.A.	Normal pregnancies of subjects with a pre-pregnant weight within 10 % of stan-dard weight for height	Not stated	60
Dieckmann	1952	U.S.A.	Hospital patients Apparently none excluded	Not stated	23,84
Humphreys	1954	U.K.	Normal healthy women—no pre-eclampsia, having normal live babies	Primigravidae Multigravidae	526 474
Bocci and Davitti	1956	Italy	Hospital subjects (i) *Controlled* 'Selected as likely to follow instructions' 12% toxaemia	{ Primigravidae Multigravidae	300 102
			(ii) *Uncontrolled* 20% toxaemia	{ Primigravidae Multigravidae	289 113
Thomson and Billewicz	1957	U.K.	Hospital patients with normal blood pressure	Primigravidae	2868
Venkatachalam, Shankar and Gopalan	1960	India	Poor class women Employed in tea plantation	Primigravidae Multigravidae	13 35

ed)

ulation of diet	Weight gain calculated from:	First weighed	Total Gain	Range	Net Gain post-partum
			lb	lb	lb
ecial diets' al advice only	Not stated	Not stated	22.28	Under 5 to over 40.	Not stated
me rationing	16–20 weeks	16–20 weeks	21.53	Not stated	Not stated
stricted for a	Not stated	Not stated	24.4	S.D. 8.7	At 3 months, 2 ± 6.3
ated	Stated pre-pregnancy weight	13 weeks	24.0	Not stated	Not stated
to limit total gain kg (15.4–17.6 lb) ains thyroid a day ected women'	6 to 20 weeks	Not stated	20.2	S.D. 8.7	Not stated
ime rationing	12 weeks	12 weeks	25.77 23.50	S.D. 8.44 S.D. 8.33	Not stated
al' diet, 3000 for overweight vith fat reduced Cal. with reduced r albuminuria food for under- hed	No data: 'for the pregnancy'	Not stated	26.8 26.5	Not stated	Not stated
	No data: 'for the pregnancy'	Not stated	30.0 32.5	Not stated	Not stated
	13 weeks	13 weeks	25.1	No data	2nd week +6.05 (unpublished)
but recognized as a poor diet	12 weeks	12 weeks	11.8 13.6	S.E. 1.67 S.E. 0.96	Not stated

Author	Year	Place	Subjects	Parity	Num
Ihrman	1960a	Northern Sweden	Consecutive hospital patients booking before 12th week	Primigravidae Multigravidae	51 49
Neser	1963	South Africa	Urban Bantu attending a clinic Those with systemic disease, toxaemia and having a baby weighing 5¾ lb or less, excluded	Primigravidae Multigravidae	95 294

of them German obstetricians, found that heavier women usually put on more weight than lighter, but recent studies, mostly from America, suggest the reverse. It is possible, and even likely, that the American findings reflect the policy of allowing thin pregnant women to eat more than the fat or obese. Thomson and Billewicz (1957) attempting to find an objective measure of the difference compared weights at the 20th week of pregnancy. With the ratio of an individual woman's weight to the median weight of all women of the same height as an 'obesity index' they found no correlation between weight and weight gain. That is perhaps not quite the same thing as a possible relation between pre-pregnant weight and weight gain but, until the question can be satisfactorily resolved by a systematic study on a large scale, it seems reasonable to assume that the influence of fatness and leanness on weight gain in pregnancy is not important.

CHARACTERISTICS OF WEIGHT GAIN
Range of weight gain

Perhaps the most astonishing finding about weight gain in pregnancy is the range that is compatible with clinical normality in pregnancy and a normal outcome. In three studies included in Table 9.1 where the standard deviation of the distribution of weight gain was calculated (King, 1949; Dieckmann, 1952; Humphreys,

ued)

pulation of diet	Weight gain calculated from:	First weighed	Total Gain	Range	Net Gain post-partum
			lb	lb	lb
tated	11 weeks to 36 weeks	9–13 weeks. Mean 11 weeks	22.44	—	3.7 days, +9.7 2 months, +4.2
ree diet and times diuretics for sive gain'	26 weeks before delivery	26 weeks before delivery	17.59	No data	6 to 8 weeks, −2.01

1954) it lay between 8 and 9 lb and indeed the limits of the range usually extend to 50 lb or more. Even when a low mean weight gain has been achieved by rigorous restriction of diet, the range has not been noticeably reduced. For example Hannah (1925), aiming at an increase of not more than 14 lb, produced in 119 primigravidae a range from − 20 to +41 lb, and in 117 multigravidae from − 25 to +35 lb.

Rate of weight gain

When the weight, or weight gain, of pregnant women is plotted against stage of pregnancy the curve is gently sigmoid in shape (Figure 9.1). In Figure 9.1 data are graphed for 2868 primigravidae whose weights were measured from the 13th week of pregnancy (Thomson and Billewicz, unpublished). Up to about the 16th to 18th week weight is gained at the rate of about 0.8 lb per week; after this there is an acceleration to a rate of a little over 1 lb per week until about the 26th to 28th week, followed by a retardation to a rate of 0.8 to 0.9 lb per week until term. There are no adequate data for weight gain before 13 weeks, but a provisional estimate is dotted into the graph. The slope is steepest, corresponding to maximum rate of gain, about or before mid-pregnancy. In Table 9.2 weights gained in 4-week intervals are shown from 8 studies in which these details were given or could be derived. The studies are widely scattered in time and place of origin, but their evidence is satisfactorily consistent. In 7 of the 8 the maximum rate of gain was between 17 and 24 weeks and in the other it was between 25 and 28 weeks.

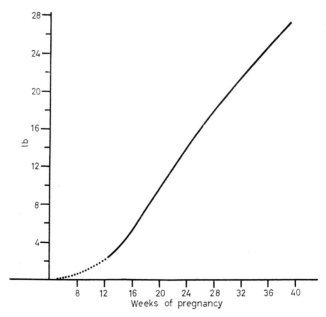

FIGURE 9.1. Mean weight gain in pregnancy of 2868 normotensive primigravidae (Thomson and Billewicz, 1957)

Net gain of weight

Not all the weight put on during pregnancy is lost during and immediately after parturition. Possible reasons will be discussed when the separate components of the weight gain are considered. At this point it will suffice to estimate the extent of the average net weight gain.

In Table 9.3 the net weight gain measured in the first two months after delivery is shown for seven studies. It ranges from a loss of 0.2 lb to a gain of 17.6 lb. The Table shows also that net gain is closely linked to total gain in pregnancy. On the average, any weight gained in pregnancy in excess of 19 lb is retained after the immediate puerperium. The average normal woman who gains 27.5 lb in pregnancy, when she leaves hospital after the lying-in period is about 9 lb above her pre-pregnant weight.

TABLE 9.2. Distribution of Weight Gain in Pregnancy.
The greatest gain in any four week period is underlined

Source	Country	No. of subjects	Weight gain in 4-week periods of pregnancy, lb						
			12–16	17–20	21–24	25–28	29–32	33–36	37–40
Plass and Yoakam (1929)	U.S.A.	48	4.4	11.0	6.6	2.2	4.4	2.2	6.6
Cummings (1934)	U.S.A.	1000	3.2	4.4	5.1	4.5	3.3	2.2	—
Stander and Pastore (1940)	U.S.A.	2324	3.46	5.06	5.04	4.64	4.02	4.04	3.36
Kuo (1941)	China	200	2.4	4.0	4.3	3.5	3.0	3.0	2.8
Robinson et al. (1942)	U.S.A.	484	1.4	3.0	3.9	4.0	3.2	3.4	3.2
Scott and Benjamin (1948)	Britain	360		4.24	4.70	3.99	3.39	3.38	2.55
Tompkins, Wiehl and Mitchell (1955)	U.S.A.	? 60	2.6	3.7	3.3	3.3	3.1	3.2	2.3
Thomson and Billewicz (1957)	Britain	2868	3.1	4.1	4.7	4.1	3.4	3.5	3.2
Venkatachalam et al. (1959)	India	130	1.94	2.37	3.24	2.06	1.94	1.72	0.73

TABLE 9.3. Net Gain of Weight in Pregnancy

| Source | Mean pregnancy wt. gain | Net weight gain post-partum | | Mean total weight gain less net weight gain |
		in second week	in second month	
	lb	lb	lb	lb
Kerwin (1926)	16.5	—	—0.2	16.7
Plass and Yoakam (1929)	37.4	17.6	—	19.8
Mauks (1939)	22.0	4.4	—	17.6
Stander and Pastore (1940)	28.3	—	9.8	18.5
Robinson et al. (1943)	24.3	—	2.0	22.3
Thomson and Billewicz (1957 and unpublished)	25.1	6.1	—	19.0
Ihrman (1960a)	22.4	—	4.2	18.2

ACCEPTABLE ESTIMATES INCLUDING A NEW ONE

Estimates of total gain

Of the assembly of 32 reports in Table 9.1 only 2 are sufficiently close to our ideal to be of value and both are of British origin. From the 12th week Humphreys (1954) weighed 1000 healthy women having normal pregnancies and Thomson and Billewicz (1957) calculated the weight gain of 2868 normotensive hospital primigravidae from the 13th week. It is unfortunate for our purpose that Thomson and Billewicz analysed their data primarily to show differences in weight between women with and without hypertensive complications, because their normotensive group includes women who had other obstetric complications. Yet, as we shall show later, these complications made very little difference to the average weight gain.

For primigravidae Humphreys found the weight gained from 12 weeks to average 25.77 lb and Thomson and Billewicz from 13 weeks calculated a mean increase of 25.1 lb. For practical purposes the difference is negligible. There is no real evidence on which we can draw for the gain before 12 weeks. Chesley (1944) quotes in his review a mean of 2.5 lb for the first trimester, taken as 13.3 weeks, and, although the information on which that estimate is based derives from statements in the literature of 'normal weight before pregnancy', it is consistent with clinical experience and is not likely to be far out. Certainly the assumption made by Humphreys and by other writers that no weight is put on during the first third cannot be accepted. In Figure 9.1 it will be seen that the mean weight is already rising steeply at 13 weeks. A sudden change from no gain at all to a gain of 0.5 lb weekly is not in accord with biological experience. We may therefore accept as an estimate of total weight gain 27.5 lb (12.5 kg) in healthy primigravidae eating without restriction.

It is interesting to see that for many of the studies quoted in Table 9.1, even where manipulation of the diet was claimed, the estimate of mean weight gain is not far from 27.5 lb. That is true in particular of more recent studies. Up to the second World War most of the published studies came from America and average weight gains were low; several were below 20 lb. Since 1940 there is much less evidence of restriction and more recent attempts to diet pregnant women have been either much less ambitious, or much less effective.

A new estimate for primigravidae

Because there is no series of measurements where the subjects fulfil all three of our criteria of acceptability we have extracted and analysed data for the required type of subject from the records of Aberdeen Maternity Hospital. Records of the prescribed sort were available only for primigravidae and we selected those of women between 20 and 29 years of age, at least 5' 3" in height, whose general physique and health were judged at their first antenatal examination to be good or excellent, and who delivered in the 39th, 40th or 41st week of pregnancy. There were 746 such women booked for confinement between 1950 and 1955, during which time no attempt was being made to regulate weight gains by dieting. Of the 746 women 486 had no major clinical abnormality; that is, there was no threatened abortion, no antepartum haemorrhage, pre-eclampsia or hypertension, and no perinatal death.

Q

Total gains of weight by these women are not strictly comparable because the pregnancies varied in length from 39 to 41 weeks. They have therefore been expressed as average weekly gains between 20 weeks and delivery. The distribution is shown in Figure 9.2.

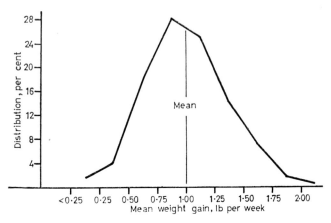

FIGURE 9.2. Distribution of mean weight gain in pregnancy for a selected group of healthy young primigravidae

The modal value for the normal group is between 0.9 and 1.0 lb weekly, giving a total gain for 20 weeks of about 19 lb, which differs only insignificantly from the average during the last half of pregnancy in much larger groups of women as calculated byThomson and Billewicz (1957) and Scott and Benjamin (1948). The Figure also shows again that the range of weight gain is very wide. Even in this highly selected group of women there are some who gained scarcely anything and others who put on more than twice the mean weight.

It is also possible to seek to establish what is a normal weight gain by finding the weight associated with the lowest incidence of abnormalities. In Figure 9.3 the incidences of three major complications are shown in relation to weekly increase of weight between the 20th week and delivery. Incidence of pre-eclampsia rises with increasing weight gain and accelerates at high weights. The incidence of prematurity is highest when least weight is put on, falls to a minimum in the middle of the distribution and rises again with higher weights, chiefly because of pre-eclampsia. The curve for perinatal death rate is similar in shape to that of prematurity.

The picture which emerges is quite clear: the best reproductive performance is associated with a weight gain of a little less than 20 lb in the last half of pregnancy. Again, this conclusion agrees with that derived from the analysis of weight gain by healthy normal primigravidae.

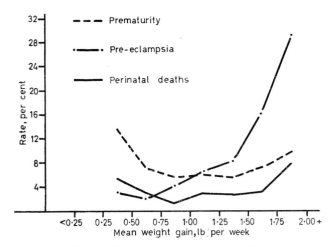

FIGURE 9.3. Incidence of three major obstetric complications by mean weight gain between 20 weeks and delivery

We have now established on a reasonable statistical and clinical basis that the average weight gain found for primigravidae by Thomson and Billewicz, namely 27.5 lb for the whole of pregnancy, and that now derived from an *ad hoc* analysis of hospital records of about 19 lb for the last half of pregnancy are acceptable norms. The same result is reached by examination of a group of healthy young women without serious obstetric complications, and from estimation of the weight at which fewest serious complications occur. Nevertheless, it remains true that healthy women with clinically normal pregnancies may put on no weight or more than twice the average. Within the limits of ordinary hospital experience no extreme has been reached which has been shown to be incompatible with a normal reproductive performance.

The norms which we have just established are derived from, and specifically refer to primigravidae. It is not possible at present to derive a corresponding estimate for later pregnancies, but the little evidence there is suggests that the average multigravida gains something like 2 lb less than primigravidae.

SUMMARY

It will be convenient for future reference to fix an average weight gained at certain points in pregnancy. We record them in both lb and kg. The following round figures fit closely the curve shown in Figure 9.1 : at 10 weeks 650 grams (about 1 lb), at 20 weeks 4000 g (about 9 lb), at 30 weeks 8500 g (about 19 lb) and at term 12,500 g (about 27.5 lb).

CHAPTER 10

Components of Weight Gain
1. The Product of Conception

In this and the following chapters we will consider the weight gained in pregnancy in terms of its major components in two groups: first, the product of conception, foetus, placenta and liquor amnii; and second, the additions to maternal structures, uterus, breasts, blood, extracellular fluid and maternal stores of nutrients.

For some of these components there are considerable bodies of data from which both average values and variation can be estimated; for others there is very little information and, for a few, only indirect evidence.

THE FOETUS

The ideal material on which to study the growth of the foetus would be a series of embryos and foetuses that had come from an ideal environment at different stages of pregnancy. In practical terms that would mean embryos and foetuses from healthy, well nourished mothers of the upper social classes, in the course of perfectly normal pregnancies. Clearly the ideal is not possible of attainment.

There is little published information about the rate of growth of the foetus because the practical difficulties of collecting enough data of the right kind are considerable. The range of individual weights at any age is wide and, in rough proportion, equally wide at all ages. Further, weights may properly be used to construct a curve of growth only if the period of gestation is accurately known for each.

EARLY PREGNANCY

There is no particular difficulty about getting approximately normal foetal weights in the early stages. Up to about the middle there are foetuses from pregnancies terminated for reasons that do not imply interference with growth. But the number of published records of such foetuses is small.

INTERMEDIATE STAGES: THE 8TH AND 9TH MONTHS

To get normal material in the second half of pregnancy, particularly for the 28th to the 36th weeks, is much more difficult. The 7 months child is regarded as viable and so pregnancies which terminate or have to be terminated between 28 and 36 weeks are, almost by definition, abnormal, and many of the conditions leading to early delivery are likely to depress foetal growth. Obviously, where intra-uterine death has occurred it is reasonable to suppose that the intra-uterine environment has not been such as to give normal growth and the stillborn should be excluded from the data. So should foetuses with congenital malformations. Short of death and deformity there are maternal conditions which are known to depress foetal growth. A relatively common cause of premature delivery, severe pre-eclampsia, as has been shown by Baird, Thomson and Billewicz (1957), may result in the birth of babies before 36 weeks which are smaller than the average for their age.

The best data available until recently were those collected by Hamilton, Boyd and Mossman (1945, 1956). That the shape of their growth curve (see Figure 10.1), was normal, particularly during the last 10 weeks of pregnancy, was questioned by Thomson (1951), who pointed out that a foetal weight gain of 0.6 kg in the last two weeks of pregnancy is not in accord with common experience. Thomson's analysis of data from Aberdeen, for foetuses without evidence of depression of growth, showed the weight curve between 28 and 36 weeks to be much steeper than that of Hamilton, Boyd and Mossman and to become less steep only in the last weeks. Subsequently, a great deal more information was collected in Aberdeen and reported briefly by Walker (1954b). Much of the data which we present here is an extension of the same Aberdeen series.

The curve for the Aberdeen data and that from the data of Hamilton, Boyd and Mossman are shown in Figure 10.1. The two curves are identical until about the 30th week, after which the curve of Hamilton *et al.* falls away and then rises steeply so that both reach approximately the same weight at 40 weeks. It seems probable that the depression in the earlier curve is not representative of normal growth, but due to the inclusion of foetuses whose growth had been inhibited; but to establish the point we must examine the collected data on which the curve is based. Hamilton, Boyd and Mossman give no information about the foetuses or embryos on which their 'personal observations' were made. Of the early writers given as sources of data, Fehling (1877) was concerned with the physiology of placental transmission and to that end studied

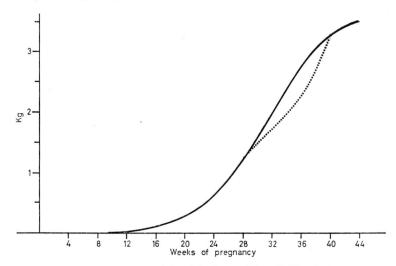

FIGURE 10.1. Growth in weight of the foetus. The solid line is the mean for selected Aberdeen material; the dotted line is based on data collected by Hamilton, Boyd and Mossman (1956)

the composition of the foetus and embryo. He analysed 21, described as 'absolutely fresh and undamaged', but in the table of composition the last three on the list are described as: stillborn; dead, macerated; prematurely born in the 9th month, died 13 days old, atrophic. It is doubtful therefore whether 'undamaged' means healthy or of normal growth. Fehling's measurements and those of Jackson (1909) who did not describe his material, are below the Hamilton curve between the ages 30 and 37 weeks. Mall's (1918) report is on 25 embryos, 19 from abortions and some described as pathological, for which weights are not recorded.

Next in chronological order come the measurements of Streeter (1920) on specimens in the collection of the Carnegie Institution of Washington which has contributed such valuable studies on the histology of the developing human embryo. Streeter's interest in length and weight was secondary to the need to know, or estimate, the age of the specimens. His descriptive account of the material may be summarized as follows. Specimens received fresh were weighed and measured in that state, but many were already fixed in formalin when received. A study was therefore made of the effect of formalin and it was found not to be consistent; distended specimens appeared too heavy, macerated specimens too light for their length. Most of the specimens belonged to the first half of pregnancy, which was 'due to the source of our material, which is chiefly from abortions . . . the larger specimens are not sent to us.' It may be concluded that the specimens on the whole were not what we should call normal and, indeed, the weights given for the second half of pregnancy are derived from values for the end of the 32nd, 36th and 40th weeks which were taken from Zangemeister (1911) and were used by Streeter to estimate age after 'increasing them by 5 per cent to make them comparable to the formalin weight of our tables'. These complicated manipulations may explain why, between 32 and 40 weeks, Streeter's weights are above the Hamilton averages. Below 32 weeks, his weights are less.

Zangemeister did not describe his material but since curves of weight are given for the major internal organs as well as foetus and placenta, there can be no doubt that it was the usual post mortem material comparable to most of what Hamilton *et al.* used.

The data given by Scammon and Calkins (1929) were for birth weights of 2904 infants born in the larger Minneapolis hospitals, reported between 1918 and 1922, and of 7282 born in other American cities and reported between 1885 and 1920. There is no description of what was included. From all that it seems fair to conclude that averages based chiefly or wholly on abortions do not represent normal healthy foetuses.

Nevertheless the main landmarks in the Aberdeen series and Hamilton *et al.* are in remarkable agreement. The average foetus weighs about 5 g at 10 weeks, 300 g at 20 weeks, 1500 g at 30 weeks and 3300 g at 40 weeks. But the normal foetus weighs 2500 g at 35 weeks; the average, mostly abnormal, foetus from the collection of Hamilton *et al.* weighed only 2000 g at 35 weeks.

The range of birth weights about the mean curve is wide. From at least the 30th week, and probably from much earlier, the biggest weight at any point is more than twice the smallest, but the data are not sufficient for analysis of the variation except at the end of pregnancy. Most of the discussion which follows refers to variation in the infant's birth weight at term.

TERM

There are many series of measurements of birth weights, but, as we will explain in the discussion of the effect of war (p. 369), some include all births, some exclude stillbirths, some exclude premature births and, to construct a curve of growth, we require as measure of normal birthweight measurements of normal infants born within a few days of 280 days of gestation. We shall discuss now the duration of pregnancy and why about 280 days, and not the longest duration, is taken as normal.

Length of Gestation

We are accustomed to speak of the length of pregnancy as 280 days from the commencement of the last menstrual bleeding, which is the only fixed point usually available from which to date the pregnancy. That extremely convenient number, divisible into 40 weeks and 10 lunar months, is in fact a reasonably good approximation to the average duration of pregnancy in European women. That it is a multiple of the conventional 28 day menstrual cycle has sometimes been taken to imply a relation of the length of gestation to the menstrual cycle, but none has been proved to exist.

The range of intervals within which a pregnancy is terminated with the birth of a child, mature by the accepted standard of 2500 g weight is wide: from as little as 32 weeks (224 days) to 52 weeks (365 days). Intervals of over 300 days from the first day of the last menstrual bleeding are common. In Hosemann's (1949a) series of 11,974 births nearly 12 per cent were born between the 43rd and 50th weeks.

Stewart (1952) in an examination of 'postmaturity' discusses the length of gestation of 135 women in whom the time of ovulation could be fixed from records of basal temperature. He says: 'The duration of pregnancy, from ovulation to the spontaneous onset of labour and delivery of a normal, full-term, living baby ranged from 250 to 285 days'. Eight of the pregnancies exceeded 300 days from the last menstrual period but none exceeded 285 days from the date of ovulation. One woman was delivered 344 days from the date of menstruation but only 278 days from ovulation; another 349 days menstrual date, but only 250 days from ovulation. One woman had a male child weighing 3900 g after 253 days, another a female child weighing 3740 g on the 279th day.

Assuming a conventional 28 day cycle, and that the range in this apparently highly selected sample of women is similar to that for women generally, the range of duration from the first day of the last menstrual period would be 264 to 299 days, or roughly 38 to 43 weeks, and the average, given by Stewart as '266 to 270' days would be 280 to 294 days, 40 to 42 weeks, which is longer than the average usually accepted. Gestations of more than 42 weeks would then be suspect of delay of ovulation.

A certain amount of support might be thought to derive from the table of distribution of gestation lengths in Aberdeen shown in Table 10.1. It might be argued that any gestation period that showed excess frequency in the poorer social classes was less than the best. If that were accepted as a valid argument, the lower limit of a complete gestation would be about the commencement of the 40th week. On the other hand, the Aberdeen data show no difference between social classes in the proportion of gestations of 42 weeks or more, suggesting delay of ovulation. If Stewart's results are confirmed by a wider survey, it would appear that a proportion of abnormally timed ovulations occur in all social classes.

Without further evidence than is afforded by Stewart's small and selected sample, it is impossible to regard these limits as more than suggestive. Obviously there is a nice question for research there. Confirmation of Stewart's findings would modify our interpretation of the foetal growth curve at ages above 42 weeks. At 44 weeks,

TABLE 10.1. Distribution of Length of Gestation in Three Social Groups
All Aberdeen Primiparae 1951–59: Single Legitimate Births

Social Class of Husband	I and II		III		IV and V	
Weeks	No.	Per cent	No.	Per cent	No.	Per cent
35 or less	22	1.7	169	3.0	81	4.4
36 and 37	40	3.1	238	4.2	86	4.7
38 and 39	215	16.8	1007	17.9	374	20.4
40 and 41	716	55.9	2913	51.8	882	48.0
42 or more	289	22.5	1299	23.1	414	22.5
Total	1282	100	5626	100	1837	100

for instance, there would be heavy babies genuinely 44 weeks old, and also babies of less age, and less weight probably, because of delayed ovulation. The flattening of the growth curve, if there is any true flattening, must be less than appears.

Birth statistics give the following representative values for length of gestation from the beginning of the last menstrual period. In Aberdeen, 1959–60, 82.5 per cent of all single legitimate births, including all birth orders, 4780 out of 5792, were born in the weeks 39, 40, 41 and 42, i.e. in 280 ±14 days. Karn (1947–49) records for the Queen Charlotte and University College Hospitals, London, that 85 per cent of births were between 260 and 304 days (37 and 43½ weeks) showing the distortion due to excess admissions of the abnormal to hospital. Hosemann (1949a) says the average time to the birth of a mature child is 281–282 days and that estimate would be accepted generally in Germany. Fraccaro (1955–56) in Italy records 276.60 ±0.37 days for male and 277.56 ±0.38 days for female children, but 'survivors' averaged a day and a half more and 'non-survivors' averaged only 256 and 254 days. Mortality was least for both sexes with a gestation of 285 days.

It is evident therefore that 280 days, for European women, is strictly speaking, neither a mean nor an optimum duration. It is a convenient point from which to make comparisons, say of birth-weight, and a useful approximation to the 'normal'.

There are interesting differences between ethnic groups. Anderson, Brown and Lyon (1943) give the mean duration of pregnancy of American (United States) white women as 279.0 days for male and 279.9 days for female children; but 274.7 and 273.3 days for negroes. The racial differences are large, far beyond the difference between social classes in the Aberdeen data quoted above (Table 10.1). Since negro infants are on the average lighter than white, weight and length of gestation correspond. It is different with Indian women. Mukherjee and Biswas (1959) give the range of gestations as 28 to 44 weeks, with 592 out of 1038 births between 39 and 41 weeks, and a corresponding mean birth weight of only 6.23 lb (2828 g). The maximum weight was attained at more than 43 weeks (over 300 days) and was then only 2992 g. The long gestation for a relatively low weight is confirmed by Balakrishnan and Namboodiri (1960) who found the highest birth weight of males at 297 days and of females at 312 days of gestation, with average durations for boys and girls of 285.6 and 286.6 days.

Almost all the statistics agree that girls are carried about a day longer than boys.

We have discussed the reported differences in birth weights (p. 253) and in twinning rates (Appendix C) of different ethnic groups. In duration of pregnancy also we find characteristic differences. About all of those more information would be welcome and a great extension of the study to cover also other groups of known different ethnic origin.

Birth weight

The fascinating history of the measurement of birth weight has been reviewed by Cone (1961). There appears to be no mention of the size at birth either in the Bible or in any of the ancient Greek, Roman or Arabic writings, and the earliest record found by Cone was in the 1694 edition of a textbook by the famous French obstetrician Mauriceau. He claimed that the newborn infant ordinarily weighed 13 lb, and since the French livre of Mauriceau's time was heavier than the standard British pound, that would give an estimate of 14 or 15 lb. This extraordinary estimate was topped in 1747 by an English surgeon, Theophilus Lobb, who quoted a weight of 16 lb 7 oz obtained for him by an 'ingenious *Surgeon*, and *Man-midwife*', of a representative baby, and the Scottish obstetrician Smellie, among others, lent his support by saying that the newborn baby weighed 10 to 12 lb, and as much as 16 lb.

It is not easy to understand how these curious estimates could have been made; Roederer, writing from Göttingen in 1753 claimed that past writers were 'hallucinating'; he himself found a mean weight of about 6 lb 12 oz for males, 6 lb 5 oz for females. Clarke who may have been the first Englishman to study birth weight, published in 1785 estimates of 7 lb $5\frac{1}{2}$ oz for boys and 6 lb $11\frac{1}{2}$ oz for girls. Systematic scientific studies of birth weight probably began in the 1830s when the remarkable mathematician, astronomer and statistician, Quetelet, measured some Brussels infants; males weighed an average of about 3200 g, females about 2900 g.

The discussion of 'birth weight' is greatly complicated by the fact that birth weight, in its most usual meaning is not the same thing as term weight, the weight in which we are interested. Statistics of birth weight will ordinarily include all infants, live or stillborn, anatomically normal or malformed and aged between

28 weeks and 44 weeks or more. Yet, because of the relatively overwhelming numbers of normal infants born alive within one or two
weeks of 280 days of age, all of these differences in the material
included make surprisingly little difference to the means for large
groups of population, or even to hospital statistics.
It would be much more satisfactory if we could discuss the
maternal and external influences on birth weight in terms of term
weight, but there are no statistics, other than our own, which permit
any clear-cut distinction between means of all, or nearly all births,
and births strictly at term.

GESTATIONAL AGE AT BIRTH
The common rough and ready measure of duration of normal
pregnancy is ten lunar months, or 280 days, from the first day of the
last menstrual period. According to some (Hosemann, 1949a) the
interval is a little longer, 281 to 282 days. Strictly speaking, the
duration of pregnancy is from conception to delivery, but the date
of conception is seldom known except when it is determined by
events such as war leave. According to Hosemann (1949a) an
analysis of 2000 such cases, where the date of conception was known
to within 3 days, had just as high a variation in duration of pregnancy as estimates based on the first day of the last menstrual
period. But the true beginning of pregnancy may be of great importance in cases where the duration appears to be abnormally, or
even impossibly, long. Hosemann's series included 266 (2.3 per
cent) where gestation was calculated to have exceeded 44 weeks.
His inclusion of cases of long duration was criticized by Daiser
(1949) and Freudenberg (1950) on the basis that the estimates were
incorrect, but from Stewart's (1952) study it is apparent that
ovulation may be greatly delayed after the cessation of menstruation, and that not all infants postmature by menstrual date are in
fact postmature. Without knowledge of conception date, the
diagnosis of postmaturity depends on clinical signs.
The upper limit of normal weight is not easy to define. Hosemann
describes the intra-uterine growth as increasing from the scarcely
weighable ovum to a mean of 3410 ±4.37 g for 11,000 'mature'
Göttingen infants. The mean of 3410 includes weights up to 5000 g
and pregnancies of 48 weeks duration. He regards both the high
weights and the long gestations as genuine. It seems possible that
they are literally genuine, in the sense that no prevarication is

TABLE 10.2. Mean

Country and Author	Date of investigation	Place	Ethnic group	Socio-economic group
CZECKOSLOVAKIA Braitenberg (1942)	1880–1940	Prague	Caucasian	No data
Fraccaro (1958)	1955	National	Caucasian	No data
GERMANY Hosemann (1949a)	1926–45	Göttingen	Caucasian	No data
Solth (1950)	1913–47 1900–48 1900–49	Berlin Würzburg Marburg	Caucasian Caucasian Caucasian	No data No data No data
ITALY Fraccaro (1955–56)	1942–51	Pavia	Mediterranean	No data
SWEDEN Mellbin (1962)	1940–60	Lapland	Lapps	No data
UNITED KINGDOM Duncan (1864–65)	No data	Edinburgh	Caucasian	No data
British Association Anthropometric Committee (1879) „ (1884)	No data	London & Edinburgh	Caucasian	Urban labouring and artisan classes
Pearson (1899–1900)	No data	Lambeth	Caucasian	No data
Brailsford Robertson (1915)	No data	Birmingham	Caucasian	No data

nt by Geographic Area and Sex

Males		Females	Total		Type of Sample
Mean weight g	Number	Mean weight g	Number	Mean weight g	
OPE					
No data		No data	25214	3298	Hospital deliveries, 'Mature' with minimum length of 48 cm and maximum of 54 cm. Stillbirths and multiple births excluded
3403	81105	3268	167676	3338	Hospital deliveries. Still and live births of more than 28 weeks gestation and above 1000 g, + all survivors for 24 hours outside these limits
No data		No data	11974	3359 (median)	All hospital deliveries where mother's last menstrual period definitely known
3301	19797	3171	41239	3239	Hospital deliveries. All single births including fresh stillbirths of over 1000 g and born 'from the 8th month'.
3250	21383	3125	44675	3189	
3339	14360	3198	29954	3274	
3239	2551	3113	5486	3180	Hospital deliveries. Abortions, malformations and twins excluded
3470	252	3320	491	3393	Born within 4 days of term
No data		No data	2053	3284	Hospital deliveries All 'mature' babies
3400	No data		No data		'Mature' babies
3230	466	3140	917	3173	,, ,,
3319	1000	3215	2000	3267	Hospital deliveries. Born at the 'normal period'. Twins excluded
3257	100	3218	200	3238	Hospital deliveries 'Normal' 'Full-time'

TABLE

Author	Date of investigation	Place	Ethnic group	Socio-economi group
				EUR
McKeown and Gibson (1951)	1947	Birmingham	No data	All births
Karn and Penrose (1951–52)	1935–46	London	Caucasian	No data
Ministry of Health (1959)	1947–50	11 Localities in England & Wales	Caucasian	Deficit of S.C. II & excess of compared to national samp
Unpublished	1950–57	Aberdeen	Caucasian	Similar to tota population
U.S.S.R. Leviant (1960)	1958	Leningrad	Caucasian	No data
Kandror (1961)	1944–46 1946–50	Tiksi No data Providentija ,, (U.S.S.R. in Asia)		No data ,,
Meredith (1952)	1896–1949	National	Caucasian Negro	See type of san
Crump et al. (1957)	1951–1956	Tennessee	Negro	'Low socio-economic statu
Connor et al. (1957)	1952–53	Hawaii	Hawaiian Puerto Rican Caucasian Chinese Japanese Korean Filipino	⎫ ⎪ ⎬No data ⎪ ⎭

ed)

Males		Females	Total		
Mean weight g	Number	Mean weight g	Number	Mean weight g	Type of Sample
ed)					
data	No data	No data	22527	3387	96.8 per cent of all births in Birmingham in 1947 Stillbirths excluded
3305	6693	3209	13730	3258	Hospital deliveries 'Normal' excluding twins, weights range down to 1 lb
3420	No data	3280	19616	3350	Infants attending health clinics before age of 2 months. 5 per cent premature by birth weight: national average of 6 per cent
data	No data		25634	3302	Total hospital deliveries of live single infants
3501	No data	3376	No data		Attenders at polyclinics, prematures, twins and extreme deviations 'from normal growth' excluded
data „	No data „		601 580	3453 3481	93 per cent of all births in the district, but excluding those under 2500 g and those whose mothers had spent less than one year in the Arctic
A. data	No data		121801 39656	3350 3230	A collection from fifteen publications Wide variety of social status but on the whole Negroes of poorer economic level than whites Dead infants and twins excluded from most studies Premature infants excluded from some
3227	874	3128	1821	3179	Hospital deliveries Premature infants excluded Twins included
3304 3239 3364 3238 3220 3276 3117	No data	3290 3122 3246 3147 3149 3175 3044	8068 687 7063 1762 9517 436 3344	No data	Data from birth certificates All births in 1952-53. 98 per cent of deliveries in hospital 'where weighing is routine and likely to be accurate'

Author	Date of investigation	Place	Ethnic group	Socio-economic group
CEYLON De Silva, Fernando and Gunaratne (1962)	1956–58	Colombo	Ceylonese	No data
CHINA Uttley (1940)	1934–39	Kowloon	Chinese (Cantonese)	No data
Lee (1948)	1945–48	Chengtu	Chinese	No data
Shan-Yah Gin (1948)	1940–41	Shanghai	Chinese	No data
INDIA Rajoo and Naidu (1944)	Not stated	Secundera-bad	Indian	No data
Namboodiri and Balakrishnan (1958–59a)	1956–57	Trivandrum	Indian	No data
Mukherjee and Biswas (1959)	1957	Calcutta	Indian	Poor class 'Paying patient
Achar and Yankauer (1962)	1954–55	Madras	Tamil and Telugo Indian	'Mostly poor' 'Well-to-do', patients
Venkatachalam (1962)	Not stated	South India	Indian	Poor 'Wealthy'
JAPAN Sagara (1961)	1949 1955	Nara	Japanese	No data
MALAYA Llewellyn-Jones (1955)	1951–52 1951–53 1951–53	Kuala Lumpur	Malay Chinese Indian	No data ,, ,,

ued)

Males Mean weight g	Females Num-ber	Females Mean weight g	Total Num-ber	Total Mean weight g	Type of Sample
EAST					
data	No data		10273	2500	From nine maternity homes run by the Municipality for normal cases living within the city No detail
3075	2654	2961	5437	3018	No data
3084	1649	2984	3550	3038	No data, but title of paper indicates 'full term' infants
3230	110	3180	228	3206	Selected from clinics as 'clinically healthy' or only 'moderately flabby' out of 4 categories of which the fourth was 'malnourished'
No data	4735	No data	10000	2897	Hospital deliveries. Infants of less than 4 lb and multiple pregnancies omitted
2904	6192	2830	12640	2868	Hospital deliveries. Stillbirths, neonatal deaths and twins excluded from about 16,000 births
2729	500	2683 }	878 / 160	2656 / 2851	Consecutive hospital deliveries
o data	No data		5176 / 512	2736 / 2985	'Mothers relatively free from pregnancy complications'
o data	No data		2777 / 1753	2810 / 3182	Born in hospitals, alive and 'at term'
3199 / 3258	1943 / 1135	3085 / 3165	4002 / 2345	3143 / 3212	No data
o data / ,, / ,,	No data / ,, / ,,		322 / 4005 / 4696	2747 / 2886 / 2644	Hospital deliveries. Hospital takes all abnormalities from a population of 500,000 and no normal case is ever 'refused admission'

TABL.

Author	Date of investiga-tion	Place	Ethnic group	Socio-econom group
				FAR ▶
Millis (1958–59a)	1950–53	Singapore	Chinese ⎱ Indian ⎰	Poor
SUMATRA				
Gamondi and Santos Reis (1960)	1957–58	Sawah Lunto	'Melano-asiatics'	No data
THAILAND				
Stahlie (1959)	1956–57	9 regions of Thailand	Thai and Chinese	No data
CONGO				
Jans (1959)	Not stated	Ituri forest area	Pygmies Bantu	No data 'Very well nourished'
			Bantu	'Well nourish◄
			Bantu	'Badly nourisl
SENEGAL				
Dupin, Massé and Corréa (1962)	1949 1954 1959	Dakar	African	No data
GHANA				
Hollingsworth (1960)	No data	Accra	African	General popu Prosperous
KENYA				
Shaw (1933)	No data	Nairobi	African Indian	No data

(continued)

Males		Females		Total		Type of Sample
Mean weight g	Number	Mean weight g	Number	Number	Mean weight g	
(continued)						
3060	22627	2983		46750	3024	Hospital deliveries Mothers in '3rd class wards' with free attention
2856	2513	2792		5166	2824	
3147	216	3080		443	3114	A hospital group. Apparently no exclusions on weight basis
3066	3531	2988		7261	3028	Reports from midwives, stationed mostly in market towns May under-represent the poorer rural areas Thought to be no exclusions

ICA

Males		Females		Total		Type of Sample
No data		No data		40	2635	Born in hospital No exclusions for weight
				No data	3026	
				No data	2965	
				No data	2850	
3051	1944	2938		4103	2997	Born in hospital Twins excluded
3145	2777	2997		5757	3072	
3180	4046	3051		8409	3117	
2985	442	2765		917	2879	Born in hospital
3210	96	3164		201	3188	
3189	363	3110		750	3153	Hospital deliveries Twins excluded together with infants 'born prematurely, with the exception of children born following induction of labour in the later weeks of pregnancy . . . for minor degrees of disproportion'
2898	107	2770		207	2830	

Author	Date of investiga- tion	Place	Ethnic group	Socio-econom group
				AF
PORTUGUESE GUINEA Janz *et al.* (1959)	1954–56	Guinea	African	No data
REPUBLIC OF SOUTH AFRICA Salber and Bradshaw (1957)	No data	Durban Pietermar- itsburg Capetown	Caucasian Coloured Bantu Indian	No data

involved, but that the length of gestation may be referable to delayed ovulation, and some of the high weights to pathology of the mother, diabetes or pre-diabetes.

Conventionally, an infant of less than 2500 g birth weight is premature, and there are no agreed signs to distinguish the truly premature and the abnormally small mature child.

COMPARISONS OF BIRTH WEIGHTS

Table 10.2 shows collected records of birth weights. In making this collection, we have not attempted to be exhaustive. The aim has been from the enormous but unevenly distributed array of papers to get a representative sample of data for different countries and ethnic groups, over such a period of time, the last 100 years, as would show a secular trend if there were any.

Not one entry in the whole published array represents what we desire to have, namely the birth weights of healthy normal infants from healthy normal mothers, born within say two weeks of 280 days from the first day of the last menstrual period. The records diverge from the ideal in so many ways that they are not strictly comparable. The final column shows the usual variation in exclusions and inclusions when they are stated. For reasons already mentioned these differences have little effect on the mean birth weights.

ued)

Males		Females		Total	
Mean weight g	Number	Mean weight g	Number	Mean weight g	Type of Sample

ued)

3490	158	3480	332	3486	Born in a maternity hospital
3443	855	3329	1757	3388	Hospital deliveries; Europeans from
3134	460	3075	931	3107	private nursing homes Abortions and multiple births excluded
3125	3742	3012	7608	3071	
2989	838	2867	1737	2930	

In order to judge what the true effect on birth weight of some of these exclusions might be, we have made an analysis of Aberdeen data, and have found, for instance, that the exclusion of prematures (infants of less than 2500 g weight) raised mean birth weight by roughly 100 g. The exclusion of postmature infants of high birth weight would lower the mean. The net effect of inclusion of weights both below and above term weight is illustrated by Hosemann's data. His mean weight at 40 weeks was 3300 g, at 41 weeks 3400 g; the median weight including 1384 (11.5 per cent of the total) of more than 44 weeks gestation, was 3359 g. The overweights are just about balanced by the lightweights. Hosemann's 40 week weight is almost the same as the Aberdeen mean at 40 weeks, 3340 g. The proportions born within two weeks of 280 days may be calculated from Hosemann's tables to be over 75 per cent; in Aberdeen it is 82.5 per cent.

McKeown and Gibson (1951) showed for all births in Birmingham in 1947 that the mean weight at 40 weeks, 3455 g was about 80 g above the overall mean birth weight of 3373 g.

Sex difference. It is well known that the average male infant is heavier than the average female. At term the difference is of the order of 100 to 140 g. (Table 10.2) McKeown and Record (1953) in an analysis of 13,020 single births found the difference established at 34 weeks, but it is not known at what stage of development the difference is first apparent. McKeown and Record's findings, with similar data from the smaller Aberdeen study, are shown in Figure 10.2. The difference between the weights increases both absolutely and relatively during the last 10 weeks of pregnancy.

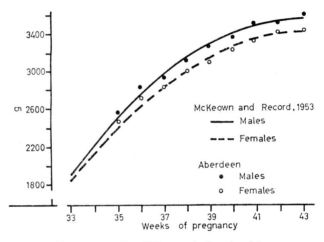

FIGURE 10.2. Sex difference in foetal weight

Secular trend. There are two major studies, one from Prague, the other from three German cities. Braitenberg (1942) in Prague collected records covering the years 1880 to 1940, and Solth (1950) in Berlin, Würzburg and Marburg for the years 1900 to 1949. These records are no doubt subject to all the inconsistencies of procedure we have described, but these would not as far as we can judge, completely obscure any significant secular change. Braitenberg claims none; Solth finds a rise of weight of about 100 g over the 49 years. It is impossible to take either claim as valid. Between 1880 and 1940, or even between 1900 and 1949 enormous changes have taken place in the economic status of both populations, and the class of patient admitted to maternity hospitals has changed. In 1880 maternity hospitals were to a large extent charities, providing shelter and some care for extremely poor working women. Nowadays, well-to-do women in increasing proportions have their babies in hospital. What these records do suggest therefore is that, where an apparent secular trend associated with a social change might have been expected, little or no change has been found.

Ethnic groups. It is not possible to quote studies of women from different ethnic groups strictly comparable in respect of social status and well-being. Table 10.2 shows that infants of American negroes are on the average lighter at birth than infants of white Americans, but then the conditions of life have in the past been widely different. There are also the studies of white, Bantu and negro infants in South Africa, of which the white were paying patients and therefore relatively well-to-do, of several ethnic groups in Hawaii, of Chinese in China, Malaya and Hawaii and of Indians in India, Malaya, Kenya and South Africa. It appears that in Hawaii Filipino infants are smaller than the others; the Chinese infant in China is lighter than European infants but the infant of the well-fed Chinese mother in Hawaii is comparable with the European. Consistently small are Indian infants, wherever they were measured: in India compared with records in general; in South Africa compared with three other groups; in Malaya compared with Chinese, and in Kenya compared with white and negro. In India the relatively small size might be due to poor diet or unfavourable environment in general, but even paying patients in Calcutta and Madras (Mukherjee and Biswas, 1959; Achar and Yankauer, 1962) had infants well below European standard and Indians in Africa are relatively well-to-do compared with the negro. The small size of Indian infants cannot be attributed to a short gestation period. Balakrishnan and Namboodiri (1960) showed that the mean length of gestation was about 286 days for male infants and about 287 for female.

The birth weight of pygmies, the smallest known ethnic group and that regarded as genetically the most uniform, is given by Jans (1959) as 2635 g.

All this seems to be good evidence of real ethnic differences in mean birth weight.

NORMAL AND OPTIMUM BIRTH WEIGHT

It seems necessary here to consider, and to set down, what we mean by 'normal' in relation to birth weight. In almost every case we shall mean either 'normal' in the statistical sense of average or representative or most likely; or 'normal' in the clinical or colloquial sense of properly made, healthy, satisfactory, or just ordinary. In neither meaning is there any implication of 'best'. We shall say that the normal infant weighs roughly 3300 g at about 280 days and we shall take that as a criterion of satisfactory intrauterine growth; but Karn and Penrose (1951–52) in their analysis of the birth weights of London infants found that the average or 'normal' birth weight was not that attended with least mortality in the first 28 days. For boys the average birth weight was 3305 g, for girls 3209 g, but to attain a mortality rate of 1 per cent a birth weight of 3566 g was required for both. Fraccaro (1955–56) in his study of birth weights in Pavia found an average birth weight of 3239 g for boys and 3113 g for girls. But least mortality to the time of discharge at 7–20 days, from their computations, demanded birth weights of 3593 and 3409 g. The bases of the two sets of calculations are not identical but the difference does not affect the conclusion that the 'optimum' baby appears to be bigger than the ordinary term baby. Evidence in the same direction comes from Hawaii (Connor, Bennett and Louis, 1957) where infant mortality, analysed by birth weight, was at a minimum for birth weights between 4000 and 4500 g.

A few years ago we made a study of the birth weight of mammals in relation to the weight of the mother (Leitch, Hytten and Billewicz, 1959). To our own surprise we found that for the whole range of mammals from the bat weighing a few grams to the whale weighing nearly 100,000 kg a close relation existed which could be expressed in a generalized equation. If we apply that equation to compute the weight (what we might call the natural or zoological weight) of the infant of a 56 kg woman, the answer is 4232 g, and is so close to the Hawaiian optimum weight that gives minimum infant mortality that we are tempted to say the mean weight of human infants at the present time is in need of improvement. The smaller the mother the greater the risk for the large child. To that extent, what appears to be optimum for a particular group will undoubtedly be a compromise between what is best for the infant and limitations imposed by the mother.

That conclusion does not, of course, mean that the heavier baby necessarily survives because it is heavier. Survival for a specified time after birth, as a criterion of merit, involves not only the health and vitality of the infant at birth, but also the standard of obstetric skill and of child care. Certainly, the health and vitality of the infant and the standard of child care are better in the upper social classes, which also produce bigger than average babies, so that the statistical segregation of a group of heavier than average infants with superior powers of survival may simply be the segregation of a fraction of superior social class.

That conclusion brings us to yet another variant to the concept of normality. There is nothing more sure than that the infant must be 'normal' for the mother. The first clear demonstration came from the well known experiment of Walton and Hammond (1938) who made the reciprocal crosses Shire stallion x Shetland mare and Shetland stallion x Shire mare. Whichever way the cross was made, the resulting foal was of a size appropriate to the dam's breed and was not intermediate. That extreme example makes it clear that the maternal intra-uterine environment, not genetic constitution, is of supreme importance in determining birth weight.

In comparison with such an experiment, and the truth of it has been confirmed in the parallel reciprocal cross of South Devon and Dexter cattle (Joubert and Hammond, 1954) and in sheep of different breeds (Starke, Smith and Joubert, 1958) the question for women is of almost academic importance. But confirmation was nevertheless sought. Donald (1938–1939) examined the variation in birth weights of the children in 454 families that had at least two, born at term after uneventful pregnancies. He calculated that 75 per cent of the variation was due to differences in the average birth weights between families, instead of 50 per cent which would be expected if sibs were not more alike than non-sibs. Compared with the family difference, the variation due to sex and birth order was almost negligible.

A much more impressive demonstration of the mother's determining influence on the size of her baby was provided by a post-war study by Morton (1955) of Japanese children. The material was collected between 1948 and 1952 as part of a study of the population of Hiroshima and Nagasaki. There were 220 pairs of twins of like sex, 40 of different sex and about 60,000 single births. In families with two or more children there were 30 pairs of maternal half-sibs, 168 pairs of paternal half-sibs and 15,000 pairs of full sibs, from which four samples were taken, 367 pairs adjacent in birth order, 654 pairs separated by one intervening sib and 153 pairs separated by two. All of the half-sibs were adjacent with respect to the common parent. There were also 442 pairs of adjacent full sibs whose parents were first cousins. The correlation between the weights of maternal half-sibs was 0.581, and between paternal half-sibs only 0.102. As the children grew the correlation between weights in the same family became less: between full sibs adjacent in birth order 0.523; with one intervening sib 0.425; with two intervening 0.363.

For twins the correlations were: like sex 0.557; unlike sex 0.655, and for adjacent sibs whose parents were first cousins, 0.481. There are other studies such as those of Robson (1953, 1954-55) which showed that there is a significant correlation between the birth weights of children of sisters, but none between those of brothers or brothers and sisters, all of which adds up to overwhelming proof that birth weight depends more on the environment provided by the mother than on any other single variable.

That being so we must consider the question of 'normality' of the child in terms of the maternal environment and seek to find whether, and to what extent, that environment may be modified to the benefit of the child, or without doing harm.

EFFECT OF AGE AND PARITY OF MOTHER

It is common knowledge that birth weight rises with birth order. The relation to age of the mother is obscured in two ways: (i) because every mother is older at each successive birth and (ii) because the age at first birth varies widely and differs with social class and convention. For these reasons we shall discuss the two together and, to avoid any confusion that might arise from the description of a woman having a first child as of 'parity 0' (not having borne a child), and of a woman having a second child as of parity 1, we shall talk of births and children, with parity number in brackets where the original account is in terms of parity.

Almost a hundred years ago an Edinburgh obstetrician (Duncan, 1864) quoted birth weights from Munich and analysed the records of Edinburgh Royal Maternity Hospital to show that the mean weight of 1011 'mature' children of first births was 7.170 lb (3255 g) and of 1042 later births 7.277 lb (3304 g). The difference was only 49 g. The Munich data with 3210 g for the weight of 'mature' first births and 3351 g for later births, gave a difference of 141 g. Of the difference Duncan says: 'If these results are subjected to some study, their apparent value almost entirely disappears. . . . The great influence producing variation in the weight of the newly-born child is not primiparity or pluriparity, but the age of the mother at the time of the birth. . . . The great majority of primiparae are young'. His analysis shows only mean weight of infant and age of mother for birth orders 1 to 7.

Much later Donald (1938–39) also in Edinburgh, reviewed the literature and concluded that birth weight increased to the third child, but changed little after the third, and that there was no relation to maternal age other than that due to the association with birth order. Only recently more rigorous analysis of the weight records of larger numbers of births have extended and clarified the picture. Karn and Penrose (1951–52) used 13,730 weights of single births between 1935 and 1946 at University College Hospital, London, to establish the correlations between weight of infant and parity, age, and length of gestation of mothers. Their conclusions were that weight rose to the third child (parity 2) and then fluctuated without definite trend, and that for each birth order (parity) weight fell as age rose.

Fraccaro made two studies on much the same pattern as that of Karn and Penrose. The first (Fraccaro, 1955–56) was of Italian (Pavia) records for the years 1942 to 1951 of 5486 single births, excluding miscarriages and therapeutic abortions and malformations. In that series weight rose linearly with birth order up to the group 7, 8, 9 (parities 6, 7, 8) and then declined. For a given parity weight bore no clear relation to age. In the second study (Fraccaro, 1958) the records of 165,874 live births in Czech territory in 1955 were analysed with the conclusion that birth weight rose from the first to the third birth (parity 0 to 2) and that thereafter there was no difference between weights. Birth weight rose also with age of mother to the age group 35–39 and then fell. Unfortunately the records were not in a form, Fraccaro says, to make possible the separation of any age effect within birth orders.

In agreement with Fraccaro's Italian study, Uttley (1940) in Kowloon and Hong Kong, Lee (1948) in west China, and Millis and You Poh Seng (1954–55) in Singapore, describe the birth weight of Chinese infants as rising with birth order to the 6th or 7th. Within parities Uttley and Millis and You Poh Seng found no more than a tendency for weight to fall with rising maternal age. In Dakar, Dupin, Massé and Corréa (1962) describe a rise in birth weight for both sexes up to the fifth parity; age was not considered. The same has been shown for Lapps by Mellbin (1962).

That birth order, and not age of mother, is the major determinant of rise of birth weight over a series of births to one woman, is confirmed for British infants by McKeown and Record (1953) and the Aberdeen data, and for Swedish infants by Abolins (1961). McKeown and Record compared the increases in foetal weight in late pregnancy, taking both sexes together, in three groups. The data are graphed in Figure 10.3. Second born babies are heavier than first born by on the average about 100 g. There is a smaller increase between second and third children. The Aberdeen data are in agreement. The difference with birth order does not appear clearly until after the 35th week of pregnancy.

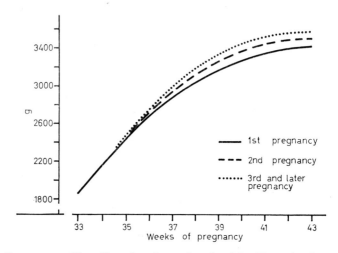

FIGURE 10.3. The effect of parity on foetal weight. From the data of McKeown and Record (1953)

It may be agreed then that birth weight rises from the first to the third child; after that what happens is obscure. There may be two reasons for the obscurity: first, that the total number of children of birth orders higher than three decreases rapidly and steadily, and second, that, in this and many other countries, relatively few women of the upper socio-economic groups have more than three children. Hence, as birth order rises, there will be represented more and more poor class women, who are smaller and less healthy, and have smaller than average infants for reasons that have nothing to do with birth order *per se*. Where there is less, or no reason to suppose such a selective effect of social class in the material analysed, the rise with birth order appears to continue to the 6th child or longer.

Within a given parity there is a tendency for birth weight to decline as maternal age rises. In general distribution the slight effect of age is covered by the greater effect of parity.

EFFECT OF STATURE AND BODY WEIGHT OF MOTHER

Tall women have slightly bigger babies than short women and heavier women than light women (Table 10.3). Aberdeen babies born between 39 and 42 weeks of gestation to women under 5′ 1″ in height were about 250 g lighter than babies born to women of 5′ 4″ or more. The difference was clearly apparent for both males and females and in all parities McKeown and Record (1954) showed that weight of first born children was strongly correlated with maternal height (r = 0.31) but not with paternal height (r = −0.03) as would be expected on the general principle that the maternal environment is of supreme importance. (See also study of Japanese children, above: Morton, 1955). For later children correlations were low and about the same for both parents. (r = 0.09 for maternal and 0.10 for paternal height).

There has been no published study of the effect of maternal body weight on birth weight. An unselected population of 4095 Aberdeen primigravidae was grouped according to height at 1 inch intervals. In each height group the distribution of weights at the 20th week of pregnancy was plotted, and smoothed curves were drawn representing the quartiles in the successive distributions. Women in the

TABLE 10.3. Effect of Maternal Height and Weight-for-Height on Mean Birth Weight in Primigravidae. Numbers of Subjects in Brackets

	Mean birth weight			
	Height			Total
Weight for height	Under 5′ 1″	5′ 1″–5′ 4″	5′ 4″ or more	
Underweight	g 2987 (237)	g 3110 (504)	g 3223 (279)	3114 (1020)
Average	3114 (460)	3228 (1025)	3396 (570)	3251 (2055)
Overweight	3201 (224)	3351 (511)	3482 (285)	3355 (1020)
Total	3101 (921)	3228 (2040)	3373 (1134)	3242 (4095)

lightest 25 per cent at any height are here described as 'underweight' and those in the heaviest 25 per cent as 'overweight' although these terms do not of course imply judgements on the degree of adiposity. Table 10.3 shows the mean birth weight of babies born to 'underweight', 'overweight', and average women in three height groups. Within each height group there is a marked increase as body weight increases; the mean birth weight for 'underweight' women of under 5' 1" in height is about 500 g less than that for 'overweight' women of 5' 4" or more in height.

EFFECT OF MATERNAL WEIGHT GAIN IN PREGNANCY

There is general agreement that birth weight of the baby is on the average related to the mother's weight gain during pregnancy. Published data are remarkably consistent and show that the average weight of a baby born to a mother who gained less than 10 lb during pregnancy is about 1 lb below that of a baby whose mother has gained 40 lb or more (Davis, 1923; Trillat, 1928; Bingham, 1932; Kuo, 1941; Waters, 1942; Beilly and Kurland, 1945; Klein, 1946; and Lysgaard, 1962). Although the women in several of those studies were subject to dietary control of weight gain they were all healthy and reasonably well-nourished (see Table 9.1) and relatively large differences in maternal weight gain occur with small differences in birth weight. The distribution of the birth weights of 3912 Aberdeen infants in 4 groups according to the weight put on by their mothers between 20 weeks and delivery is shown in Figure 10.4. The average birth weight rose by altogether 3/4 lb as the average weekly weight gain of the mothers rose by 1/2 lb, but in each group there are birth weights below $3\frac{1}{2}$ and above $9\frac{1}{2}$ lb.

THE EFFECT OF SMOKING

Seven recent studies are in agreement that babies born to mothers who smoke cigarettes during pregnancy are smaller than those of non-smokers. Evidence about the quantitative relations is not clear. (Simpson, 1957; Lowe, 1959; Frazier et al. 1961; Herriot, Billewicz and Hytten (1962); Savel and Roth (1962); Järvinen and Österlund (1963); Zabriskie (1963)). The mean weight difference at term is between 150 and 200 g and the effect is apparent from before 34 weeks of gestation. The relation holds for all parities, social groups and maternal heights, and is all the more important in that almost half of all pregnant women smoke. The

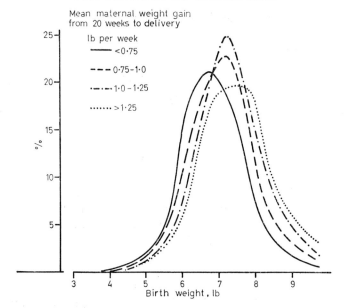

FIGURE 10.4. Distribution of birth weights of 3912 Aberdeen infants related to maternal weight gain in the second half of pregnancy

incidence has a social gradient; in Aberdeen the proportion of women smoking during pregnancy rises from 38 in Social Classes I & II to 44 per cent in Social Class III and 57 per cent in Social Classes IV & V. (Herriot *et al.* 1962).

SOCIO-ECONOMIC IMPLICATIONS

The several causes of variation of birth weight which we have just discussed, do not bear equally on all sections of the community.

Mean length of gestation is slightly less in the lower socio-economic groups because of a higher proportion of unexplained early labours (Table 10.1). The mean length of gestation in American negroes is roughly 274 days; in the white population about 279 days (Anderson, Brown and Lyon, 1943).

The effects of age and parity are not easily disentangled from socio-economic effects. The poor breed earlier and more frequently but the benefits in terms of birth weight of youth and higher parities are more than offset by the handicaps of general ill-health and poor growth.

S

In addition to all these disadvantages of physique, as if they were not enough, the poorer class women smoke more during pregnancy. In view of all those handicaps to the production of a large and healthy child, handicaps which are more frequent among the poor but all too common in all socio-economic classes, it seems eminently likely that improvement of the physique of mothers would improve the prospects for the children.

MULTIPLE PREGNANCY

The product of conception may include more than one foetus. Whether multiple pregnancy should be considered as 'normal' and physiological is arguable; it is certainly attended by more obstetric difficulty and the foetal losses are relatively high. Twins are discussed in detail in Appendix C.

THE PLACENTA

Before we discuss the growth of the placenta and the contribution it makes to a woman's weight increase in pregnancy, it would seem sensible to define what we mean by 'placenta', which is the more necessary that there is surely no other anatomical organ about which the same need could arise. If we speak of the heart or liver or kidney there would be no need to define, but in relation to the placenta there appear to be two schools of thought.

There can be no doubt about the name 'placenta'. It means a flat cake and the allusion is certainly to the human afterbirth as that with which human beings would be most familiar. There are placentae of many different shapes and also placentae that are not shed as afterbirth, but the human afterbirth has the shape of a flat cake. A dictionary definition is: 'The structure that unites the unborn mammal to the womb of its mother and establishes a nutritive connexion between them', which is sound description and evades the question of origin. Kellar (1957) says: 'It is of great importance to remember that although colloquially the afterbirth is called the *placenta*, yet this in reality only represents the foetal part. Biologically the placenta is an organ developed by mother and child in symbiosis and can be defined anatomically as the chorion frondosum, the decidua basalis and the chorio-decidual space or blood lake between.' The physiologist Amoroso (1958) says: 'The mammalian ovum . . . is retained for a longer or shorter period in the uterus, where, by special modifications of the uterine mucosa and a part of the ovum, a placenta is formed . . .'. It is, of course, perfectly reasonable to speak of the uterine mucosa as being specially modified, but the outgrowths of the chorion which form the cotyledons of the placenta are not modifications of any previous structure but are *sui generis*, constitute a highly individual organ, and in the early stages grow much faster and mature much earlier than the foetus itself.

In contrast with those writers Dancis (1959) in a review says: 'As early as the second week after implantation, villi have formed from the trophoblast (chorionic epithelium). . . . By continuous branching and invasion of the decidua (endometrium), the placenta increases in size and complexity. Erosion of maternal vessels produces small pools of blood which coalesce to form the maternal lake or intervillous space. . . . And so, at term, the placenta consists of innumerable richly vascularized fetal villi dipping into a maternal lake of blood . . .' Not perhaps so clearly stated that the exponents of the dual nature of the placenta could not claim it in their own support, but, let us say, certainly capable of the interpretation that the placenta is foetal and that the villi invade the endometrium. And here finally is what the embryologists Hamilton, Boyd and Mossman (1945) say: 'In general it can be said that any tissue or structure developed from the ovum which does not form part of the embryo proper is an *embryonic membrane*. This, of course, includes such structures as the placenta and umbilical cord which are not, strictly speaking, 'membranes', but convenience and custom have sanctioned this broad use of the term'. Crawford (1959), did not define, but the whole sense of his description of the beautifully dissected, weighed and measured human placenta is that the placenta is an organ, consisting of about 200 cotyledons, which is produced by the embryo. In reply to our request for a definition he wrote: 'The placenta represents an extra-corporeal extension of the foetal capillary bed'.

It seems to us that clinician and physiologist have somehow allowed function and purpose to cloud morphology. The embryologist and anatomist properly regard the placenta as the tissue or structure developed by the embryo to anchor it to the wall of the uterus, to procure from the maternal blood the means of living, and to return to the maternal blood the waste products of its metabolism.

We would cheerfully call that structure 'the afterbirth' and so avoid the issue, were it not that, in much of the literature we shall be quoting, the structure in question is called the placenta, and for most of the time in which we are interested it is not an afterbirth, but a busily functioning tissue. When considering function and chemical exchange between mother and foetus we shall speak in terms of supply in the maternal blood (for after all, the blood in the uterus during pregnancy is not a separate 'compartment' but part of the general circulation), and transmission across a foetal membrane to the foetal circulation. Both anatomically and functionally maternal blood and foetal chorionic structures are distinct.

When the placenta (afterbirth) is weighed it contains remnants of maternal decidua and clotted maternal blood trapped between the villi. That is to say, the weight is not all foetal weight, which is what we wish to measure, but the error involved is small and can be neglected. There are other sources of confusion. Usually the placenta is weighed with the cord and other membranes; occasionally without. Also the weight depends on the length of time that elapses between delivery of the child and the tying of the cord, if blood from the placenta is allowed to drain into the child in the interval. We shall take as standard measurement the weight with cord and membranes at delivery, without drainage.

Figure 10.5 shows the growth in weight of the placenta, so measured, from over 8000 births in Aberdeen, and the almost identical values for about 5000 placentae recorded by McKeown

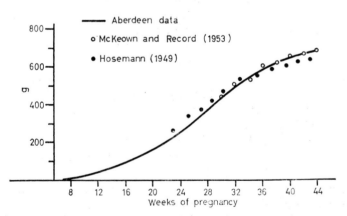

FIGURE 10.5. Growth in weight of the placenta

and Record (1953) from the 30th week of pregnancy. Hosemann (1949b) presents data for nearly 12,000 placentae. His curve of growth is above the British to the 34th week and below it thereafter, with a difference of 50 g at 40 weeks. Differences may be due to differences in method of delivery and in the time at which the umbilical cord is tied.

The mean weight of the placenta from the two concordant sets of data is about 20 g at 10 weeks, 170 g at 20 weeks, 430 g at 30 weeks and 650 g at 40 weeks. The rate of growth declines towards the end of pregnancy, as it does in the foetus, but growth continues at least to 44 weeks.

FOETAL AND PLACENTAL WEIGHT

When foetal and placental weights are compared it appears at once that the relation of foetal to placental weight changes during the course of pregnancy. The placenta weighs more than the foetus until about the 16th week, which is some time after growth in the number of cotyledons is complete, at 12 weeks (Crawford, 1959). After the 16th week the placenta forms a progressively smaller proportion of total foetal tissue. At the end of pregnancy the weight of the placenta is related to the weight of the foetus, but not as closely as might be expected of two parts of the same organism. From the Aberdeen data, the correlation coefficients are 0.538 for females and 0.558 for males. Sex differences between placental weights are less than between foetal weights; indeed, in the Aberdeen data there was no consistent difference between male and female. McKeown and Record (1953) found average male placentae to be consistently heavier than female to 42 weeks, when the difference disappeared. The two sets of data taken together suggest that male foetuses have relatively smaller placentae than female, or, as McKeown and Record express it, males make greater use than females do of a given weight of placenta.

According to McKeown and Record (1953), the weight of the placenta is less for first born than for later births taken together; there is no clear effect of maternal age.

LIQUOR AMNII

There is no shortage of estimates of the volume of liquor amnii at term, but few measurements. Textbooks of obstetrics give a range of normal volumes varying from between half and one litre to between one and two litres.

Direct measurement is difficult; the only satisfactory method would be to remove all the liquor at caesarean section and measure it. Guthmann and May (1930) attempted to do that in 15 subjects at term and found a mean volume of 1800 ml. More recent evidence suggests that their estimate is much too high although it is difficult to see where a recurrent error could have been made. Hutchinson et al. (1955) have shown that liquor amnii is turned over at a rate of more than 600 ml per hour in the intact amniotic sac and it is conceivable that the rate might be greatly increased when the sac is opened and liquor is removed. If this were to happen then some liquor might be secreted during the time taken to remove it from the open uterus at operation, how much it is impossible to guess. More recently the volume of liquor amnii has been measured in the intact sac by dilution methods but unfortunately the aim seems to have been to compare tracer substances, or the experiment was incidental to other investigations, so that there is no means of knowing how far the subjects were representative of normal clinical material. Hutchinson et al. (1955) measured liquor amnii in 20 women with D_2O as the tracer; twelve of the subjects were arbitrarily assumed to be normal and had volumes ranging from 385 to 1420, with a mean of 788. Hanon (1957) in a review of the literature gives the normal range as 400 to 1200 ml.

Recently Elliott and Inman (1961) measured the liquor volume by dilution of Coomassie blue dye in 59 normal pregnancies near term. The volume declined steadily from a maximum level of about 1 litre at 38 weeks to about 200 ml at 43 weeks; at 40 weeks the mean was about 800 ml. Numbers of subjects at each week of gestation were naturally small and there was a wide range of values so that these figures can be no more than approximations. Unpublished figures from Aberdeen by Dennis and Cheyne who used congo red dye suggest similar volumes of liquor amnii at term, also with much variation.

The best estimate we can make at present for the volume of liquor at term is 800 ml, but a great deal more information is needed.

Some more direct information is available for early pregnancy. Guthmann and May (1930) collected liquor by syringe at operations for termination of pregnancy at or before $4\frac{1}{2}$ months in about

15 women and Monie (1953) measured liquor amnii in 66 early pregnancies. Only 9 of Monie's specimens were obtained at hysterotomy; the rest were from 53 abortions and 4 extrauterine gestations. For his 'normal' figures he included only 14 where there was no abnormality of the foetus and no maceration, and where the actual menstrual age was within 1½ weeks of the foetal age estimated from foetal length. There are more recent estimates collected by Wagner and Fuchs (1962) from 45 women whose pregnancies were terminated between 10 and 20 weeks. Monie's normal values are shown in Figure 10.6 with the average figures published by Guthmann and May and by Wagner and Fuchs. There is good

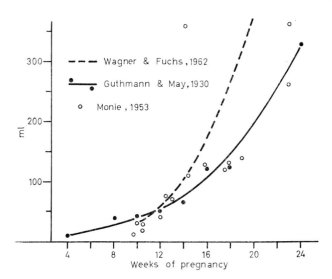

FIGURE 10.6. The volume of liquor amnii in the first half of pregnancy

agreement between these series in the early weeks and we can with some confidence select 30 ml as representative for 10 weeks. There is a wide spread of results about 20 weeks and a value of about 250 ml is tentative only.

Between about the 24th week and term few measurements have been made. Guthmann and May measured the volumes during 2 caesarean sections at 28 and 32 weeks and found 1000 and 1200 ml. Those values seem high and their findings by the same technique of an average of 1800 ml at term suggest a technical fault leading to overestimate.

The clinical impression is that there is not much less liquor at 30 weeks than at term and an estimate of 600 ml is not likely to be very far out.

The specific gravity of liquor amnii is sufficiently close to unity to allow these average volumes to be considered as weights. Tentative estimates of the weight of liquor amnii at 10, 20, 30 and 40 weeks can therefore be taken as 30, 250, 600 and 800 g.

SUMMARY

Table 10.4 summarises the weights of the total uterine contents at four points in pregnancy.

TABLE 10.4. Weight of The Product of Conception

| | Weeks of Pregnancy | | | |
	10	20	30	40
Foetus	g 5	g 300	g 1500	g 3300
Placenta	20	170	430	650
Liquor	30	250	600	800
Total	55	720	2530	4750

As a proportion of the total weight gained by the mother, the product of conception rises from about 8 per cent at 10 weeks to 18 per cent at 20 weeks, 30 per cent at 30 weeks and about 38 per cent at term.

CHAPTER 11

Components of Weight Gain
2. Changes in the Maternal Body

STRUCTURAL

The uterus

Very few data have been published on the growth in weight of the pregnant uterus. When one considers the mass of post-mortem material which has been available this is surprising; and regrettable, because to-day when death during pregnancy and at delivery is rare there is little opportunity to accumulate measurements.

The only growth curve has been published by Gillespie (1950) and is shown as the continuous line in Figure 11.1. It was based on only 16 uteri at the Carnegie Institution of Washington and must therefore be a much smoothed line. Actual weights are not given and there is no information about the subjects. From a non-pregnant weight of about 50 g the uterus grows to a weight of about 200 g at 10 weeks and then, rapidly, to a weight of about 700 g at 20 weeks. During the same time the thickness of the uterine wall averages between 8 and 9 mm and the increasing size of the uterus is an expression of growth of the muscle. After mid-pregnancy the rate of growth *in weight* slows down; the uterus weighs about 900 g at 30 weeks and about 950 g at term. During the second half of pregnancy there is a great increase in the size of the uterus which is brought about in large measure by stretching with thinning of the muscle to under 6 mm at term.

The general pattern of early hypertrophy and later stretching is given considerable support in the literature and the general shape of Gillespie's curve is probably valid. A final weight of 1000 g is, however, almost certainly too low, although that estimate is supported by early literature reviewed by Stieve (1932). Robles, Pratt and Starr (1961) found that the uterus weighed about 10 per cent less after fixation in formalin which may in part explain Gillespie's curve. Stieve himself had weighed a large series of term uteri and found the range to be 1080 to 1420 g; the mean was about 1200 g. He did not define what he measured so that we do not know whether the Fallopian tubes or the cervix or both were included. Eight term uteri with cervix but without tubes measured recently in Aberdeen give a range of about 850 g to 1250 g. There is no doubt about the gross weight of the non-pregnant uterus. Stieve (1932) describes the nulliparous uterus as weighing 40–50 g and the parous uterus 60–70 g, so that a starting weight of 50 g may be assumed. The weight reached at 10 weeks, about 200 g, agrees with our own experience of a number removed at that stage. The intermediate figures are more shadowy and we can do little at this stage but accept Gillespie's estimates. On the assumption that his final figure is too low we would suggest a higher terminal phase to the curve ending at 1050 g (Figure 11.1). Thus the best estimates we can make for the gross weights of uterus at 10, 20, 30 and 40 weeks are 200, 700, 950 and 1050 g, giving increases during pregnancy of 150, 650, 900 and 1000 g.

The crude weight of the pregnant uterus, measured after its

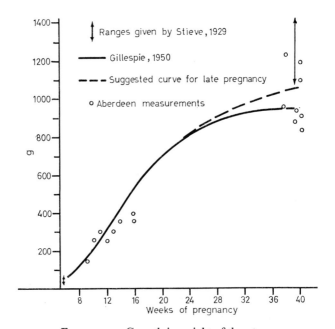

FIGURE 11.1. Growth in weight of the uterus

TABLE 11.1. Increase in Weight of the Uterus

	Weeks of Pregnancy				
	0	10	20	30	40
Gross weight	g 50	g 200	g 700	g 950	g 1050
Contained blood	5	20	70	95	105
Blood free uterus	45	180	630	855	945
Increase above non-pregnant weight of blood free uterus	—	135	585	810	900

removal, will include the blood contained in its vessels and, since the increased blood volume of pregnancy is to be considered separately, the estimate we need for the uterus is for the blood-free organ. Estimates based on the amount of contained haemoglobin in the Aberdeen specimens suggest that about 10 per cent of the weight of the uterus as removed may be contained blood. We may therefore summarize the weight gain of the uterus alone as set out in Table 11.1.

It need hardly be said that there is no published evidence to show whether differences in uterine growth are associated with such possible influences as age and parity.

The breasts

No direct measurement of increase in weight of the breasts can be expected, and indeed none may be possible. Even if removed puerperal breasts were to be weighed—and it would be impossible to define precisely the extent of the tissues which constitute the 'breast'—the non-pregnant gland is so variable that one could not estimate the increase due to pregnancy.

The only data available are indirect measurements of increase of breast volume estimated by a water-displacement method (Hytten, 1954b). While such a measurement is bound to lack the precision of a weight, the numbers available, 143 primigravidae and 73 multigravidae, give acceptable average values. Breast changes are discussed also in Chapter 7. For present purposes we need give only a summary.

The mean volume of the primigravid breast in early pregnancy (9–12 weeks) was about 565 ml; it rose to about 665 ml by 20 weeks and 775 ml at term. There were not sufficient data from which to draw a curve of the increasing volume, but from a few repeat measurements and from clinical observation, it is probable that little growth takes place in the last 10 weeks of pregnancy. The multiparae measured began pregnancy with a somewhat greater breast volume of about 590 ml and reached a mean of 780 ml at term.

Taking the two groups together it seems reasonable to suggest, at least provisionally, that some 75 ml are added to each breast between 10 and 20 weeks, a further 100 ml between 20 and 30 weeks, and little, say 25 ml, thereafter. Subjectively, many women experience considerable swelling and tenderness of the breasts in the first few weeks of pregnancy before our measurements were begun; the cause is almost certainly a vascular response which appears to regress by 10 or 12 weeks and the permanent gain is probably small. A small gain of 25 ml during early pregnancy seems realistic, and gives a total gain of about 250 ml for each breast, 500 ml for both.

There is a decline in the amount of breast enlargement as maternal age increases (Chapter 7). The estimates we have made are reasonable averages for young women.

The measured increase in breast volume includes more than increase in mammary gland; there is contained blood and possibly a small proportion of fat, although little if any subcutaneous fat appears to be added to sites above the waist.

TABLE 11.2. Increase in Weight of the Mammary Glands:
Both Breasts Together

	Weeks of Pregnancy			
	10	20	30	40
Gross weight	g 50	g 200	g 400	g 450
Blood	5	20	40	45
Gland-tissue	45	180	360	405

We have no information from which we can gauge the quantity of contained blood. We can only say that clinically the breast appears to be highly vascular in pregnancy, and the assumption that about 10 per cent of the weight of gland substance is blood is certainly not an overestimate.

We can now summarize the increase in size of the two breasts (Table 11.2). These estimates, originally derived from volume changes, are already the result of many approximations and it would be absurd to sophisticate them further by making an assumption about the specific gravity of the tissue. It will be sufficiently close to unity for them to be regarded henceforth as weights.

Blood

The increase in blood plasma and red cells is treated in detail in Chapter 1. There is much individual variation but the averages presented here can be regarded as characteristic of healthy young women. For present purposes it is enough to say that the plasma volume is increased above the non-pregnant level by probably 50 ml in the first 10 weeks, 550 by 20 weeks and 1150 at 30 weeks. A peak of some 1300 ml above the non-pregnant mean is reached at about 34 weeks and is followed by a fall to about 1000 ml above the non-pregnant at term.

The volume of red cells is probably not increased appreciably at 10 weeks, but is up by an average of about 50 ml at 20 weeks, 150 ml at 30 weeks and 250 ml at term.

Other sites

It has often been suggested that there may be increases in other organs and tissues. There is some evidence from experimental animals that liver and intestinal mucosa may enlarge in pregnancy. We have no evidence for man and we will discuss below reasons why we believe other significant changes to be unlikely.

COMPOSITIONAL

In the next sections we will consider changes in the composition of the maternal body as a whole, rather than in specific organs, but before we do so it is necessary to discuss the methods of estimation on which the information is based.

Principles and techniques of measurement

BODY WATER

Compartments. The total body water is generally considered to be in two major compartments: (i) water inside cells or intracellular water; (ii) the remainder which is extracellular and is often further subdivided into intravascular or plasma water and extravascular extracellular water made up of water in lymph, 'interstitial' fluid, cerebrospinal fluid, eye humors, serous and glandular secretions.

That concept of the water space appears simple and as Manery (1954) said 'it has brought order and rationale to many data difficult to interpret', but the simplicity is illusory and can be seriously misleading. There are two overwhelming difficulties. First, the water compartments so defined are not capable of precise measurement; and second, of more importance, they are not rigid but highly elastic, swelling and shrinking, together, independently, or one at the expense of the other in response to a wide variety of physiological stimuli. Even the 'normal' total water content of the living body can never be more than a concept. Water is lost continuously to the environment and replenished or over-replenished at intervals. There is no way of knowing what is the normal or even the mean level of this fluctuating quantity. The estimate of a water space will therefore be blurred, not only by the inevitable error of the laboratory process, but also by the fact that at any one moment the measurement is a snapshot of a moving scene.

Tracer techniques. Techniques of estimation will be discussed first. In all the methods, an estimate is made of the dilution experienced by a known quantity of a tracer substance in the unknown volume of the compartment to be measured. For such an indirect measurement to be valid certain basic requirements must be met: (i) the tracer should behave in the same way as the substance it is tracing; i.e. it should remain evenly distributed only in the space it is measuring; (ii) the concentration of the tracer substance should be easily measurable at the concentration reached and (iii) the equilibrium characteristics should be such that there is a reasonably flat time-concentration curve which gives a plateau where the concentration changes slowly so that the time of sampling is not critical.

The last two requirements are satisfied by most of the tracer substances commonly used; the first requirement is never met completely and variation in the extent to which different tracers meet it is responsible for many of the difficulties that arise in the interpretation of results.

TOTAL BODY WATER

Only for total body water can indirect estimates by the dilution technique be checked by the direct method of drying, and it is surprising that no such check has been made for many of the tracer substances, even with small animals. Substances commonly used are: urea, thiourea, sulphanilamide, antipyrine, N-acetyl 4-amino antipyrine (NAAP) and more recently water itself labelled with a hydrogen isotope, deuterium or tritium.

Antipyrine and its derivative NAAP, which is believed to be better, are probably the most widely used and in normal persons give results closely similar to estimates made with labelled water. They underestimate the total water when there are abnormal deposits as in oedema (Faller *et al.* 1955). The estimation has two major sources of error. Antipyrine is broken down at rates which vary between 1 and 17 per cent per hour (Soberman *et al.* 1949) and there is some localization by binding to plasma protein and possibly to tissue protein. It appears that, in the average subject, these two errors tend to cancel each other but evidence will be presented later to show that this happy accident does not occur in pregnancy.

Water labelled with a hydrogen isotope, deuterium or tritium, should theoretically be almost the perfect tracer and indeed seems to be so, although there is a slow exchange with the hydrogen of other substances, particularly protein, and so it slightly over-estimates body water by an amount estimated as about 1 per cent (Schloerb *et al.* 1950, Pinson, 1952). The main disadvantage in practice is the difficulty of measurement. Deuterium oxide is only 10 per cent heavier than water and its detection in a final concentration of about 0.2 per cent in body water requires highly sensitive physical methods (Hytten *et al.* 1962). None of these can be applied casually; the apparatus must be maintained with great care and requires a technician with skill and experience. Tritium is radioactive, but its radiation is not easily measured by simple methods of detection; the services of an experienced physicist are needed. With the careful use of water labelled with either isotope repeated studies on the same person will give estimates which will not vary by more than 2 or 3 per cent from the mean.

EXTRACELLULAR WATER

Some parts of the extracellular water are of little interest in the present context, namely cerebrospinal fluid, serous secretions, eye humors and gland secretions. The more important parts of extracellular space are the plasma water and the water of lymph and interstitial fluid in which ions and small molecules can diffuse readily, easy to define in these terms but morphologically vague. The greater part of it, the interstitial water, is probably continuous with plasma water and lymph at the capillaries and bathes every body cell in a fine film; the water of hydration of connective tissue and bone is less free. As a buffer between the body's transport system, the plasma, and the cells which depend upon it the interstitial component of the extracellular water appears to be an extremely flexible compartment capable of buffering large shifts of water into and out of cells in response to osmotic and other influences of which we are still lamentably ignorant. The concept of interstitial water as a large vaguely defined and fluctuant mass cannot be related to histological findings; it must remain a physiological image.

A tracer substance suitable for the measurement of extracellular water must distribute itself evenly throughout the space and remain completely outside cells. No such substance has been found and extracellular water as we have defined it has never been measured. Indeed its measurement is theoretically impossible, because it is incapable of anatomical definition.

In spite of these serious limitations, estimates of extracellular water are made with a variety of tracer substances and of necessity their concentration in plasma is taken as characteristic of extracellular fluid generally. Only the briefest summary of an extensive literature can be given here. The tracer substances fall into two main groups: those which resemble sodium or chloride in their distribution, such as isotopes of sodium and chlorine, thiocyanate, sulphate, thiosulphate, bromide and iodide; and larger nonelectrolytes, which readily escape from the blood but do not, apparently, enter cells, such as mannitol, inulin, sucrose and raffinose. The first group overestimate the extracellular space since they all penetrate cells to some extent and sodium, for example, also accumulates in bone. The bigger molecules give a smaller estimate of the space but they probably fail to penetrate to the furthest recesses of the extracellular space; there is relatively little information about the exact distribution.

Thiocyanate, one of the more popular of the ionic group, may be cited as an example of the confusing behaviour of these substances. It becomes attached to plasma albumin and up to 30 per cent of it is present in that non-diffusible fraction. On that account the concentration in plasma is much higher than in extracellular water generally and extracellular water is underestimated on the basis of plasma dilution. That is compensated to an unknown extent by the entry of thiocyanate into red cells and possibly other cells; and its concentration by up to 20 times in intestinal secretions (Kaltreider *et al.* 1941; Elkington and Taffel, 1942; Moister and Freis, 1949). Thus, as with antipyrine, a physiologically sensible answer is obtained only because two gross errors tend to cancel. Scheinberg and Kowalski (1950) have suggested formulae which may be used to correct for the effect of plasma albumin, but the elimination of one in a complex of errors will give only a spurious impression of greater accuracy. Quite clearly such estimates made under differing physiological conditions are incapable of rational interpretation.

The failure of all these substances to act as true tracers for extracellular water is acknowledged by the use of such terms as 'sodium space' or 'inulin space' to describe the compartment studied, which in the present state of our ignorance has much to commend it.

INTRACELLULAR WATER

At present, intracellular water can be estimated only by difference when total body water and extracellular water have been estimated. It will be obvious from what has been said about those measurements that any estimate of intracellular water can be no more than a first approximation. The possibility of estimating small differences in, say, cell hydration by such means is out of the question.

BLOOD AND PLASMA WATER

Methods of estimation of blood and plasma water are discussed in Chapter 1.

SOLID CONSTITUENTS

Measurement of the major non-water constituents of the body is of fundamental importance in any study of body composition but the techniques available are extremely circuitous and involve several

T

assumptions; almost nothing is known about their use in pregnancy.

Methods of estimating body composition are discussed in detail by Siri (1956). In all current methods the body is considered to be made up of four basic substances: water, lipid, protein and inorganic mineral, and estimates of body composition rely on measurements of body water or body density or both. The measurement of body water has just been discussed. Body density has usually been estimated in one of two ways. The original and most used method has been to weigh the subject in air and then under water, so that body volume can be calculated from water displacement. This simple plan is technically difficult to realize because gas in the body gives a falsely high volume. The lung gas content can be estimated separately but it is not possible to account for intestinal gas. In a somewhat more convenient method, developed by Siri (1955), body volume is calculated by displacement of air in a tank; the air volume before and after the subject enters the tank is measured by helium dilution. In pregnancy Siri's method would be considerably simpler than underwater weighing but it still requires complex apparatus and is not without technical difficulties.

When body water alone is known then body fat and the 'lean body mass', or body weight minus fat, has been calculated by assuming that water is a fixed proportion of the lean mass, usually 72 per cent. The proportion appears to be relatively constant in small animals but is undoubtedly less constant in man. In pregnancy the proportion will change because the non-fat weight added in pregnancy has a water content of over 90 per cent.

It is known that body density decreases as fatness increases and body fat has been estimated from density measurements alone. But such an estimate must assume that the composition of the fat-free body is constant; it is therefore only a crude guide in the non-pregnant subject and almost without value in pregnancy. When both body water and body density are estimated, then the body fat can be calculated with much more confidence. In these circumstances the only assumption which need be made is of a constant relation between the protein and mineral constituents of the lean mass. Whether constant or not the ratio will have only a slight effect on the calculation of fat. Very little is known about the application in pregnancy of these methods, which appear to have been used only by McCartney, Pottinger and Harrod (1959).

A more direct measurement of body fat is possible with the use of tracer substances which are selectively absorbed in fat. Two such substances are cyclopropane and ^{85}krypton. The results have proved encouraging in animal experiments but use of those tracers in man is just beginning (Hytten, 1964). No attempt has yet been made to apply them in pregnancy.

Recently an attempt has been made to estimate lean body mass by calculating the ^{40}K content of the body by whole-body scintillation counting (Forbes, Gallup and Hursh, 1961). There is evidence that the potassium content of the body is related to lean mass but the magnitude of the ratio has to be assumed in each case and the method is therefore no more reliable than the measurement of body water for estimating body composition. It has not been used in pregnancy.

Some minor constituents of the body can be measured by the dilution technique. We have just seen that body K can be estimated by whole body scintillation counting of the naturally occurring isotope ^{40}K; more commonly the so called 'exchangeable K' has been calculated from the dilution of introduced ^{42}K. 'Exchangeable sodium', similarly, has been estimated from the dilution of introduced isotopes, ^{22}Na or ^{24}Na, and exchangeable chlorine from the distribution of the bromine isotope ^{82}Br.

The 'exchangeable' pool of an element is simply that quantity of it in which the tracer can move and exchange freely; it cannot be defined physiologically but is generally assumed to represent the whole body content, both in and out of cells, which is in solution and osmotically active. It is known that something like one third of the sodium in the body is held in bone salts and that two thirds of it are not readily exchangeable; it exchanges slowly and there is a gradual increase in the sodium space after a first rapid phase of equilibration. It is therefore essential that when comparison of sodium space or total exchangeable sodium are made they must represent equilibration over the same time interval.

Physiological variations of body fluids

We have already said that the difficulties of estimating body composition in pregnancy are likely to be due at least as much to the continuous physiological adjustments which occur as to the uncertainties of the technical procedures. If estimates for different subjects, or for the same subject at different times, are to be comparable then they must be performed, as far as is possible, under the same physiological conditions. Relatively little is known about fluid changes, except for blood volume, and these are discussed in Chapter 1. Deviations outside the normal inevitable fluctuation in the total body water of a healthy subject are probably uncommon. Dehydration, in the sense of hydration appreciably below the normal mean level, can presumably result from big losses of water, for example in sweat, but the order of change is not known. Mean body water is presumably less after a night's sleep, during which water is lost continuously, than during the day when it is replenished frequently. Overhydration is probably even less common but can undoubtedly occur when a lot of fluid is drunk quickly.

In late pregnancy, when oedema of the lower limbs is common, there may be relatively big diurnal differences in total body water. The oedema, which may involve 1 or 2 litres of water, often disappears after a night's rest in bed and then reappears during the day; the change may be partly a matter of redistribution, but there is often nocturnal diuresis. Also in late pregnancy the diuretic response to a water load is considerably reduced, and the increase of body water after drinking is therefore prolonged (Chapter 4).

There is almost no information about variations in the proportions of extracellular and intracellular water, for reasons which will be plain from a consideration of the methods for their estimation. If, for example, one wanted to know the effect of pregnancy on extracellular water volume, to measure the thiocyanate space would be simply to beg the question. An increase in the measurement means only that the thiocyanate ion is apparently distributed in a bigger volume. It might be penetrating the cells more easily so that the increased volume would not be in the extracellular space as we understand it. The method is valid only if one can be sure that pregnancy has not affected the mode of distribution. The effect of pregnancy, or indeed of any other physiological state, on the distribution of extracellular water tracers is not known.

In present circumstances, when so little is known about changes in body water distribution, the conditions of measurement can be standardized only within limits. Measurements which are to be compared should at least be made at the same time of day and in the same relation to rest and food. During equilibration water turnover should be kept to a minimum by a comfortable environment and rest.

Changes in body composition in pregnancy

Changes in body composition during pregnancy, as measured, usually involve the product of conception; changes in the maternal body cannot be measured in isolation. That is true of total body water and to a greater or less extent, depending on the tracer, of extracellular water. When body fat is computed from body water and density, or measured by fat-soluble gas, then foetal fat also is measured. Most measurements of blood volume, on the other hand, are of maternal blood only because neither plasma albumin labelled with Evans blue dye nor labelled red cells have been shown to cross the placenta; only when carbon monoxide is used to label red cells does the tracer cross to the foetus. This may be obvious, but it is often forgotten and can lead to confusion in calculations.

TOTAL BODY WATER

Total body water increases continuously during pregnancy, but few satisfactory measurements have been published. Because there are wide individual differences in the amount of body water, isolated measurements have little meaning and changes during pregnancy can be judged only where serial estimates have been made. Even then different series of measurements seldom span the same period of pregnancy and are therefore not comparable. The best we can do is to take, where it is possible, differences in body water between late pregnancy and the post-partum period. For some of these the post-partum measurement has been made some weeks after parturition when the body water has returned to the early pregnancy or pre-pregnancy value, but other workers have made the post-partum measurement only a week after delivery when there is still some excess body water resulting from the pregnancy.

Table 11.3 shows the results. All that can be said about these figures is that when D_2O is used as a tracer there is reasonable agreement about the average quantity of water retained in pregnancy. Considerable individual variation is typical of almost all physiological changes in pregnancy but how much of the variation shown here is real and how much accidental cannot be guessed. The extremes may well be due to technical errors; but that there

TABLE 11.3. Increment of Total Body Water in Pregnancy
Measured as the Difference Between the Volume Post-partum
and that in Late Pregnancy

Author and Subjects	Tracer used	Measurements made:		Difference in total body water	Mean
		post-partum	late pregnancy		
				litres	litres
Haley and Woodbury (1956) 3 subjects	D$_2$O	8 weeks 3 weeks 8 weeks	'during labour' ,, ,, ,, ,,	5.3 3.2 7.4	5.3
Hutchinson, Plentl and Taylor (1954) 4 subjects	D$_2$O	1 week 1 week 1 week 1 week	36 weeks 38 weeks 37 weeks 36 weeks	6.9 2.7 7.3 5.7	5.7
McCartney, Pottinger and Harrod (1959) 5 subjects	D$_2$O	7 days 7 days 8 days 7 days 8 days	37 weeks 37 weeks 38 weeks 38 weeks 39 weeks	4.1 5.7 9.1 14.2 0	6.6
Seitchik and Alper (1956) 4 subjects	Anti-pyrine	6 weeks 7 weeks 7 weeks 7 weeks	37 weeks 37 weeks 39 weeks 39 weeks	14.8 13.0 15.1 7.3	12.5
Hytten and Thomson (unpublished) 34 subjects	D$_2$O	Serial measurements during pregnancy (see text and Table 11.4)			6.96

should be no change in body water between 39 weeks of pregnancy and 8 days post-partum as shown by one of McCartney *et al*'s subjects, is scarcely possible.

Estimates made with antipyrine as a tracer are of a different order. It was pointed out in the discussion of methods that in normal persons antipyrine gives estimates which are similar to those of D$_2$O because two large errors, fixation to plasma albumin and metabolic destruction, tend to cancel. In pregnancy, plasma albumin concentration is reduced and destruction of antipyrine may very well be increased in the generally raised metabolic turnover; both changes, by reducing the plasma concentration of anti-pyrine will cause overestimation of body water.

Data from Aberdeen (Hytten and Thomson, unpublished) on changes in body water in 34 primigravidae, support the published studies where D_2O was used, and in addition allow a distinction to be made between subjects with and without oedema. The study of gain of total body water is complicated by the need to account for oedema. There seems to be little doubt that pitting oedema often occurs in pregnancies which from all other points of view are to be regarded as clinically normal, and there is reason to believe that increased hydration of some maternal tissues is physiological rather than pathological. In a large series of normotensive primigravidae, oedema of the feet or ankles was recorded in 30.5 per cent, and more generalized oedema (e.g. the hands and face) in a further 4.7 per cent (unpublished Aberdeen data). In the series of 34 'clinically normal' primigravidae in whom deuterium space was measured at intervals during pregnancy, the proportions in whom oedema was noted are different: 9 (26.5 per cent) had oedema of ankles or feet, and 10 (29.4 per cent) had generalized oedema. The proportion with generalized oedema is in part attributable to more careful recording in subjects who were undergoing special investigation, but it is probable that by chance the group of women selected in early pregnancy later had an exceptionally high incidence; three of them had quite gross oedema. In neither of these series were any steps taken to prevent or treat oedema by diet or by diuretics.

Table 11.4 gives the mean increases in body water in the 34 women classified according to severity of oedema. The averages for all 34 subjects are 3.80 litres from 12 to 30 weeks and 3.28 litres for 30–38 weeks; extrapolating the last value to 40 weeks we obtain an average gain from 12 to 40 weeks of 7.90 litres. If the figures in the table are weighted in accordance with the incidence of oedema noted in a large representative population, we obtain average gains of 3.55 litres from 12 to 30 weeks, 2.57 litres from 30–38 weeks and 6.76 litres from 12 to 40 weeks. This last series of weighted means is thought to be more representative than the unweighted averages for purposes of further calculation, but the unweighted averages may be borne in mind as possible maxima. Both averages are plotted in Figure 11.2.

There is no information about the amount of body water stored

TABLE 11.4. Mean Increase in Total Body Water (Deuterium
Space) in 34 Clinically Normal Primigravidae
(Hytten and Thomson, unpublished)

Increase in body water, litres	No oedema (15)	Ankle oedema (9)	Generalized oedema (10)	Total mean (34)	Weighted mean (see p. 283)
12–30 weeks	3.44	3.65	4.46	3.80	3.55
30–38 weeks	2.28	2.78	5.24	3.28	2.57
38–40 weeks (extrapolated)	0.57	0.70	1.31	0.82	0.64
0–12 weeks (guessed)	0.20	0.20	0.20	0.20	0.20
Total 0–40 weeks	6.49	7.33	11.21	8.10	6.96

before 12 weeks. It seems unlikely to exceed about 200 ml and we have added this to our measurements which brings the total weighted average, for the whole of pregnancy, to 6.96 litres.

For the fixed points which we will use in later calculations we can say on present evidence that the average primigravida has gained about 1500 ml of water by 20 weeks, 3750 ml by 30 weeks and 7000 ml at term.

In Table 11.5 is listed the water content of all the components added during pregnancy which we have discussed above. The totals at 20, 30 and 40 weeks are compared to the average of the measured increments of total body water (See also Figure 11.2). There is reasonable agreement at 20 and 30 weeks. The synthetic totals are above the estimates obtained by direct measurement, but since many assumptions have been made in the construction of the table and since the estimates of total body water are tentative no significance can be given to differences of the order shown. All that can be said with some confidence is that up to 30 weeks there is no excess water in pregnancy which cannot be accounted for in the product of conception and added maternal blood and tissue.

At term the discrepancy is bigger and in the opposite direction. That is, there appears to be about 1200 ml of water in the body which cannot be accounted for in the usual sites. The difference is

TABLE 11.5. Water Component of Weight Gain

	Weeks of Pregnancy								
	20			30			40		
	Weight	Water	Water	Weight	Water	Water	Weight	Water	Water
	g	%	g	g	%	g	g	%	g
Foetus	300	88	264	1500	79	1185	3300	71	2343
Placenta	170	90	153	430	85	366	650	83	540
Liquor amnii	250	99	247	600	99	594	800	99	792
Blood free uterus	585	82.5	483	810	82.5	668	900	82.5	743
Blood and fat free mammary gland	180	75	135	360	75	270	405	75	304
Plasma	550	92	506	1150	92	1058	1000	92	920
Red cells	50	65	32	150	65	98	250	65	163
			1820			4239			5805
Measured increment of water			1500			3750			7000

(handwritten annotations on Placenta row: 20 weeks "53%"; 30 weeks "19.7"; 40 weeks "1278")

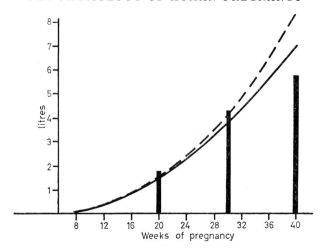

FIGURE 11.2. Increase in body water in pregnancy. The two curves represent the mean values measured in 34 normal primigravidae (Hytten and Thomson, unpublished); the dotted line is the unweighted mean, the solid line has been weighted for a more representative incidence of oedema (see text). The vertical bars represent the amount of water calculated to be present in the product of conception and added maternal tissues (Table 11.5)

almost certainly real, if not numerically precise, and probably represents oedema fluid.

EXTRACELLULAR WATER

More estimates have been made of extracellular water than of total body water. The most popular tracer substance has been sodium thiocyanate. Chesley (1943) used it in a cross-sectional study of 442 pregnant women and calculated the mean increase between early and late pregnancy to be about 6.3 litres; Caton *et al.* (1949) found a mean increase of 6.0 litres in a serial study of 7 subjects and Röttger (1953–54) a mean of 6.9 litres in a cross-sectional study of 95 women between the second and tenth months of pregnancy. Unpublished data from Aberdeen have shown a mean increase of about 6 litres.

Somewhat smaller estimates have been made with other tracers. Seitchik and Alper (1954) used mannitol and found in 4 women a mean increase of 5.2 litres and McCartney *et al.* (1959) a similar change in two women when ^{22}Na was used as tracer.

Friedman, Goodfriend, Berlin and Goldstein (1951) and Gray and Plentl (1954) describe increases of a different order. Gray and Plentl used ^{24}Na in a study of 8 women and found a mean increase of 3.1 litres; Friedman *et al.* estimated the bromide space in late pregnancy to be about 3 litres above the mean non-pregnant average.

It would be easy to accept the majority opinion from these estimates and conclude that extracellular water increases by about 6 litres during pregnancy but the detailed records do not inspire confidence. The individual range is huge and in those subjects where both total body water and extracellular water were measured simultaneously there was often little correspondence. It is, in fact,

TABLE 11.6. An Estimate of Extracellular and Intracellular Water Added During Pregnancy

	Total water	Extracellular	Intracellular
Foetus[1]	2343	1360 *58%*	983 *42%*
Placenta[2]	540	260 *48%*	280 *52%*
Liquor amnii	792	792	0
Uterus[3]	743	490 *66*	253 *34%*
Mammary gland[4]	304	148 *49%*	156 *51%*
Plasma	920	920	0
Red cells	163	0	163
Extracellular extravascular water	1195	1195	0
	7000	5165	1835

[1] Extracellular space = 41.2 per cent of body weight (Fellers *et al.* 1949)

[2] Assuming 48 per cent of water to be extracellular as in liver (Harrison, Darrow and Yannet, 1936)

[3] Assuming 66 per cent of water to be extracellular (Hawkins and Nixon, 1958)

[4] Assuming 49 per cent of water to be extracellular as in 'viscera' (Harrison *et al.* 1936)

characteristic of extracellular water measurements that they show unaccountable, often large, fluctuations during pregnancy.

The theoretical problems involved in the measurement of extracellular water have been discussed above and it was stated that the effect of pregnancy on the behaviour of extracellular water tracers is unknown. That their behaviour may be modified is suggested by the fact that the thiocyanate space, which is normally between 85 and 90 per cent of the bromide space (Goudsmit and Louis, 1942; Fellers *et al.* 1949) is as great as or greater than the bromide space in pregnancy (MacGillivray, unpublished). Little is known about the penetration of these tracers into the uterine contents. Most workers have assumed that thiocyanate, for example, enters the product of conception freely. In fact the thiocyanate level in foetal blood reaches about 80–90 per cent of the maternal blood level after 3 or 4 hours and the level in the liquor amnii reaches only about 50 per cent after equilibration. The extracellular water in the product of conception is therefore systematically underestimated (Hytten and Cheyne, 1962).

With present methods it is difficult to be optimistic about the value of extracellular water measurements in the study of body composition during pregnancy and there is great need for further research.

In Table 11.6 an estimate is made of the additional extracellular water at the end of pregnancy in terms of the components discussed above. It suggests that the added volume is little more than 5 litres, and that the usual methods of measuring extracellular water may overestimate the increment.

We are now in a position to make a final accounting of the weight gained in pregnancy and this is done in Table 11.7.

The final row of figures represents the weight gained during pregnancy which has not been accounted for in the structures we have discussed in these last two chapters. The residual weight gain will now be discussed.

MATERNAL STORES

The mother makes a net gain of about 4 kg (9 lb) which is not in any of the tissues directly concerned with reproduction and which contains no water. We will show that this is almost certainly depot fat. Before discussing the evidence for fat storage it is necessary to dispose of some widely held but misleading notions.

TABLE 11.7. Analysis of Weight Gain

Tissues and fluids accounted for	Increase in weight up to:			
	10 weeks	20 weeks	30 weeks	40 weeks
	g	g	g	g
Foetus	5	300	1500	3300
Placenta	20	170	430	650
Liquor	30	250	600	800
Uterus	135	585	810	900
Mammary gland	34	180	360	405
Blood	100	600	1300	1250
Extracellular extravascular water	0	0	0	1200
Total	324	2085	5000	8505
Total weight gained	650	4000	8500	12500
Weight not accounted for	326	1915	3500	3995

Protein. Almost every authority who has written on the metabolism of pregnancy has accepted that the pregnant woman stores protein. In Marshall's standard work on the Physiology of Reproduction, for example, Newton (1952) states 'There is no doubt that, on an adequate diet, considerable storage of N takes place.' The evidence for this goes back to Hoffström (1910) who, from a continuous nitrogen balance on a woman from the 17th week of pregnancy, found a total accumulation of 109.8 g of nitrogen. Only a part of it could be accounted for in the product of conception and the mother's reproductive organs; what remained was considered to have been 'stored'.

Since Hoffström's pioneer work, bigger and bigger estimates have been made. Wilson (1916) studied 2 women for long periods in pregnancy; one of these was estimated to have accumulated 419 g of nitrogen between the 16th and 35th weeks, the other 336 g between the 24th week and term. Wilson made estimates of the nitrogen content of the product of conception, uterus, breasts and extra maternal blood and concluded that these two women had stored 284 and 211 g of nitrogen outside these specified sites; he could not say where.

A similar picture was described by Coons and others (Coons and Blunt, 1930; Coons and Coons, 1935) but the inflationary trend reached its peak with the massive studies in Detroit by Macy and her co-workers (for example Macy and Hunscher, 1934; Hunscher *et al.* 1935; Hummel *et al.* 1937). A summary paper based on 954 daily balances in pregnant women (Macy and Hunscher, 1934) shows an *average* total accumulation from the 4th to the 10th months of pregnancy of 515 g of nitrogen. This huge total leaves about 370 g after the usual allocations to known sites. More recently, Heller (1955) extrapolating from a number of 4-day balance studies, concluded that the mean storage of N was 140.84 g in the 8th month, 165.66 g in the 9th month and 177.40 g in the 10th month, a total of 483.9 g for the last 3 months of pregnancy.

Generally, the problem of where such a quantity of nitrogen could be put has been avoided. Wilson (1916) admitted this: 'In regard to the place of storage and the form assumed by this nitrogen, it is of course quite impossible to make any positive statement . . .'. The Detroit workers ignored it altogether: 'This surplus must serve as a maternal reserve to take care of the losses encountered during labour and parturition and, in addition, to prepare the maternal body for meeting the physiologic needs of lactation' (Macy and Hunscher, 1934), and in reference to a later study '. . . a maternal reserve of 250 g of nitrogen for future dissipation or enrichment of the maternal body at termination of the reproductive cycle.' (Hunscher *et al.* 1935).

Newton (1952) also avoided the issue, although the work of Poo, Lew and Addis (1939) is quoted as showing N accumulation in the liver and alimentary tract of pregnant rats.

To illustrate the problem, we may consider the more moderate estimates of 250 g of nitrogen stored in the non-reproductive tissues. This represents about 1600 g of dry protein. Storage of protein is thought to be accompanied by storage of associated water. In the liver, where protein can be stored, Kaplan and Chaikoff (1936) found a close relation between protein and water in dogs in a wide range of nutritional states. The ratio of water to protein averaged 4.3 with little variation. If the same ratio holds for other tissues also, then the 1600 g of protein would carry with it about

6900 g of water, giving a total accumulation of about 8500 g (nearly 19 lb). The subject of Hunscher *et al.* (1935) who was estimated to have stored 'a maternal reserve of 250 g of nitrogen' made a total gain in weight during her pregnancy of over one kilogram less than the necessary 8500 g. The average of 370 g nitrogen quoted by Macy and Hunscher in 1934 would give 12.3 kg (about 27 lb) of protein and water. It must be quite clear that estimates of nitrogen storage on this scale are absurd.

It is now recognized that the balance experiment is in general one of the least reliable tools of investigation. Nitrogen balances in animals, except the most recent, have shown the same sort of excess retention as we have here. Not until the results were tested against carcase analysis were the errors recognized. Now it appears that, in addition to errors in analysis, in collection of excreta and recording of intake, there is considerable loss of volatile nitrogen compounds, in particular ammonia. Meticulous attention to detail and collection of all excreta in acid are tedious, but they do give results that check with carcase analysis (Duncan, 1964). We may assume therefore that a large part of the 'stored' protein in recorded balances, in excess over what can be accounted for in maternal gains and the foetus, is likely to be explained in the same way and may be discounted. It is suggestive that the subject studied by Hummel *et al.* (1937) who was in a metabolic ward throughout her balance period of 65 days in late pregnancy stored only 86 g N in that time. That total is not grossly different from our calculated increment of about 60 g for that period. The fact is that the normally nourished body has little capacity for storage of protein (Peters and Van Slyke, 1946).

Allison (1961) discussing the question of protein reserves in general says that there is no storage of protein in discrete compartments, as there is of fat, and that the only reserve protein to be called upon in time of dire need is probably plasma albumin (or a proportion of it), plasma amino acids, and such part of intracellular protein as may normally exchange with the amino acid pool. On that statement if the pregnant woman wished to increase her store of reserve protein she would be expected to raise or at least maintain the concentration of plasma albumin; instead a spectacular decrease occurs early in pregnancy before there is any question of dilution in the increased plasma volume, and the low concentration is maintained with a maximum total increase of about 30 g.

It is generally believed that storage of protein, presumably in excess of measured increases in maternal structures and foetus, occurs in experimental pregnant animals. In default of any convincing quantitative evidence of similar storage for man, we propose to assume that no more protein is laid down than we have accounted for in the foetus and maternal tissues and fluids.

Fat. It seems always to have been recognized, although vaguely, that pregnant women accumulate fat. Zangemeister (1916) in one of the early discussions of the composition of weight gained in pregnancy said that 'about a considerable increase in the fat layer in pregnancy nothing is really known', and Slemons and Fagan (1927) used the accumulation of fat as a threat to prevent their patients gaining what was regarded as excessive weight. It is part of folklore that many women become progressively fatter with childbearing: Sheldon (1949) gives a number of examples, and Karn (1957–58) in an analysis of women's measurements for the Clothing Council found that married women who had borne children were, on the average, heavier than single women of the same age. Almost no quantitative data exist. The only published attempt to measure body fat was made by McCartney, Pottinger and Harrod (1959). They measured body density by weighing under water, and body water with deuterium oxide, in forty pregnant women at different stages of pregnancy; sixteen of them had normal pregnancies. Unfortunately most of the women were measured only once or twice and individual variation in body composition is so great that means of small groups are not necessarily comparable. Table 11.8 shows the estimates of total body fat for the only 2 women who were measured three times in pregnancy. Subject FV had stored 1.1 kg of fat in a total weight gain of 8.25 kg between 15 and 38 weeks;

TABLE 11.8. Total Body Fat
(McCartney, Pottinger and Harrod, 1959)

Subject	Weeks of Pregnancy					
	15–16		30		37–38	
	kg	%	kg	%	kg	%
FV	14	25.4	15.1	23.1	15.1	23.8
KF	18.5	26.5	22.43	29.1	23.44	28.7

KF had stored nearly 5 kg of fat in a total weight gain of 11.87 kg between 16 and 37 weeks. As far as it is possible to say when differences are small and the experimental error likely to be substantial, most of the fat was stored before 30 weeks.

Two other women first measured at 20–21 weeks put on 1.16 and 5.65 kg of fat with weight gains 6.17 and 6.83 kg in the next eleven weeks. Of two others measured at about 30 weeks and again near term one put on 1.8 kg of fat with a total weight gain of 3.85 kg; the other lost nearly 4 kg of fat with a total weight gain of 0.9 kg, while the product of conception would be expected to double its weight.

Obviously, no great reliance can be put on these few figures, but as far as they go they fit the theoretical picture we have derived which showed a storage of about 4 kg of fat before 30 weeks and little gain thereafter.

Seitchik and Alper (1956) made estimates of body fat solely from measurements of body water. They measured body water by dilution of antipyrine and, as we have seen, the method grossly overestimates body water in pregnancy. The seven women in their study apparently gained more water than body weight: only one woman was reckoned to have gained fat, 3.6 kg; the rest lost up to 12.5 kg during the pregnancy. These figures are against all common sense and experience and they can be attributed solely to the distortion by pregnancy of the method for measuring body water.

An index of subcutaneous fat storage can be derived from measurements of skinfold thickness. The method of measuring the thickness of a double fold of skin by calipers which exert a standard pressure is well established, but it seems rarely to have been used in pregnancy. Taggart (1961b and unpublished) has made serial measurements during pregnancy of skinfold thickness at a number of sites in the body. Over the abdomen, the back and the upper thighs there is a progressive increase in skin thickness up to about 30 weeks of pregnancy, after which there is little or no further increase. Over the arms and the lower part of the thigh there is no increase in thickness and in many subjects there is actual loss of skin thickness. Over the abdomen where the gain is greatest, skin thickness increases by about 40 per cent, over the back and upper thighs by about 20–30 per cent. This pattern of distribution may be characteristic of pregnancy.

It is interesting that in an animal experiment in which fat storage in early pregnancy was measured (Beaton, Beare, Ryu and

U

McHenry, 1954) rats gained fat between the 8th and 16th days of pregnancy, but lost it again by the end of pregnancy.

Non-pregnant obese women have been shown by Edwards (1950) to decrease their skinfold thickness proportionately all over the body when they lose weight by dieting, so that a decrease of 50 per cent in abdominal skinfold thickness would be accompanied by a decrease of 50 per cent in the thickness of skinfolds all over the body.

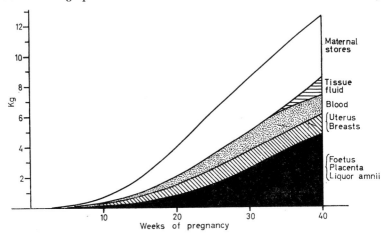

FIGURE 11.3. The components of weight gain in normal pregnancy

There is no way of estimating total body fat from skinfold measurements and, indeed, there is evidence that changes other than fat accumulation may influence the thickness. For example about one third of the increased skinfold thickness in pregnant women is rapidly lost after delivery, and the fall may be due to loss of accumulated water or to regression of the greatly increased blood supply which is characteristic of pregnancy.

There is a great deal more that we should like to know about accumulation of fat in pregnancy, particularly in women who gain much or very little weight, but present methods of measurement are unsatisfactory. A more direct dilution method for the measurement of total body fat is needed.

We have discussed the accumulation of the fat store as if it were pure lipid. Keys, Anderson and Brozek (1955) estimated that the composition of weight gained by 'simple overeating' contained little more than 60 per cent fat; the remainder was extracellular water and cell mass. The weights gained were big; they averaged 10.6 kg over six months and ranged up to 22.3 kg. Entenman *et al.* (1958) have analysed excised subcutaneous adipose tissue before and after weight reduction in obese subjects. In one subject the fat content of the adipose tissue fell from 79.2 per cent to 62.3 per cent in association with a loss of body fat estimated to be about 8 kg; in the second subject the fat of adipose tissue fell from 89.1 to 78.9 per

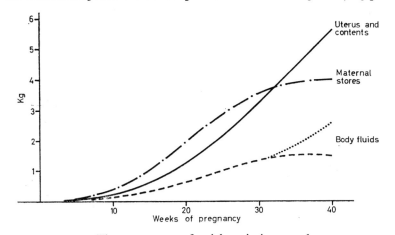

FIGURE 11.4. The components of weight gain in normal pregnancy

cent while about 4.5 kg of fat was lost. As fat was lost from adipose tissue the proportion of water and non-fat solids rose. There is little doubt that the fat cells of adipose tissue are easily capable of storing pure fat in much greater quantities than that stored by the average pregnant woman.

We are now able to account for all the weight gain in pregnancy and Figures 11.3 and 11.4 show the changing pattern. The accumulation of fat is shown separately in Figure 11.4 and it can be seen that it dominates weight gain in the first half of pregnancy. As the product of conception makes its final spurt of growth in the last 10 weeks, maternal storage slows down.

THE PURPOSE OF MATERNAL STORAGE

The obvious role of stored fat in pregnancy is as an energy bank and we will be discussing the whole weight gain in terms of energy later (Chapter 13). It is enough here to say that the store amounts to over 35,000 kcal, almost half the total calorie requirement specific to pregnancy. Our average woman therefore enters the last third of pregnancy with a very considerable buffer against deprivation of food. In Western society, the healthy pregnant woman probably needs no such safety measure, but many, possibly the majority of the world's pregnant women do manual labour until the day they have the baby; in many societies the agriculture of a community may depend upon them. Food may be scarce and in these circumstances the increasing energy demands of late pregnancy can be met in large part from the fat which has been stored in early pregnancy. An interesting example of this mechanism is discussed in Chapter 14.

A further use for the stores which remain at the end of pregnancy is as a subsidy for lactation where energy requirements are considerably greater than those of pregnancy.

THE STIMULUS TO FAT STORAGE

The suggestion has been made (see, for example, the review by Kosterlitz and Campbell, 1957) that progesterone may be important for the storage of early pregnancy. There are no more than straws in the wind from animal experiments (Galletti and Klopper, 1962) but we have seen an example in Aberdeen which supports the suggestion. A primigravida had her body water measured at intervals from the 7th week of pregnancy and weekly measurements were made of pregnanediol and oestriol in urine. Her hormone production is shown in Figure 11.5. At the 27th week she was delivered of a stillborn macerated foetus which did not appear to be more mature than 20 weeks. Oestriol production has been shown by Cassmer (1959) to be governed by foetal metabolism and it is apparent from the oestriol curve, which dropped below the normal line at 12–14 weeks, that the foetus was then abnormal. The placenta, to judge by the pregnanediol excretion, continued normally until 20 weeks when it began to die. Thus the subject was under the influence of high progesterone production, without oestrogen, at least up to 20 weeks. During that time she gained 2.5 kg in weight but her body water fell slightly; at 27 weeks when abortion occurred her weight and body water volume were the same. Allowing for errors of water measurement it is likely that this woman gained no appreciable water and that the 2.5 kg of weight was almost all fat. An increase in skinfold thickness up to 20 weeks, but not thereafter, supports the probability.

The idea that progesterone is antagonized by oestriol in respect of fat storage is entirely speculative, although antagonism has been shown for other functions (Edgren, Elton and Calhoun, 1961). If it were correct, the abrupt rise in oestriol secretion in the last 10 weeks

	9 weeks	19 weeks	27 weeks	9weeks post-partum
Body weight, kg	54·3	56·9	56·9	56·8
Body water, kg	32·0	30·3	31·2	30·9
Dry weight, kg	22·3	26·6	25·7	25·9
Increase in mean skinfold thickness, mm		3·6	2·9	2·9

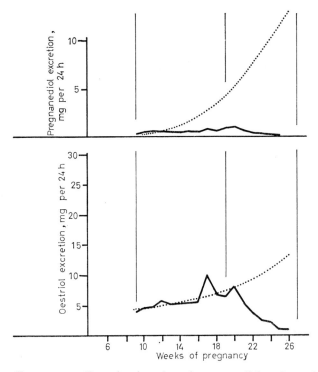

FIGURE 11.5. Excretion in urine of pregnanediol and oestriol in a subject where a normal output of pregnanediol was accompanied by an excessively low output of oestriol. Gain in body weight appears to have been mostly fat.

of pregnancy (see Chapter 6) when progesterone secretion is increasing much more slowly would explain the decrease of fat storage after 30 weeks. The difficulty about postulating any hormonal agent as responsible for fat storage is the fact that when the mother stops accumulating fat, the foetus starts. The idea of a progesterone-oestriol antagonism is nevertheless extremely attractive and, since the foetus controls the output of oestriol it is itself putting the brake on maternal storage at a time when its own requirements for nutrients are increasing rapidly. The ratio of the two hormones may well be different in maternal and foetal blood. Here there is a great field for research.

MINERALS

What has been said above about nitrogen storage in pregnancy can be said also about mineral storage. Estimates based on balance studies are usually very much larger than estimates made by isotope dilution or than can be accounted for in known sites of storage.

We will deal here only with three that have seemed important clinically or nutritionally: sodium, potassium and calcium; iron will be considered later.

Sodium. Two long term balance studies have been published by the Detroit group (Hummel, Sternberger, Hunscher and Macy, 1936; Hummel, Hunscher, Bates, Bonner and Macy, 1937). In the first study a woman in her fourth pregnancy, living at home, stored 81 g (3500 mEq) of sodium between the 135th and 280th day of pregnancy. In the second study a primigravida living in a metabolic ward apparently stored 7.26 g (316 mEq) in the final 65 days of her pregnancy, which is one fifth the rate of the first subject.

Several studies of total exchangeable sodium have been made. Gray and Plentl (1954) estimated exchangeable sodium at intervals during pregnancy in 8 normal women. The average body content was 2289 mEq in early pregnancy and 2816 mEq in late pregnancy, a difference of 527 mEq. Davey, O'Sullivan and Browne (1961) found an increase of about 460 mEq between 16 and 36 weeks, and MacGillivray and Buchanan (1958) found a larger difference of 773 mEq: 2248 mEq in a group of women in early pregnancy compared with 3021 mEq in another group in late pregnancy.

The sodium contents of tissues added to the mother during pregnancy are listed in Table 11.9. Many of these figures are

TABLE 11.9. Storage of Minerals During Pregnancy

	Na	K	Ca
	mEq	mEq	g
Foetus	280	154	28.0
Placenta	57	42	0.65
Liquor amnii	100	3	negligible
Uterus	78	49	0.22
Breasts[1]	35	35	0.06
Plasma	140	4	0.12
Red cells[2]	5	24	0.38
Oedema fluid	155	5	0.15
Total	850	316	29.56

[1] Taken as of average viscera, 200 mg/100 g for Na and K; 15 mg Ca (Documenta Geigy, 1956)
[2] 21 mEq per litre of Na; 95 mEq per litre of K (Documenta Geigy, 1956)

approximations but the total of about 850 mEq is of a similar order to that found by MacGillivray and Buchanan (1958) and in the one balance study of Hummel *et al.* (1937). The widely quoted figure found in the early balance study is presumably a product of technical error.

Potassium. The same story can be told of potassium. The earlier Detroit subject is reputed to have stored 207 g (5300 mEq) in 145 days while the second subject stored at less than one hundredth of that rate: 0.5 g (13 mEq) in 65 days. Neither estimate makes sense.

MacGillivray and Buchanan (1958) estimated exchangeable potassium in their cross-sectional study but unfortunately their subjects in early pregnancy were of low average body weight and it is not easy to make comparisons. Compared to the non-pregnant woman with 2370 mEq of potassium the late pregnancy value of 2541 shows an increase of 171 mEq, but compared to the very early pregnancy group with 1982 mEq the increase is 559 mEq. Estimates shown in Table 11.9 suggest that the average stored may be about 300 mEq.

Calcium. A number of balance studies were made in the 1930s. In

Detroit, Macy, Hunscher, Nims and McCosh (1930) studied 3 women at intervals during pregnancy. The week to week variation in calcium storage ranging from a loss of 1.276 g daily to a gain of 0.278 g daily makes it impossible to draw any conclusion other than that balance studies are difficult. The two later balances indicated gains of 52.9 g between the 135th and 280th days of pregnancy (Hummel *et al.* 1936) and 46.29 g in the last 65 days (Hummel *et al.* 1937).

Coons and Coons (1935) studied one woman during the last 101 days of pregnancy and found average daily gains between 0.098 g and 0.215 g. In 1930 Coons and Blunt decided, on the basis of balance studies of 9 women that the positive calcium balance almost exactly coincided with foetal requirements.

Table 11.9 shows that the calcium increment which can be calculated from known sites of storage is probably under 30 grams; the foetus for which direct analyses are available (see Chapter 12) accounts for almost all of it and the estimate is unlikely to be much in error. From analyses of the skeletons of animals, for instance the ewe (Benzie, Boyne, Dalgarno, Duckworth, Hill and Walker, 1955), it seems to be established that calcium is stored in pregnancy in excess of the needs of the foetus, and in amounts to supply part of the much greater demand of the following lactation. There is every reason to suppose that there will be storage also in human pregnancy but no information to show to what extent. It is impossible even to hazard a guess regarding the possible amount, but it is safe to say that the estimate above will be an underestimate of the amount stored in normal pregnancy.

Altogether it appears that more and better studies of mineral storage are needed. Balance studies are extremely difficult in human subjects and anything less than a most exacting technique, which almost certainly implies residence in a metabolic ward, is likely to give wildly unlikely answers.

CHAPTER 12

The Gross Composition of the
Components of Weight Gain

We intend, in this chapter to deal only with major constituents or those of particular nutritional interest.

THE FOETUS

The analysis of a whole foetus presents considerable technical difficulty and it is surprising that so many analyses have been made. In 1951 Kelly *et al.* published data collected from the literature for 95 foetuses and in the same year Widdowson and Spray (1951) published analyses of 19. All that follows is based on these two papers, with unpublished individual figures kindly supplied by Dr Widdowson for the foetuses in her paper.

The assembled data provide a remarkably consistent pattern of chemical development and the general picture is probably reliable. But we must be cautious about accepting the detail for physiological purposes because many, possibly most, of the foetuses which have been analysed were to some extent abnormal. Ideally, the foetus should have developed normally to within a short time of its death so that, for the early picture, foetuses removed at hysterotomy are likely to be the best material; spontaneous abortions where the foetus may or may not have suffered some nutritional deprivation before death are less satisfactory. For larger, viable infants, the best one can hope for is a history of sudden death from a condition which is unlikely, as far as can be known, to have interfered with normal development. For example, of the six infants of over 3000 g in Widdowson and Spray's series only two came within this category with histories, one of presumably traumatic death associated with breech delivery and one probably quick death associated with placenta praevia. But of the other four, one was hydrocephalic and therefore had a gross anatomical abnormality, one died following eclampsia in the mother and the cause of death in two was 'unknown'. Many babies who die for obscure reasons at term are believed to have suffered from some 'placental insufficiency' and if so, then their chemical development is not necessarily normal. [Compare what was said of the growth of the foetus, Chapter 10, pp. 233-236].

WATER

The water content of the foetus falls throughout its development (Figure 12.1). In the smallest foetuses, of under 10 g weight, water content is between 92 and 94 per cent. It falls to about 90 per cent for a 100 g foetus and to 82 to 84 per cent at 1000 g. The decline is less rapid in the later stages of development and for the term foetus of 3000 to 3500 g the mean water content is between 70 and 72 per cent. We have fitted the following regression equation to the published data for foetal weights between 100 g and 4000 g.

Water, per cent $= 90.3094 - 8.1911\,w + 0.7936\,w^2$

where w = weight in kg.

FAT

Figure 12.1 contrasts the fat content with the water content. The values are for percentage of body fat in 42 foetuses from the collection made by Kelly et al. and 16 from Widdowson and Spray. Up to the weight of about 500 g the proportion of fat in the body remains approximately constant at between 0.5 and 1.0 per cent of body weight; this is presumably structural fat. Beyond that weight there is an increasing proportion of fat in the body as depot fat is accumulated. The rise of fat content is particularly steep as the baby nears term, and there is great individual variation. Clinically it is obvious that big babies at term have a lot of body fat but there are few analyses. There were only three foetuses of over 3000 g in the collection made by Kelly et al. the largest 3348 g. Widdowson and Spray added six more and one of these was above 4000 g. That one baby, a hydrocephalic of 4375 g had 1238 g of fat; the next highest amounts of body fat were 573 g and 555 g in babies of 3767 and 3994 g. The upper end of the curve must therefore be in doubt; body fat is undoubtedly increasing quickly but it is doubtful whether anything much above 600 g could be considered normal in our sense.

Fat seems to be the most variable of the body components. For example, four of the foetuses with body weights between 3048 and 3105 g contained amounts of fat varying from 341 to 479 g and

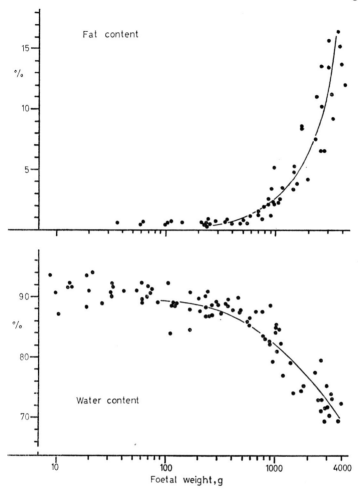

FIGURE 12.1. Fat and water content of the foetus. From the data of
Kelly *et al.* (1951) and Widdowson and Spray (1951)

three foetuses between 2616 and 2683 g in weight contained from
177 to 358 g of fat. We have no means of knowing how much of this
variation is 'normal' and how much may have been contributed by
interference with nutrition *in utero*. It is likely that the proportion of
fat may be more closely related to maturity than to weight itself
but there are no data available to test the point.

A regression line fitted by us to the data for body fat content gives the formula:

Log fat content (g per kg body weight) $= -2.7462 + 1.3870$ W where $W = $ log body weight in grams.

NITROGEN : PROTEIN

Protein, as such, has not been measured in the foetus and all published figures are derived from estimates of nitrogen. It is surprising, when the accurate measurement of nitrogen is a relatively simple chemical procedure, that nitrogen was measured in so few of the foetuses analysed. Estimates for 16 of the Widdowson and Spray series and 23 of the bigger collection by Kelly *et al.* are plotted against body weight in Figure 12.2. The two sets of data are in complete agreement and the calculated regression line for foetuses over about 500 g is sigmoid, not as Widdowson and Spray suggested a straight line.

The sigmoid shape was to be expected. The first inflexion occurs between the foetal weights of 500 and 1000 g, at which stage there is a rapid decrease of body water content but no great increase of

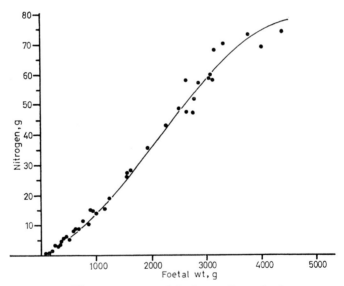

FIGURE 12.2. Nitrogen content of the foetus. From the data of Kelly *et al.* (1951) and Widdowson and Spray (1951)

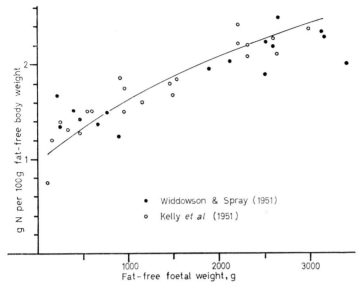

FIGURE 12.3. Nitrogen content of the fat-free foetal body

body fat. There seems to be a condensation of protoplasm here which continues throughout development. In Figure 12.3 the nitrogen content of the fat-free body is shown to increase continuously from about 1 per cent for the smallest foetuses to almost 2.5 per cent for the biggest.

The decrease in slope (Figure 12.2) occurring gradually above a foetal weight of 3000 g is due to the rapidly increasing proportion of body fat, which exceeds the increase of nitrogen content.

It has been customary to convert nitrogen to protein by multiplication with the factor 6.25. The assumption that the average protein contains 16 per cent of nitrogen is a useful simplification which has been widely applied to food proteins. But the foetus contains an enormous variety of N-containing substances which include a considerable proportion of scleroproteins, such as collagen with a low N-content. From the published analyses, when the fat and total ash are deducted from the total dry weight, the remaining dry weight contains between 13 and 15 per cent of nitrogen. It is true that some of the dry weight will be carbohydrate, but a rough estimate from figures in Shelley's (1961) review suggests that the carbohydrate is unlikely to exceed 50 g and, until better evidence is available, we can accept that the nitrogen content of 'average' foetal body protein is more nearly 15 per cent than 16 per cent. The use of any single factor for such a conglomeration of N-containing compounds gives an answer which is bound to be inaccurate in terms of protein, but for what it is worth 6.7 is nearer the truth than 6.25.

ASH

The total ash is of little interest in itself except to make the picture of changing body composition complete. It rises, with considerable individual variation, from about 5 g in a 300 g foetus to about 40 g in a 1500 g foetus and about 85 g in a term foetus of 3300 g.

Many constituents of the ash have been separately estimated; they include calcium, magnesium, sodium, potassium, phosphorus, chlorine, iron, copper, zinc and iodine. We propose to examine only a few of these.

Calcium. The relation to body weight is almost linear. There is little more than 1 g in a foetus of 300 g, about 10 g in a foetus of 1500 g and about 28 g in a term foetus of 3300 g. With increasing calcification of the skeleton, as well as growth, the concentration of calcium in the body increases progressively from under 2 g per kg for the smallest foetuses to over 8 g per kg at term.

Leitch and Aitken (1959) estimated the regression of calcium content on weight from a scatter diagram of the six foetuses of more than 3000 g weight in the array of Widdowson and Spray, term infants in the collected series of Hamilton and Moriarty (1929) and one term infant analysed by Iob and Swanson (1934). The calcium contents of infants of 3300 and 3500 g were judged to be 27.3 and 28.5 g. We will use the convenient figure of 28 g.

Sodium. For sodium and potassium the estimates of Widdowson and Spray are above earlier estimates and what follows is based on their material. All published analyses were made before the introduction of modern flame-photometric methods and we have no means of knowing which figures are more reliable. The sodium content of the foetus rises progressively to about 6 or 7 g at term. There is a smooth increase with weight since the sodium concentration per 100 g of fat-free tissue remains almost constant at 230–240 mg during most of foetal development. Constancy is maintained by changing the distribution of sodium; there is a relative fall of the sodium contained in extracellular water as the water content of the foetus falls, counterbalanced by an increasing deposit of sodium in the calcifying skeleton. The total sodium in the foetus at term is not equivalent to the total 'exchangeable' sodium of the living infant. Of the sodium built into the skeleton, possibly as much as 30 per cent is not in a dissociated form and will not be measured by dilution techniques.

Potassium. The potassium content also rises smoothly with foetal growth, to a level of about 6 g at term. The concentration per 100 g of fat-free tissue also rises throughout development, from 160–170 mg in the smallest foetuses up to 200–210 mg at term. Potassium is mostly intracellular and its increased concentration in the body reflects cell growth. Potassium is almost entirely 'exchangeable' and measurements by dilution methods of potassium in the living infant should be comparable with measurements by direct analysis of the dead foetus.

Iron. The analyses of Widdowson and Spray show great variation in the total iron content of the term foetus. For the six foetuses weighing more than 3000 g the total iron content ranged from 200 mg in a foetus weighing 3994 g to 374 mg in a foetus weighing 3767 g. It seems that the earlier estimates, 400 to 600 mg by Garry and Stiven (1935–36) and 400 mg by Fullerton (1937) for example, may have been too high.

We have no information about what might cause the variation of iron content in the foetus. There has been a deal of speculation about the possibility that iron deficiency in the mother might hinder iron storage in the foetus, but the evidence is poor. There is much room for research into iron metabolism in pregnancy.

THE PLACENTA

Despite the fact that the placenta is probably the most readily available of all normal organs it has seldom been analysed. Fortunately, at least for the major components there is a close agreement in the analyses that have been made. From published accounts it is seldom clear just what has been analysed. We have already explained, in relation to the weight of the placenta, that the afterbirth will have maternal decidual tissue and clotted maternal blood trapped between the villi, and that the amount of foetal blood in the placental vessels will depend on the technique of tying the cord. Some investigators have washed the placenta before analysing it, which will get rid of some or most of the maternal residues, but no washing, not even perfusion, will remove all the blood in the foetal vessels. The main effect will be to increase the water content of the placenta itself. The umbilical cord is usually removed before the placenta is analysed, which is a pity, but does not make a great deal of difference.

WATER

The water content of several hundred term placentae analysed in Aberdeen (Hytten, unpublished) was almost invariably within 1 or 2 per cent of 83 per cent, which is similar to the average found by Mischel (1957–58a) and McKay *et al.* (1958) but below the averages given by Pratt *et al.* (1946a) and Widdowson and Spray of about 85 or 86 per cent. The difference is small but probably real, because of the very narrow range of values found in our series, and could easily result from difference in timing of tying the cord.

Pratt *et al.* rinsed their placentae in distilled water and as would be expected, the water content is high; two of these placentae with 92 per cent and 94 per cent of water are well outside the limits of anything we have seen (see Figure 12.4).

There is a suggestion in both Mischel's and Widdowson and Spray's data that the smaller and less mature placentae have a higher water content, which is confirmed by McKay *et al.* (1958), who found the mean in a few placentae before 20 weeks of pregnancy to be about 90 per cent. There are not sufficient data for us to plot the developmental trend, but 90 per cent up to 20 weeks, 85 per cent at 30 weeks and 83 per cent at term can be accepted tentatively as a fair approximation. It is of interest that the final water content is similar to that of foetal fat-free tissue. For example the nine foetuses above 3000 g weight in the two series of Kelly *et al.* and Widdowson and Spray had a mean water content of about 82.5 per cent of the lean tissue with a narrow range from 81.5 to 83.9 per cent.

NITROGEN:PROTEIN

Figure 12.4 shows the remarkably close relation of total placental nitrogen to placental weight for 159 placentae. These are mostly unpublished Aberdeen data but include also those of Widdowson and Spray, and Pratt *et al.* The regression indicates a constant proportion of about 2.3 g N per 100 g of placenta, at least for placentae

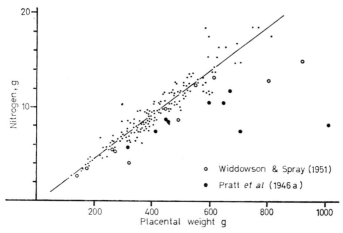

FIGURE 12.4. Nitrogen content of the placenta. Unpublished Aberdeen data with data published by Pratt *et al.* (1946a) and Widdowson and Spray (1951)

of more than about 200 g weight. Below that weight water content is high and the nitrogen content may be less than 1.5 per cent. The same arguments can be applied to the conversion of N to protein as presented on p. 305 for foetal nitrogen. There is always a considerable discrepancy in the dry weight when the factor 6.25 is used to convert N to protein. If we assume a round value of 2 per cent of placental weight to account for ash, fat and glycogen (see below) then 2.3 g of N is equivalent to 15 g of protein, giving a conversion factor of about 6.5.

LIPID

The placenta contains very little lipid and in remarkably constant proportion. Of the twenty-one analyses made by Widdowson and Spray and Pratt *et al.* (1946b), 13 gave between 0.5 and 0.7 per cent; the overall range was from 0.24 to 1.0 per cent. An average of about 0.60 per cent can be accepted with confidence.

GLYCOGEN

Glycogen has been estimated in placentae by Szendi (1934) who published only a graph of his results. The very early placenta, about the first two months, contains per 100 g about 500 mg glycogen. There is a rapid fall in concentration during the third and

X

fourth months to about 150 mg and the average amount at term is of the order of 100 mg.

ASH

The total ash content of term placentae probably averages about 1 per cent but is immensely variable because of differences in calcium content. Mischel (1957–58a) has shown a steady rise from about 0.5 per cent at 2 months.

Calcium. Areas of calcification occur so frequently in the mature placenta that it is difficult to arrive at an average value for calcium content which has much meaning. Masters and Clayton (1940) found that in 21 placentae delivered more than 2 weeks before term the average calcium content was about 30 mg per 100 g with a range of from 7 to 76; in 24 placentae delivered within 2 weeks of term the mean was 98 with a range of 14 to 510, and in 16 placentae delivered more than 14 days after term a mean of 123 with a range of 28 to 404.

Mischel (1957–58c) found a mean content of 86.4 mg per 100 g in 30 term placentae. In Widdowson and Spray's small series all the placentae up to 32 weeks had contents per 100 g under 30 mg, one at 34 weeks had 151.5 mg and three near term from 27 to 48. McKay *et al.* show their results only in a graph. While most of the values seem to be within the range found by other workers, one placenta at term had a calcium content of almost 300 mg per g of dry weight. This is equivalent to about 5 per cent in fresh placenta and such a highly exceptional figure would represent a total of about 25 g of calcium in a placenta of average size.

It is clearly impossible to give a neat conclusion from this range of results. The best we can do is to give representative figures which will be useful for future calculations per 100 g: 25 mg up to mid-pregnancy, 30 mg at 30 weeks and 100 mg at term.

Sodium. Widdowson and Spray found the sodium content per 100 g to be about 250 mg in early placentae and about 200 mg at term. These estimates must include a proportion of sodium contained in trapped blood and the high water content of these placentae suggests that trapped blood may have had a considerable influence on the results. Mischel (1957–58b), who corrected for contained blood, found the Na content per 100 g of the placenta itself to fall from about 140 mg in early pregnancy to about 100 mg at term.

Potassium. Only Widdowson and Spray have published estimates of potassium. The results are variable but lie for all stages of pregnancy between 120 and 190 mg per 100 g. Although the presence of blood is likely to have a much smaller effect on the K than on the Na content, it is difficult to know what significance can be attached to these figures.

Iron. Mischel (1957–58d) found the mean total Fe content of 29 term placentae to be 11.1 mg per 100 g; in the blood-free organ it was 4.15 mg per 100 g. Estimates for early stages of development were lower. Up to about 30 weeks the mean total iron content was about 6 mg per 100 g of fresh placenta. The estimate of non-haemoglobin iron, which varied from 5.25 mg for one placenta at 2 months to a mean of 0.8 mg for 3 placentae at 5 months seems unlikely to be reliable and suggests a technical error.

McCoy, Bleiler and Ohlson (1961) estimated the iron content of 46 placentae and cords which contained the foetal blood left when the cord was ligated after pulsation had ceased. Their mean placental weight was 560 g and the mean iron content 75.7 mg, with a range of 34.5 to 170 mg.

A graph in the paper by McKay *et al.* suggests that the non-haemoglobin iron in placentae from the first half of pregnancy is variable, ranging from under 20 to more than 200 μg per g dry weight (equivalent to 0.2 to 2.0 mg per 100 g total weight) and falling to a mean of about 60 μg per g dry weight (about 1 mg per 100 g total weight) with a much smaller range of variation near term.

McKay *et al.* suggests on slender evidence that there is a rise in mid-pregnancy. A fall in mid-pregnancy was claimed by Mischel. Estimation of iron is notoriously subject to error because of contamination and we have no means of knowing how to choose between these two estimates. From the nutritional point of view, and it is only in this context that we will be considering iron, the recent figure of 75 mg for the placenta and its blood is likely to be a safe one.

LIQUOR AMNII

The puzzle of where and how liquor amnii is formed has inspired a great many chemists to estimate a great many substances in it; the relevance and meaning of much of the work is not clear and we do not propose to explore the composition in detail. A fairly comprehensive list of results is given in a review by Hanon (1957) and the following estimates are mostly taken from it. They have been confirmed by unpublished analyses in Aberdeen.

Liquor amnii is about 99 per cent water. Protein accounts for about 0.25 per cent and its protein pattern suggests that it is a dialysate of maternal serum protein (Abbas and Tovey, 1960). There is about 0.05 per cent total fat and about 0.03 per cent sugar. The sodium content of liquor is a little below maternal serum level at about 125 mEq per litre and potassium is a little above at about 4 mEq per litre (Battaglia *et al.* 1959). The amounts of calcium and iron are negligible.

THE PRODUCT OF CONCEPTION

At this point it may be useful to reduce this mass of data to a more assimilable form. It is obvious that all the material we have been able to find is less than ideal and the deductions we have made from it can be regarded only as tentative. Any rounding off of averages in the summary which follows is in the interests of simplicity and such adjustments as we make are well inside the limits of confidence in the final figure.

The average analyses below refer to the product of conception at 10, 20, 30 and 40 weeks and for the average weights of components as given in Chapters 10 and 11.

PROTEIN

Table 12.1 shows the mean protein contents. For the foetus and placenta protein is calculated by multiplying the nitrogen content by 6.70; for liquor amnii the factor used is 6.25.

FAT

At 10 weeks the fat content of the product of conception is negligible. From mid-pregnancy the averages are as shown in Table 12.2.

CALCIUM

From the nutritional viewpoint calcium and iron are the two most important minerals, or at all events they are the only two commonly discussed in terms of dietary deficiency. The accumulation of calcium in the product of conception is shown in Table 12.3.

TABLE 12.1. Protein in the Product of Conception

	Weeks of Pregnancy			
	10	20	30	40
Foetus	g 0.3	g 27	g 160	g 435
Placenta	2	16	60	100
Liquor	0.08	0.5	2	3
Total	2	44	222	538

TABLE 12.2. Fat in the Product of Conception

	Weeks of Pregnancy		
	20	30	40
Foetus	g 2	g 80	g 430
Placenta	1	3	4
Liquor	0.1	0.4	0.5
Total	3	83	435

TABLE 12.3. Calcium in the Product of Conception

	Weeks of Pregnancy			
	10	20	30	40
Foetus	Negligible	g 1.5	g 10	g 28
Placenta	Negligible	0.05	0.13	0.65
Liquor		Negligible		
Total	Negligible	1.5	10	29

IRON

There are not sufficient data for us to construct a table for a developmental trend in iron content of the product of conception. The greatest amount of iron found in a term foetus by Widdowson and Spray was 374 mg and an estimate of the placental iron, including that in its contained blood, is 75 mg. Altogether a total of 450 mg provides a safe basis for calculation of requirements.

THE MATERNAL COMPONENTS OF THE PREGNANCY WEIGHT GAIN

Uterus

We can find almost no published information about the chemical composition of the uterus. Hawkins and Nixon (1958) in a study of uterine electrolytes measured the water content of biopsy samples of muscle taken at hysterotomy from nine subjects between 10 and 20 weeks of pregnancy and from a number of subjects during caesarean section at or a little before term. They found an average water content of about 83 per cent for both groups and stated that the fat content of their samples was generally less than 0.5 per cent.

Slemons (1914) reported the analysis of a uterus weighing 850 g removed at caesarean section. It had a water content of 70 per cent and contained 38.75 g of nitrogen, about 4.6 g N per 100 g.

We ourselves have been able to analyse nine whole uteri removed at term and twelve others removed between 9 and 18 weeks of pregnancy. The water contents were in a narrow range between 80 and 84 per cent with a mean value closely similar to that of Hawkins and Nixon. The fat contents were almost all below 0.5 per cent, average about 0.4 per cent. All uteri had total nitrogen contents close to 2.4 per cent. With the factor 6.25 the protein content is 15 per cent. The contents of water, fat and protein should add up to almost 100 per cent of the weight and it is probable, again, that the protein factor is too low. The considerable quantity of connective tissue in the uterus makes this likely. A nitrogen content for total uterine protein of between 14 and 15 per cent would raise the protein to a more likely content of 16.5 per cent. We cannot explain Slemons's curious finding which is so grossly out of line with our own analyses and indeed with the composition of any other muscle tissue.

For the purposes of future calculations, the following estimate of gross percentage composition of the uterus is likely to be near the truth for all stages of pregnancy: water 83, protein 16.6 and fat 0.4.

But as we have already said, about 10 per cent of the gross weight of the uterus is contained blood. The composition of the added maternal blood is to be treated separately so that to avoid double counting we must consider here only the blood-free uterus. The adjustment is a small one and the final percentage composition of blood-free uterus becomes: water 82.5, protein 17.1 and fat 0.4.

Hawkins and Nixon (1958) estimated the electrolyte content of the uterus. At term the values given in mEq per 100 g dry weight were: Na 48.3, K 30.4 and Ca 6.7.

Breasts

For the composition of the breast tissue added in pregnancy we have nothing but our imagination to guide us.

We have suggested that the increase in subcutaneous fat is likely to be negligible. Here we are concerned only with the blood-free glandular tissue which, for both breasts at the end of prgenancy, may be estimated as 405 g (see p. 272). Pancreas, another largely glandular tissue, has a water content of about 75 per cent, a protein content of about 20 per cent and a fat content of about 3 per cent (Documenta Geigy, 1956). Breast tissue is probably not grossly different and until we have some better information we will adopt these figures for breast tissue.

The accumulation of protein and fat in the uterine and breast tissue is summarized in Tables 12.4 and 12.5.

TABLE 12.4. Protein in the Added Uterine and Breast Tissue

	Weeks of pregnancy			
	10	20	30	40
Blood-free uterus	g 23	g 100	g 139	g 154
Blood-free mammary gland	9	36	72	81
Total	32	136	211	235

TABLE 12.5. Fat in the Added Uterine and Breast Tissue

	Weeks of pregnancy			
	10	20	30	40
	g	g	g	g
Blood-free uterus	0.5	2.3	3.2	3.6
Blood-free mammary gland	1.4	5.4	10.8	12.2
Total	1.9	7.7	14.0	15.8

Maternal blood

For present purposes we will summarize only the water, protein and fat contents. Plasma composition has been treated more fully in Chapter 1.

PLASMA (Serum)

Analyses are made sometimes on plasma, sometimes on serum. It is possible only to make a composite statement.

The water content of plasma is slightly above normal during pregnancy (Paaby, 1959, 1960). It rises irregularly and with considerable individual variation from about 91.5 per cent in early pregnancy to 92–92.5 per cent in late pregnancy. We will use the round figure of 92 per cent.

It is generally agreed that the protein content of the serum falls during pregnancy (Chapter 1). For the purposes of our calculations we will take 6.6, 6.2, 6.2 and 6.5 g per 100 ml for 10, 20, 30 and 40 weeks of pregnancy.

There are more marked changes in the fat content of the serum. According to de Alvarez et al. (1959) there is no real change from a normal level of 700 mg per 100 ml until after mid-pregnancy when the fat content in mg per 100 ml rises steeply, reaching about 950 at 30 weeks and about 1050 at term.

RED CELLS

The water content of red cells is given as 65 per cent in Geigy's Tables (Documenta Geigy, 1956). Most of the solid must be protein since haemoglobin accounts for about 33 g in every 100 ml of red cells. The fat content is negligible and for the gross composi-

TABLE 12.6. The Increase in Circulating Protein Due to the Expanded Blood Volume

	Weeks of pregnancy			
	10	20	30	40
	g	g	g	g
Plasma	0	13	51	52
Red cells	0	17	51	85
Total	0	30	102	137

TABLE 12.7. The Increase in Circulating Fat due to the Expanded Plasma Volume

Weeks of pregnancy			
10	20	30	40
g	g	g	g
0.4	3.9	17.4	19.6

TABLE 12.8. The Components of Protein Storage in Pregnancy

	Weeks of pregnancy			
	10	20	30	40
	g	g	g	g
Foetus	0.3	27	160	435
Placenta	2	16	60	100
Liquor	0	0.5	2	3
Uterus	23	100	139	154
Breasts	9	36	72	81
Blood	0	30	102	137
Total	35	210	535	910

TABLE 12.9. The Components of Fat Storage in Pregnancy

	Weeks of pregnancy			
	10	20	30	40
Foetus	g negligible	g 2	g 80	g 430
Placenta	negligible	1	3	4
Uterus	0.5	2.3	3.2	3.6
Breasts	1.4	5.4	10.8	12.2
Plasma	0.4	3.9	17.4	19.6
Maternal Stores	365	1915	3500	3995
Total	367	1930	3613	4464

tion a round value of 34 g of protein per 100 g of red cells is close enough. The increase in haemoglobin has been considered in Chapter 1.

Table 12.6 shows the increment of protein in the mother's circulating blood due to the expanded blood volume and Table 12.7 the increment of fat in the increased plasma volume.

The total increments of protein and fat which will form the basis of the discussion of requirements for protein and energy in Chapter 13 are shown in Tables 12.8 and 12.9.

Adaptations of Metabolism and Nutrient Requirements

Much of what will be said in this chapter is based on observations and computations described in earlier chapters; in particular data on the volume and composition of the blood (Chapter 1) and on the components of weight gain and their composition (Chapters 10, 11 and 12) will be used.

It is necessary to begin by considering some peculiarities of metabolism in pregnancy that seem to be essential to the satisfactory nutrition of the foetus and, to some extent, affect the pattern of requirements. Then calculations will be made of nutritional requirements arising from the growth of the product of conception and changes in the composition of the maternal body, such as we have ourselves measured. To these will be added observations on requirements of some other nutrients for which estimates have been made elsewhere. Finally, representative records of the food consumption of pregnant women in different regions and social spheres will be summarized and compared with standard allowances proposed by official authorities.

ADAPTATIONS OF METABOLISM IN PREGNANCY

It is generally accepted that metabolism in normal pregnancy is anabolic. Not only are extra materials acquired and retained in the product of conception, but certain additions are made to maternal tissues. Pregnancy is a period of gain. The idea is clear, simple and appropriate in terms of balance sheets; not so easy to interpret in terms of metabolic processes. The idea of anabolism implies that there is a change, favouring absorption, retention and construction of tissues. But the usual processes of catabolism do go on, and interpretation of the term anabolism requires answers to two questions: is there a change of balance favouring retention and, if so, how is it obtained?

A change from equilibrium, characteristic of the non-pregnant adult, might be achieved in a number of different ways, singly or together. First, absorption might be improved.

Absorption

In respect of absorption from the gut, the main nutrients fall into two groups. For instance, sodium and potassium, chlorine, iodine and fluorine, when they are liberated by digestion, pass freely into the body. Sugars also are freely absorbed, though possibly with some difference in rates of absorption. They need not be further discussed here. It is otherwise with 'protein' (by which is meant the digestion products of protein), calcium, phosphorus, magnesium and iron. Absorption from the gut depends in the first place on the nature of the food eaten. Digestion is less easy and percentage absorption is less from foods with a high percentage of fibre. Absorption depends also on the pH of the contents of the small intestine and on the presence or absence of adjuvant or interfering substances which form soluble or insoluble complexes with the components to be absorbed. It is unlikely that pregnancy could have any effect on the purely physico-chemical side of digestion and absorption. On the other hand, it might well affect the production of digestive enzymes. The evidence set out in Chapter 5 is that the secretory activity of the stomach is not enhanced, but reduced.

The first control over absorption from the intestine is exerted at the gut surface. Absorption depends closely on demand, as is amply demonstrated in deprivation-rehabilitation experiments and in growth studies after treatment of disorders of absorption, such as coeliac disease (Prader, Tanner and Harnack, 1963). In so far as demand controls absorption, pregnancy would be expected to improve absorption, but it is not easy to demonstrate that it does.

If the diet before pregnancy was adequate in, say, protein or calcium, then an increase in quantity of food eaten would not, of itself, 'improve' absorption in the sense of raising the percentage absorbed. On the other hand, the increase of demand in pregnancy might produce a rise of percentage absorbed if there was little or no increase of food eaten. It is unfortunate that balance experiments on pregnant women have not been so planned as to show whether capacity to absorb is changed; almost all such experiments have been made with intakes so high that percentage absorption tended to fall. The question was discussed in Chapter 5 and the case was described of the woman with only 3 feet of small intestine who had two successful pregnancies. There can be no doubt in that case of a great increase of total absorption, or of a true increase of absorption per unit of gut surface. But, because there was a large increase of food eaten, it can not be said with certainty whether the percentage absorbed of digested food rose, or the total increase was due to the greater concentration of products of digestion in the gut, or both changes occurred.

The second possible means to establish an anabolic balance is by improving the use made of absorbed nutrients.

Use of absorbed nutrients

Better use of absorbed amino acids or sugar, for example, might imply faster removal from the mother's bloodstream to her tissues, or the tissues of the foetus, so that less would be lost through the kidney. The evidence is directly opposed to such an idea. Sugar tolerance tests show a 'lag' curve with delayed return to normal, explained in part at least by reduced sensitivity to insulin. Not only so, but glomerular filtration rate is raised (as explained in Chapter 4), so that filtered glucose may exceed the capacity of the tubules to reabsorb, and glucose spills over into the urine.

Amino acids too are lost, not because improved absorption from the gut has raised the concentration of free amino acids in blood, but in spite of the low concentration of amino acids in blood. Table 13.1, abbreviated from Christensen *et al.* (1957) shows, for 3 non-pregnant women and 3 in the third or fourth month of pregnancy, the concentration in plasma, loss in urine computed to mg per 24 hr, and renal clearance of 8 essential amino acids out of the total of 19 measured. With the sole exception of *iso*leucine (and asparagine, of the 11 not reproduced) renal clearance and loss in urine by pregnant women were greater by up to 4 times than in non-pregnant controls, with a total loss for those measured of about a gram a day.

The work was done on only three pregnant women, one convalescent from hyperemesis, one with recently threatened abortion and the third with fibroids. It would be important to confirm the analysis on normal women at all stages of pregnancy. As far as it goes, it confirms earlier work by Wallraff *et al.* (1950) who found a significantly greater loss of 7 of 14 free amino acids tested. The ratios of loss by pregnant women to that by the non-pregnant for

TABLE 13.1. Amino Acids in Blood Plasma and Urine (Adapted from Christensen et al. 1957)

Amino acid	In plasma: μg/ml		In urine: mg/24 hr		Renal clearance: mg/min/1.73 m²		
	Non-pregnant	Pregnant	Non-pregnant	Pregnant	Non-pregnant	Pregnant	Ratio
Threonine	15.7	18.2	1.88	48	0.8	1.8	2.3
Glycine	31.9	9.5	18.3	220	4.5	16.6	3.7
Methionine	3.7	2.6	5.2	9.1	1.1	2.4	2.2
Isoleucine	7.4	6.4	13.1	10.4	1.4	1.2	0.9
Leucine	13.2	11.7	5.4	8.9	0.3	0.6	2.0
Tyrosine	7.7	4.7	10.5	18.4	1.1	2.8	2.5
Phenylalanine	7.9	6.2	8.5	8.8	0.8	1.0	1.2
Lysine	20.4	19.9	8.8	36.5	0.3	1.3	4.3

the 7 amino acids lost in excess were: histidine 3.3, tyrosine 2.3, arginine 1.6, phenylalanine 1.6, serine 2.9, threonine 8.0 and tryptophan 2.7. The pattern of loss of amino acids in pregnancy, as shown in those studies is quite different from that recorded by Cusworth and Dent (1960) in chronic renal failure and a number of other conditions associated with loss of amino acids in urine. We may conclude that the spillage of amino acids in pregnancy is not due to any disability of the kidney, but is part of the normal adaptation of metabolism. Page *et al.* (1954) from a study of histidine in urine in pregnancy, ascribed one-half of the excess loss to increase of glomerular filtration rate, one-fourth to reduction of tubular reabsorption and one-fourth to failure of removal from the blood to maternal intracellular space.

The meaning of changes in composition of the blood

The carrying capacity of maternal blood is raised by increase of volume. The level of components in the expanded volume is not simply the result of dilution. Of some, the concentration is less but the total carried is more. For instance, there is more haemoglobin in circulation and the total is adjusted with some precision to the increased demand for oxygen. Not all components of blood conform to one pattern. The concentration of ionised calcium for example must be maintained within very narrow limits, in pregnancy as in the non-pregnant. The total carried in blood therefore becomes greater in proportion to increase of blood volume, but there is no change in the pressure-head. The implication is that the control of absorption of calcium by demand, in the first place, and the minute-by-minute regulation of plasma ionised calcium level by the sensitive reaction of the parathyroid gland to that level, are so intimately adjusted at all times that there is no need for change. Since calcification of the foetal skeleton is progressive from the beginning of the third month, it may be taken that the foetal parathyroid is active from then also.

A third, entirely different, pattern is shown by blood copper. Both free copper and copper bound in coeruloplasmin show a continuous slow rise throughout pregnancy (Humoller *et al.* 1960; Johnson, 1961). One of the functions of copper is to keep stores of iron mobile so that they can be used for formation of haemoglobin when erythrocytes have to be replaced, or the supply increased. The rise of plasma copper in pregnancy may be to prevent the immobilization of maternal stores and ensure greater and more prolonged mobility, for the benefit of the foetus.

It seems possible that the nature of the change in level of inorganic components of the blood is closely related to function. The loss of iodine in urine was discussed in Chapter 4.

Metabolism of vitamins

There is not much evidence on which to judge the pattern, or patterns, of change in metabolism of the vitamins in pregnancy. We may speculate that the metabolism of vitamin D will undergo little change because it is so intimately related to absorption of calcium and calcification of bone (Leitch, 1964). Bro-Rasmussen (1958) regards the metabolism of riboflavin as closely related to that of protein, and so to energy metabolism, as is also the metabolism of thiamine, nicotinic acid and pyridoxine. About the metabolism of most other vitamins in pregnancy there is little information. There are important studies, of vitamin B_{12} and folic acid, arising from the function of those vitamins in blood formation and the occasional occurrence of megaloblastic anaemia in pregnancy.

Hellegers *et al.* (1957) describe an oral load test on pregnant and non-pregnant women with vitamin B_{12}. When 1000 μg was given the peak level in serum was half as great again in the pregnant as in the non-pregnant. The result was interpreted to mean greater absorption by the pregnant. It might equally well mean slow removal from maternal serum, a view that is supported by the parallel study in rats with labelled vitamin B_{12} in which 60 per cent of the injected vitamin was found in the foetuses, and pregnant rats had much less activity in livers and kidneys than non-pregnant controls. Since the concentration of vitamin B_{12} in serum is less in pregnant than in non-pregnant women, vitamin B_{12} metabolism changes in much the same way as metabolism of amino acids (Killander, 1957; Sadovsky *et al.* 1959).

In a series of studies of megaloblastic anamia in pregnancy the evidence of Thompson (1957) and Giles and Shuttleworth (1958) suggests a relation to the poverty of industrial workers living in municipal housing estates, with diets that had little green vegetable. Folic acid was curative. Forshaw *et al.* (1957) in their study thought that a defect of folic acid metabolism might be involved since megaloblastic anaemia recurred in some of the patients in a second pregnancy. Such a recurrence might, of course, be due to repetition of the same type of diet, but there are now two investigations of folic acid metabolism in pregnancy which offer another and more satisfactory explanation. Chanarin *et al.* (1959) estimated the rate of disappearance of folic acid from the blood, after intravenous injection, in 250 pregnant women grouped by stage of gestation at 3-week intervals. A similar study was made by Hansen and Klewesahl-Palm (1963) on 86 pregnant women, with 20 non-pregnant controls. The two studies are in perfect agreement and the results are shown in Figure 13.1. The non-pregnant women had a

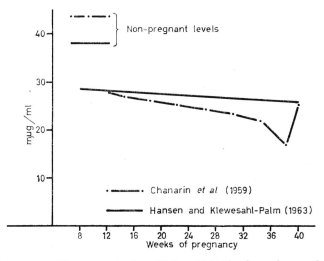

FIGURE 13.1. The concentration of folic acid in blood 15 minutes after an intravenous injection of folic acid

concentration of folic acid in blood of roughly 40 mμg per ml 15 minutes after the intravenous load. At the earliest stage of pregnancy at which the test was made, 13–16 weeks in the first and 8 weeks in the second study, the blood folic acid had fallen to about 25 mμg per ml 15 minutes after the injection and the low level was maintained to the end of gestation. There, as in so much else that is written of metabolism in pregnancy, the fall of concentration of folic acid in maternal serum was attributed to the demand of the foetus. It is forgotten or ignored that at 8 weeks the foetus weighs 3 g, and contains 250 mg total solids; at 10 weeks, 5 g and 400 mg. Competitive demand can scarcely be the explanation, and indeed the graph shows clearly that there is no correlation whatever

Y

between size of the foetus and the clearance of folic acid from maternal serum. The only likely explanation, still to be confirmed experimentally, is that folic acid is spilled in the urine when the glomerular filtration rate rises, as it does in early pregnancy. To return to the clinical observations, it is now clear that small individual differences in renal clearance may be sufficient to determine which pregnant women will spill so much of a not too liberal supply that there is not enough left for the maturation of their own blood cells. The course of events is comparable with that described in Chapter 6 for iodine. Loss through increased renal clearance and reduced tubular reabsorption of iodine and of folic acid produces a state of maternal deficiency shown in each case by the characteristic reaction. There is no reason to implicate the foetus, either as a cause or as likely to suffer in consequence.

The demands of the foetus

In Chapter 8, where the passage of nutrients from mother to foetus was discussed, it was shown that the transfer is not directly from maternal to foetal blood, often against a concentration gradient, but from maternal blood to placental syncytium which is a busy chemical laboratory, elaborating a multitude of essential complexes. Of those complexes some, like progesterone and the oestrogens, appear to serve both mother and child; others, primarily nutrients, are specifically for the foetus. It is, we suggest, to the demands of the foetus, through the placental syncytium, and to the rate of formation of complexes there, that the supply of nutrients in maternal blood must be adjusted.

If there were any appreciable rise in the concentration of nutrients in maternal blood there would be pressure on her tissues to remove the surplus. And since the receptive area of her own tissues may be much greater than that of the placenta, in spite of the doubtful possibility that microvilli increase its absorbing surface, it seems right and necessary that adaptation to supplying the foetus should involve some means of damping down transmission from maternal blood to maternal tissues. There is direct evidence for this view in insensitivity to insulin, ensuring longer carriage of sugar in the blood. Peripheral thyroid activity is reduced, so saving on the turnover in maternal tissues of a number of metabolites. Muscle generally is relaxed, saving the cost of maintaining high tonus. The evidence, in fact, is that there is a general quiescence of metabolism in maternal tissues. Further support for the view that transfer to maternal tissues is controlled is that, while the concentrations of plasma globulins, many of which act as carrier proteins, are maintained at or above their usual levels, plasma albumin, which Allison (1961) regards as part of the meagre system for storage of protein, falls both relatively and absolutely.

Loss through the kidney is wasteful of nutrients and we have no means of knowing, at present, whether the increase of glomerular filtration rate is purposeful in respect of all nutrients spilled. But we suggest that the prodigal use of nutrients may be the price to be paid for diversion of incoming nutrients from maternal stores to meet foetal requirements.

To complete the picture it is only necessary to recall that all of the major changes in maternal physiology take place at an early stage when there is no question of any significant demand on the part of the foetus. Most are well established before the end of the first trimester: the increase of cardiac output, the drop in arterial carbon dioxide (pCO_2) caused by overbreathing, the fall in plasma albumin, the change in renal clearance, and the deposition of fat in peripheral stores have been described in earlier chapters. They are manifestly not adaptive to any accomplished major change, but are anticipatory, directed to the *future* needs of the foetus.

In view of all this, and to return to the questions asked at the beginning of this chapter, we must say that the metabolism of the mother in normal pregnancy is anabolic as far as acquisition of nutrients is concerned; anabolic within her body in respect of temporarily inert stores of fat and possibly of calcium for later use; relatively quiescent in the turnover of nutrients in her own cells; and, in order that she may maintain a flow of nutrients available to the foetus, prodigal of many nutrients by loss through the kidney. Much more information on renal clearances and the magnitude of those losses is required.

THE SPECIFIC REQUIREMENTS OF PREGNANCY

Calculations in this chapter are based on a standard woman corresponding to an average Aberdeen primigravida: age 24 years, height 163 cm, weight before pregnancy 56 kg. Adjusted for local

TABLE 13.2. Mean Daily Increments of Protein and Fat and
Total Increments in Foetus and Maternal Body

Weeks of pregnancy		0–10*	10–20	20–30	30–40	Cumulative Total
Protein	g	0.63	2.5	4.64	5.36	910
Fat	g	6.55	22.3	24.0	12.3	4464

* For the first 10 week period total increment is divided by 56 since pregnancy is dated from the last menstrual period.

temperature and humidity her basal metabolic rate is 1400 kcal
daily (Quenouille *et al.* 1951).

The organic components of the foetus and added maternal
tissues are simply and conveniently grouped as protein and fat.
Table 13.2, adapted from the summary tables 12.8 and 12.9, shows
the mean daily increments of protein and fat for the four quarters
of pregnancy, and the total increments for pregnancy.

TABLE 13.3. The Cumulative Energy Cost of Pregnancy Computed from the
Energy Equivalents of Protein and Fat Increments and the Energy Cost of
Maintaining the Foetus and Added Maternal Tissues. The Last Figures are
Derived from Oxygen Consumption Figures (See Table 3.2) assuming an
RQ of 0.90

Weeks of pregnancy	0–10*	10–20	20–30	30–40	Cumulative Total
	Equivalent, kcal per day				kcal
Protein	3.5	14.0	26.0	30.0	5096
Fat	62.3	212.1	228.4	115.5	42409
Oxygen consumption	19.9	65.6	122.3	174.4	26475
Total net energy	85.7	291.7	376.7	319.9	73980
Metabolizable energy (Total net energy + 10 per cent)	94	321	414	352	81378

* For the first 10 week period total increment is divided by 56 since pregnancy is dated from the last menstrual period.

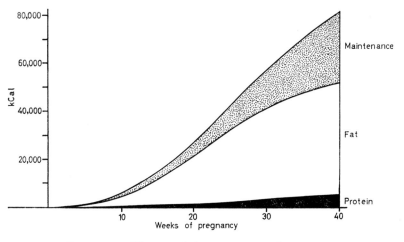

FIGURE 13.2. The cumulative energy cost of pregnancy

Table 13.3 and Figure 13.2 show the net energy equivalents of those increments as their heats of combustion, and the net energy cost of maintaining the foetus and added maternal tissues, computed from their oxygen consumption as set out in Chapter 3. In the last line of Table 13.3 the total net energy is converted to metabolizable energy, in terms of which the energy of food is usually expressed. The efficiency of conversion is not known; we have allowed 90 per cent as a reasonable approximation.

Protein

The biological value of a protein is now regarded as determined by the mixture of amino acids it carries. The idea is embodied in Block and Mitchell's 'chemical score' (1946), in the amino acid pattern used by FAO (1957a) and in the 'ideal aminogram' devised by Allison (1961). Much work has been done recently to compare such amino acid scores with biological values measured by different criteria in the living animal or its carcase. By such procedures, in agreement, the common animal proteins rank above plant; egg and milk compete for first place and provide the reference value 100. Of plant proteins there are not many values for man above 80 and a few, those for legumes, such incomplete proteins as zein, and the protein of cassava, rank below 50. Biological values of mixed diets depend on the combination of the amino acids provided. That of the present United Kingdom diet is reckoned to be 80, of diets that derive their protein mainly from cereals and legumes about 60, and of the poorest diets, especially those with any considerable proportion of cassava, about 40.

That is to say, for our standard woman and measured in terms of the average United Kingdom diet, the food protein equivalent of the specific requirement of pregnancy is less than 7 g daily during the time when the rate of gain is greatest. For emergent countries, with smaller mothers and smaller babies, for instance of birth weight 2700 g (Chapters 10 and 14), the reduction of specific requirement is a little more than compensated by the lower biological value of the protein supply, and the food protein requirement is about 7.5 g daily. For still smaller mothers with the poorest diets and their babies, weighing 2500 g, the specific requirement would be 4 g and the diet protein to correspond 10 g.

Fat and energy

The additional requirement for energy specific to pregnancy comes from two demands, as shown in Table 13.3, and Figure 13.2. There is the protein and fat accumulated by the foetus and the fat stored by the mother, their energy measured as heats of combustion; and the added cost of the metabolism of the foetus and new maternal tissues, measured as oxygen consumption. There is no known requirement for fat, as such, except as a vehicle for the carriage and possibily the absorption of fat-soluble vitamins and possibly some other substances; and an unmeasured need for highly unsaturated fatty acids, thought to be useful in prevention of cardiovascular disease. Apart from small quantities of structural carbohydrate in brain, cartilage, connective tissue, and enough, with deaminated protein, to prevent ketosis, there is no requirement for carbohydrate as such. It will be assumed that any diet taken habitually by a large number of people contains enough fat and carbohydrate for special purposes. Consumption of fat for fuel varies widely; in diets with a high proportion of animal foods it is usually higher than in diets of plant food, and is often considered excessive. Where food supplies and purchasing power are adequate, the proportion of fat to carbohydrate depends on habit and preference; where supplies are less than adequate or purchasing power low, carbohydrate rises at the expense of fat. Consumption of the two together is, or ought to be, dictated by energy expenditure.

In terms of oxygen consumption, the specific increment due to the respiration of the foetus and added maternal tissues, with the extra work of maternal heart and respiratory effort, over the last 140 days is about 150 kcal daily. The daily cost of materials in foetus and maternal tissues, as their heats of combustion, is about 250 kcal in the third quarter of pregnancy, when the combined rate of increase is greatest. Cost of construction materials is productive energy, not normally to be met in adult allowances above resting expenditure. If the conventional allowance of 2300 kcal for the FAO standard woman with a resting metabolism stated as 1260 kcal, be taken as illustration, the margin for activity is 1040 kcal and both extra oxygen consumption and cost of materials, as computed here for the third quarter of pregnancy, are equivalent to only 40 per cent of the activity expenditure envisaged for the non-pregnant woman.

TABLE 13.4. Mean Daily Energy Intake and Activity in 4 Weeks of Pregnancy (Taggart unpublished)

I. 13 primigravidae

Week	10	20	30	38
Energy intake: kcal	2100	2320	2340	2250
Activity: hours				
Walking, outdoors	1.2	1.1	1.1	0.7
Strenuous work	0.6	0.6	0.6	0.5
Light work	5.4	5.3	5.0	4.9
Sitting	7.5	7.3	7.4	7.2
In bed	9.3	9.7	9.9	10.7

II. 9 multigravidae

Week	10	20	30	38
Energy intake: kcal	2190	2320	2210	2320
Activity: hours				
Walking, outdoors	0.8	0.8	0.6	0.5
Strenuous work	0.4	0.6	0.5	0.4
Light work	6.8	6.4	6.6	6.5
Sitting	6.1	6.7	6.3	6.4
In bed	9.9	9.5	10.0	10.2

We have recalculated the probable resting metabolic rate of the FAO standard woman on the basis of mean weight for height in British women (Kemsley, Billewicz and Thomson, 1962) and the tables of basal metabolic rates of Quenouille *et al.* (1951). With a weight of 55 kg her height would be 162.5 cm and, at temperature 50°F and age 25 her basal metabolic rate would be 1380 kcal, which is not significantly different from that computed for our standard woman at 1400. On this basis the margin for activity is 920 kcal, still more than twice the specific energy requirement of pregnancy. The energy costs of pregnancy could be met without increase of food intake by economy of activity, and economy of activity is characteristic of pregnancy in both animals and man.

In an attempt to see how such a saving might be made, an 'activity diary' study of 13 primigravidae and 9 pregnant women with one or two small children to care for (Taggart, unpublished, 1963) was made during four weeks in which a diet survey also was made. The results are shown in Table 13.4 and Figure 13.3. All activities but particularly more strenuous activities were reduced in favour of rest in bed. But to translate the time-table into terms of energy expenditure would require an *ad hoc* study of the cost of

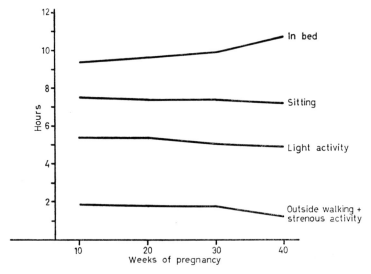

FIGURE 13.3. The changing pattern of daily activity in pregnancy. Unpublished data for 13 primigravidae

activities. Theoretically all walking activities of the pregnant woman should cost more as her weight rises, but, in fact, the cost of motion in the relatively relaxed state of pregnancy, and possibly with changed tempo, is not known. Some studies by indirect calorimetry of pregnant women performing their ordinary tasks, not standardized exercise tests to which they are not accustomed, is the next step to elucidate energy balance in pregnancy. See also Chapters 2 and 3.

Calcium

The specific increment of calcium in pregnancy is only 2.5 per cent of the calcium in the maternal skeleton and can be provided from that store if necessary. Indeed, the requirement of the foetus will be met, with diminishing success, in a succession of pregnancies even if the result is osteomalacia in the mother and foetal rickets. At the opposite extreme, the foetal skeleton may be calcified while the maternal store of calcium, if not already replete, is itself strengthened. Since the daily demand for calcium is much greater in successful lactation than it is in pregnancy, it may be assumed that some addition to the maternal skeleton during pregnancy is a natural preparatory measure, and to be desired. The daily amount required for the standard foetal skeleton can be calculated from Table 13.5 to be about 250 mg over the last quarter when the demand is highest. We shall see that such a demand is high in relation to the amounts supplied by many common diets, or absorbed from them.

TABLE 13.5. Specific Increments for Pregnancy of Calcium, Phosphorus and Iron Compared with Content of Maternal Body Before Pregnancy

Component		Specific increment	Maternal content	Increment per cent
Calcium	g	29.56	1120	2.5
Phosphorus	g	21.5	630	3.4
Iron, total	mg	740	3600	21
Iron in foetus and blood loss	mg	500	3600	14

Phosphorus

Since 85 per cent or more of the phosphorus in the body is combined with calcium in bone, what has been said of the specific requirement for calcium may also be said of phosphorus. What is not in the skeleton is concerned in the enzyme reactions of energy metabolism and varies independently of that in bone. The total specific increment is about 3.4 per cent of the total in the maternal skeleton. The amount required daily during the fourth quarter of pregnancy is calculated from Table 13.5 to be 200 mg. The supply of phosphorus from food is less often short than that of calcium, because most foods, especially staple plant foods, contain more phosphorus than calcium in relation to their energy value.

The specific requirements of both calcium and phosphorus, like that of protein, are less for smaller women and smaller babies.

Iron

In relation to the total iron content of the maternal body, the specific increment of pregnancy is high, 21 per cent (Table 13.5). That estimate includes the iron in the mother's expanded blood volume, 290 mg out of the gross requirement of 740 mg. But the total of 3600 mg iron in the mother's body before pregnancy includes about 1000 mg of iron stored in ferritin and haemosiderin. Of that amount about threequarters is ferritin and is regarded as an easily available reserve from which the iron required for the normal turnover of erythrocytes is derived, and to which iron is returned when erythrocytes are destroyed. If the normal intake of iron is sufficient to replace the small losses that occur in the turnover of erythrocyte iron, it should be ample to maintain the minute turnover on the additional 290 mg of erythrocyte iron. To aid in such maintenance there is a saving of iron loss in menstruation, estimated as 120 mg on the average for a pregnancy (Cheyne and Hytten, 1963 and unpublished).

The true specific requirement, iron that is lost to the maternal body at parturition, is therefore that in the foetus, placenta and blood lost. The product of conception has an average content of about 450 mg, and blood loss is generously assessed as 50 mg iron, making a total of 500 mg, almost all to be acquired during the second half of pregnancy. As a percentage of maternal iron content it is still high, 14 per cent, and as a quantity to be provided daily it represents 3.6 mg, or more towards the end of pregnancy.

Sodium and Potassium

The specific requirements for sodium and potassium are assessed (Table 11.9) as 850 and 316 mEq (about 20 g and 12 g). The supply of potassium is abundant for all needs in any known diet, and more abundant in diets predominantly of plant foods. In relation to potassium, plant foods provide less sodium than do animal foods and there is a natural urge to balance the two by adding salt (sodium chloride) to food. So long as there is unrestricted access to sodium chloride, there is no likelihood of shortage. Many believe that more salt is taken with food than is required or desirable, and many pregnant women have a craving for salty foods. Shortage of either sodium or potassium is not likely.

Other inorganic substances

So far, specific increments of pregnancy have not been computed for other inorganic components but there must be a specific increment for each of the essential elements. There is some information about the effects of deficiency of many of them in animals, but with the exception of iodine, none to suggest that a close study in man would be worth while.

Vitamins

Much has been written about requirements in pregnancy, chiefly to show that it is easier to induce deficiency during pregnancy than in the non-pregnant, the difference being attributed to the demands of the foetus. There is little or no information about specific requirements, and no attention has been paid to the possible effect of the raised glomerular filtration rate.

Little is known about the requirements of any of the fat-soluble vitamins and observations are obscured by the indiscriminate use of them in clinical practice. About four of the B vitamins, thiamine, riboflavin, nicotinic acid, and pyridoxine it is safe to assume that, during pregnancy as in the non-pregnant, requirement is related to energy expenditure.

DIETS OF PREGNANT WOMEN

The snags and pitfalls that beset the path of those who attempt to make accurate estimates of what people eat are countless. To

TABLE 13.6. Mean Daily Inta

Place	Subjects	Calories Kcal.	Protein g	Calc g
				Che
Chicago and Oklahoma	15 housewives	2497	70	1.25
				D
England and Wales	26 professional class	2498	80	0.90
	21 artisan class	2700	82	0.80
	20 wives of employed labourers	2389	73	0.60
	32 wives of unemployed miners in Gateshead	2138	66	0.60
	21 wives of unemployed miners in Wales	2081	54	0.50
	16 poorest class	2211	60	0.50
Edinburgh	35 housewives. Husbands in Armed Forces or skilled artisans	2550	91	—
Bristol	111 primigravidae, 'better type of woman in poor and middle classes'	2400	90	1.20
Aberdeen	489 primigravidae:			
	101 in social class A	2633	80	1.20
	109 in social class B	2521	78	1.10
	279 in social class C	2354	72	0.90
Potsdam, Germany	89 women: 5th and 8th month	2753	77	0.81
				Dietary re
Philadelphia	382 white and 132 negro clinic and private patients	2013	66	0.70
Mexico City	101 women, low economic status	2114	72	0.78
Tennessee	2046 hospital patients, low to moderate income, 3rd trimester of pregnancy net gain 20 lb	2020	70	1.00

ents by Pregnant Women in Different Surveys

in Thiamine mg	Ribo- flavin mg	Nicotinic acid mg	Ascor- bic acid mg	Reference
is of duplicate servings				
—	—	—	—	Coons, 1933–4
quantities weighed				
—	—	—	—	
—	—	—	—	
—	—	—	—	McCance *et al.* 1938
—	—	—	—	
—	—	—	—	
—	—	—	29–56	Roscoe and McKay, 1946
1.25	1.70	10.0	81	Hobson, 1948
1.22	2.05	12.0	79	Thomson, 1958
1.18	1.89	11.4	65	
1.16	1.74	11.6	61	
1.57	1.85	15.1	79	Gräfe, 1961
ities in household measures				
1.02 (median)	1.30	—	53 (median)	Williams and Fralin, 1942
1.33	1.17	8.6	49	Anderson, Robinson, Calvo and Payne, 1946
1.40	2.30	11.0	55 (median)	Darby *et al.* 1953

Place	Subjects	Calories kcal.	Protein g	Cal g
				Dietary h
Glasgow	100 women, low economic status with full-term infants	1946	72	1.22
New York	38 white and 32 negro women, with full-term infants	2520	91	1.43
Iowa	62 students' wives	2535	75	1.14
	288 wives of labourers	2463	60	0.53
Holland	270 women, mostly rural, in mid-pregnancy	2770	78	0.98
S. India	100 women, poor	1815	44	0.37
	352 women, poor	1410	38	0.32
Netherlands	498 women: 1st trimester	2620	79	0.85
	2nd trimester	2720	80	1.08
	3rd trimester	2620	76	1.00
Israel	370 women, low economic status	2050	72	0.83
Calcutta	150 women, poor	1920	48	—
	50 women, well-to-do	2760	86	—
Malaya	Rural smallholders	1812	49	0.57
	Urban workers	1966	40	—
Chile	800 working class women	2130	74	0.74

* Not including carotene

estimate the total food eaten by a population or group of people is, in some ways, simpler than to estimate the food eaten by a family, which is again less arduous and complicated than to estimate for a single individual.

In finding estimates of diets eaten by pregnant women the same *nued)*

nin	Thiamine mg	Ribo-flavin mg	Nicotinic acid mg	Ascorbic acid mg	Reference
nnaire or unstated method					
	—	—	—	—	Cameron and Graham, 1944
	1.50	2.70	11.6	112	Speert, Graff and Graff, 1951
	1.76	2.18	—	97	Jeans, Smith and Stearns,
	1.58	1.46	—	73	1952
*	1.38	1.57	14.0	114	den Hartog, Posthuma and de Haas, 1953
	—	—	—	—	Pasricha, 1958
	—	—	—	—	Venkatachalam, 1962
*	1.32	—	—	123	
*	1.30	—	—	120	
*	1.30	—	—	122	Van der Rijst, 1962
	—	1.45	—	—	Poznanski, Brzezinski and Guggenheim, 1962
	—	—	—	—	Bagchi and Bose, 1962
	—	—	—	—	
	0.6	0.4	9.0	30	Llewellyn-Jones, 1962
	0.6	0.6	9.5	20	
	1.11	1.70	10.3	92	Valiente and Muñoz, 1962

difficulty arises as in finding valid estimates of normal weight gain, and for the same reason: there are few centres where women are not subject to dietary advice, so that what they eat does not necessarily reflect their inclinations or even physiological needs. The finding by the Vanderbilt team (McGanity *et al.* 1954) that women with pre-eclampsia ate less than normal pregnant women is almost certainly due to the fact that women showing early signs of pre-eclampsia are often dieted.

Because the estimation of diet in pregnancy is, of necessity, estimation for individuals, the total number of such surveys is small. The number of surveys in which the food eaten was weighed is still less and only one is recorded in which duplicate servings were chemically analysed. It has been shown elsewhere (Morrison, Russell and Stevenson, 1949; Thomson, 1958) that the results of questionnaire or diet history surveys tend to be inaccurate and misleading. In spite of that, there is little difference between the averages reported for pregnant women.

The composition of recorded diets

In Table 13.6 is reproduced a summary of published estimates. Leaving aside for the moment the estimates from poor populations, it is astounding how uniform the picture is, regardless of whether the foods were meticulously weighed, or recorded by some easier process of measurement or by guess. We may therefore discuss the table as a whole.

It is clear that food intake rises with economic class in Britain and the Far East (McCance *et al.* 1938; Thomson, 1958; Bagchi and Bose 1962), as we know it does for families and populations everywhere. There is not much difference shown in the Table between the three trimesters of pregnancy, which may be explained in part by the finding (p. 128 and Figure 11.4) that appetite rises and fat is deposited in pregnancy, before the foetus exercises any perceptible demand, so that the load of acquisition is spread the more evenly over pregnancy. The decline of activity towards the end of pregnancy offsets part of the foetal demand when it is highest.

In view of comparisons to be made in Chapter 14 of secular changes in indices of health in pregnant women, and of reproduction in sophisticated and emergent populations, Table 13.7 was prepared to compare the survey of pregnant women's diets made by McCance, Widdowson and Verdon-Roe (1938) with that of Thomson (1958). The outstanding difference between the two is that, in 1938, working class families included many from depressed areas with high unemployment rates and many multiparae. Thomson's groups, surveyed in 1950-53, were of primigravidae only and there was little or no unemployment. In McCance's series,

TABLE 13.7. Comparison of intakes. Thomson's (1958) survey and that of McCance et al. (1951)

Class[1]	kcal	kcal per kg body wt	kcal per cm height	Protein Animal g	Protein Total g	Fat g	Carbo-hydrate g	Calcium g
Thomson								
A	2633	40	16.3	46.7	80.4	112	349	1.19
McCance et al.								
VI	2498	41	15.2	55	80	108	284	0.94
V	2781	46	17.3	55	86	121	317	0.75
Thomson								
B	2521	40	15.9	44.3	78.4	108	329	1.06
McCance et al.								
IV	2471	42	15.3	46	75	95	315	0.75
III	2194	39	14.0	37	66	86	273	0.52[2]
Thomson								
C	2354	38	14.9	40.4	71.8	100	312	0.88
McCance et al.								
II	2155	37	14.0	36	64	86	267	0.53[2]
I	2211	35	14.2	28	60	88	281	0.51[2]

[1] Thomson's A, B and C classes as follows:
Class A: Registrar-General's Classes I and II (professional, managerial and generally well-to-do) and 'white-collar' occupations from Class III.
Class B: Registrar-General's Class III (skilled occupations, mainly manual) less 'white-collar' occupations.
Class C: Registrar-General's Classes IV and V (semi-skilled and unskilled manual occupations) (Registrar-General, 1951)

McCance et al. based their classification on income (less rent) per head of the family per week: I less than 6/-, II 6/- to 9/-, III 9/- to 15/-, IV 15/- to 25/-, V 25/- to 40/-, VI Over 40/-.
The classes as grouped above are taken to be roughly comparable in terms of occupations. Incomes are, of course, widely different.

[2] Including free milk. Averages without free milk 0.24 to 0.33 g.

the multiparae had on the average about 200 kcal daily less than primigravidae.

In both surveys there is the usual gradient with economic class. There is little difference between the better-off groups, except for calcium intake, which in the post-war series exceeded by nearly 40 per cent that in 1938. Poorer classes compared with the better-off at the earlier date ate less, in a straight comparison or in relation to weight or height. They had less protein, especially animal protein, and a lower proportion of energy from protein. They had much less calcium, even although some were given supplements of free milk. In respect of calcium intake, Thomson's poorest group was better off than any except the top economic group in 1938 and the working class women not receiving free milk in 1938 had about one third of the calcium intake of their near counterparts at the later date. Differences of similar type and much the same magnitude have been found between the diets of working class families in 1937–39 and 1955–58; there were corresponding differences in

TABLE 13.8. Mean Nutritive Values of Daily Diets Taken by Tall, Medium and Short Primigravidae (from Thomson and Billewicz, 1961)

	Tall (5 ft 4 in. and over)	Medium (5 ft 1 in.– 5 ft 3 in.)	Short (Under 5 ft 1 in.)
Calories (kcal)	2595	2475	2229
Protein (g)	80.0	75.1	69.2
Calcium (g)	1.08	0.99	0.85
Thiamine (mg)	1.24	1.18	1.08
Riboflavin (mg)	1.95	1.86	1.67
Nicotinic acid (mg)	12.1	11.7	11.0
Asorbic acid (mg)	76.5	63.8	56.9
No. of subjects*	133	239	117

* Not representing the true distribution by height of the population investigated.

height and weight of children (Baines, Hollingsworth and Leitch, 1963).

What is not evident from Table 13.6 is the extent to which food intake depends on the stature and weight of the women studied. It was shown by Thomson and Billewicz (1961) that both quantity and quality of diet parallel the height of the women studied but, when diets were classified into three groups in terms of weight-for-height, there was no difference in either quantity or quality between underweight, average and overweight women (Tables 13.8 and 13.9).

It is difficult with the meagre information given about height and weight of the women in the Far East surveys to compare the

TABLE 13.9. Mean Nutritive Values of Daily Diets taken by Women in Three Weight-for-Height Groups. 'Overweight' signifies that the Women were in the Heaviest 25 per cent of Subjects at each Height, and 'Underweight' signifies that they were in the Lightest 25 per cent. 'Average Weight' covers the Intermediate 50 per cent (from Thomson and Billewicz, 1961)

	Underweight	Average weight	Overweight
Calories (kcal)	2400	2460	2456
Protein (g)	72.7	75.4	75.5
Calcium (g)	0.96	0.97	0.98
Thiamine (mg)	1.13	1.19	1.19
Riboflavin (mg)	1.83	1.83	1.83
Nicotinic acid (mg)	11.6	11.7	11.5
Ascorbic acid (mg)	68.4	65.5	62.4
No. of subjects*	94	204	114
Mean weight at 20th week of pregnancy (kg)	49.9	56.5	65.6
Mean height (cm)	158.0	158.2	158.5

* The weight-for-height standards were derived from a large representative sample of Aberdeen primigravidae.

recorded intakes with intakes in the United Kingdom. We have therefore made a purely hypothetical case as follows.

(i) We have assumed that our standard woman with a resting pre-pregnant energy expenditure of 1400 kcal and an extra resting energy expenditure specific to the second half of pregnancy of 150 kcal daily (Table 13.3) has a diet of value 2475 kcal, corresponding to the average diet of women of medium height as described by Thomson and Billewicz (1961). That is to say, consumption in kcal would be roughly 60 per cent above resting energy expenditure.

(ii) Taking a small Indian hill woman, as measured by McLaren (1955), to represent small women in the Far East, height 148 cm, weight 40 kg, with baby of average birth weight 2500 g, we have computed her resting pre-pregnant metabolism as 1080 kcal (Quenouille *et al.* 1951) and the increment of pregnancy, proportional to the weight of the baby, as about 115 kcal daily. If the sum of those values be then increased by 60 per cent, her food consumption in kcal would be 1910. That is to say, food energy values of the order of those shown in Table 13.6 for the Far East bear the same relation to resting energy expenditure of small women producing small babies, as do diets in this country with bigger women and bigger babies, with margins of between 600 and 800 kcal daily for construction and activity. The only exception to that statement is the record by Venkatachalam (1962) of only 1410 kcal from diet which would leave only 235 kcal for construction and activity.

Before comparing the food habits of pregnant women with the recommendations made and allowances prescribed for them by committees whose task it is to review all the evidence, a few notes on unusual diets and odd ideas about diet may be appropriate.

Vegetarian diet

The diet of a high proportion of the world's population is almost entirely of plant foods. We have quoted typical studies of such diets as taken by pregnant women. The adequacy of such diets is in doubt for several reasons. Techniques may be less than adequate to the task of procuring accurate information; and a proportion, possibly a high proportion in some areas, are restricted in quantity by poverty. Our information about the people themselves, and about their diets, is far too meagre to permit separation of the effects of underfeeding from any there may be of vegetarian diet. If we look to the west for more accurate information, none of the studies so far made is altogether satisfactory. That of Hardinges and Stare (1954) was by diet history. They found no pregnant woman taking an exclusively plant diet, but 26 lacto-ovo-vegetarians whose diets they compared with those of 28 non-vegetarians, the two groups matched for height and weight. The vegetarians ate less (kcal 2650 against 3010), and had less total and animal protein (97 and 56 g against 111 and 81 g) and less nicotinic acid (14 against 18 mg), but more calcium (1.8 g against 1.5) and all other nutrients measured, so that on a crude chemical basis they had diets of better quality with adequate energy value and more than sufficient protein.

Wokes, Badenoch and Sinclair (1955) are of the opinion that amenorrhoea and other disorders are more frequent in 'Vegans' (vegetarians who eat no food of animal origin) than in women on mixed diets, but the fertility of populations in underdeveloped countries, even those on the poorest diets, lends no support to such an idea. At the opposite extreme, the fertility of the Eskimo on their natural diet mostly of animal flesh, is judged to have been low (Rabinowitch, 1936).

Habits and taboo

There are many habits and prohibitions peculiar to diet in pregnancy. Abnormal appetite in western women has been touched on in Chapter 5. Some of the habits and restrictions in less developed peoples are almost certainly beneficial, such as the practice of adding crude salts, with sodium, calcium, iron, cobalt, to vegetable food, especially women's food, or the habit of the Masai whose diet is mainly of milk, meat and blood, of sending 'the pregnant women into the bush to eat berries' (Orr and Gilks, 1931). On the other hand, there are taboos which appear more likely to be harmful than beneficial. For instance Mollor (1961) describes the customs of several tribes in Tanganyika; eggs and meat and fish are most often forbidden and some legumes also are taboo. That might suggest a low protein intake, but the estimates of protein intake by women in Kenya (Orr and Gilks, 1931) are high. More information is needed.

TABLE 13.10. Allowanc

| | Standard woman | | | | | |
	Height cm	Weight kg	Weight increase kg	Energy kcal	Protein g	Calc g
(USA) Nat. Acad. Sci. National Research Council (1958)						
Non-pregnant	163	58	—	2300	58	0.8
Pregnant: second half	163	—	9	2600	78	1.5
FAO: Energy (1957b) Protein (1957a) FAO/WHO: Calcium (1962)					Minimum (Reference)	
Non-pregnant	—	55	—	2300	19.25	0.4–
Pregnant	—	—	10 ± 2	—	—	1.0–
Canadian Council on Nutrition, 1948 (1950)						
Non-pregnant:						
Sedentary	—	54.5	—	2125	55	0.55
Moderate activity	—	54.5	—	2400	55	0.55
Pregnant, second half,						
Sedentary, up to:	—	—	—	2615	80	1.55
Moderate activity,						
up to:	—	—	—	2900	80	1.55
British Medical Association (1950)						
Pregnant: first half	—	—	—	2500	93	0.8
second half	—	—	—	2700	102	1.5
(Netherlands) Commissie Voedingsnormen (1961)						
Non-pregnant:						
Sedentary	—	—	—	2200	60	1.0
Moderate activity	—	—	—	2400	60	1.0
Heavy work	165	60	—	3000	75	1.0
Pregnant, last three months if active or not fully grown				+300	+20	1.5
Russian standards (Jarusova, 1961)	—	—	—	—	—	

on-pregnant and Pregnant Woman

Vitamin A I.U.	Vitamin D I.U.	Thiamine mg	Riboflavin mg	Nicotinic acid, or equivalent mg	Vitamin B_6 mg	Vitamin C mg
5000	400	1.0	1.5	17	—	70
6000	400	1.3	2.0	20	—	100
—	—	—	—	—	—	—
—	—	—	—	—	—	—
As carotene						
4000	—	0.65	1.0	6.5	—	30
4000	—	0.75	1.1	7.5	—	30
6000	—	0.80	1.2	8.0	—	30
6000	—	0.90	1.3	9.0	—	30
6000	400	1.0	1.5	10	—	40
6000	600	1.1	1.6	11	—	40
mg 0.45+ carotene	—	0.9	1.4	9		50
1.80	—	1.0	1.5	10		
	—	1.2	1.8	12		
0.55+ carotene 2.50		1.2	2.0	12		75
6600	not more than 500	2.5	3	20	4	100
	750	3.75	—	—	—	150

	Standard woman					
	Height	Weight	Weight increase	Energy kcal	Protein g	Cal g
	cm	kg	kg			
Nutrition Division, Inst. Med. Res., Malaya (Llewellyn-Jones, 1962)	—	50	—	2185	70	1.5
National Inst. Nutrition, Tokyo (Yanagi *et al.* 1951)						
Non-pregnant	150.1	48.5		2140	70	
Pregnant, up to 5th month				2400	85	
From 6th month				2700	95	

OFFICIAL RECOMMENDED ALLOWANCES FOR PREGNANCY

The stated aims of 'allowances' and 'dietary standards'

In the United States, the National Academy of Sciences—National Research Council (NRC) says of the allowances it proposes: 'Recommended dietary allowances have been provided to serve as a guide for planning adequate diets for normal healthy populations or individuals'; and also that the allowances aim to cover: 'needs of those with greatest requirements, and providing a substantial margin of sufficiency for the majority of individuals'. They are concerned more with individuals who deviate upwards from the mean than with specific needs for any particular function such as growth or pregnancy.

The expressed aim of the Canadian Council on Nutrition (1950) is different. The Canadian dietary standard 'is recommended as a scientific basis for planning food supplies for individuals or groups, . . . in terms of probably physiological requirements. The figures can further be used to indicate a 'nutritional floor' beneath which maintenance of health in people cannot be assumed'.

The British Medical Association (1950) Committee on Nutrition says: 'In dealing with *nutritional needs* (sic) the Committee took only conditions of health into account . . . it believes that the needs of representative individuals in each group are met. . . .'

Many other authorities have formulated standards, often without

Vitamin A I.U.	Vitamin D I.U.	Thiamine mg	Riboflavin mg	Nicotinic acid, or equivalent mg	B_6 mg	C mg
6000	400	1.1	1.8	20	—	100

defining aim or purpose; and, possibly to avoid awkward questions about the relation of proposed standards to needs, the practice has been adopted, more and more widely, of describing recommendations as allowances.

It will be seen in Table 13.10 that specification of aims can lead to confusing discrepancies. For the second half of pregnancy the NRC complete cover allowance, for the 58 kg woman putting on 20 lb weight, is 2600 kcal daily; the Canadian 'floor', computed for a woman of about the same weight, as non-pregnant need plus up to 500 kcal (the permissive allowance) comes to as much as 2625 for a sedentary woman and 2925 for one doing moderate work; the BMA recommendation (no weight stated) is about half way between the sedentary and moderate-work Canadian standards. The NRC complete cover allowance is the least.

In fact, physiological information is insufficient to define needs in respect of all the variations that occur in ordinary life, or indeed in respect of most of them. To cater for the largest requirement must be prodigal of resources since all the population below the top few will have a surplus; and the surplus is not likely to be of any benefit to individuals in general. The establishment of a minimum, below which maintenance of health cannot be assumed, ought to be based firmly on needs specific to the task in question, and ought further to be checked against the composition of the diets of people who are healthy and efficient in the task studied. But, as Hytten and Thomson (1961) wrote in their discussion of the needs of lactation, 'planning for a healthy society cannot await the acquisition of a complete and detailed knowledge of metabolism . . .. There is no need to appeal to physiology when devising allowances intended as social targets . . . Such allowances may be specified by reference to the diets of persons known to be healthy. Allowances derived empirically in this way will be both practical and safe, because they are derived from real diets taken by people who are observed to be healthy.'

Recommended allowances in practice

A list of allowances approved by authorities is shown as Table 13.10. It includes the pregnancy allowances from the very widely used, United States, National Research Council (1958) scheme and the latest revisions of allowances by the Food and Agriculture Organization of the United Nations (FAO, 1957b). Both of these schemes, as a whole, are applied to measure the *proportions* of populations undernourished or malnourished, or the *degree* to which a population as a whole is underfed or illfed in one respect or another, and the National Research Council allowances are seldom or never applied outside the United States as complete-cover allowances; indeed, when they are used to estimate proportions or degrees of failure to meet the standards, 'margins of safety' are apt to be added.

NATIONAL RESEARCH COUNCIL

The National Research Council made no allowance for the first half of pregnancy. The 'calorie cost' they say 'is small and tends to be compensated for by a corresponding decrease in physical activity. It is important that the relatively greater need . . . be met in the second half of pregnancy. For this reason it is proposed that calorie allowances be increased by 300 calories per day during this interval. This is of particular concern for the active, young, and immature woman undergoing first pregnancy. Other women, however, may so reduce physical activity during this period that the extra demands for calories may be largely compensated for without addition of food calories.' The Council goes on to say that diet must be controlled by physician, nurse or nutritionist, according to pre-pregnant weight and desired gain.

The pattern of distribution of extra food, and the implied pattern of activity, in respect of the average pregnant woman are not in accord with normal behaviour. Normally the appetite of the pregnant woman increases in early pregnancy, more food is eaten, activity is unaltered, and fat is laid down. It is true that if the total weight gain is limited to 20 lb, no fat will be laid down in the maternal body and the addition of 300 kcal daily during the second half will be more than adequate to meet the specific needs.

The ordinary protein allowance for adults is 1 g per kg body weight; the extra allowance of 20 g daily for the last five lunar months is based on metabolism experiments about whose validity we have grave doubts, already set out in Chapter 11. It should be compared with our estimate of 7 to 10 g food protein of biological values 80 to 40, according to physique of mothers and type of diet, and a possible small addition to allow for the spillage in urine, perhaps of the order of a gram of amino acids daily.

The allowance of calcium for the reference non-pregnant woman is 800 mg daily and that during the second half of pregnancy, 1500 mg. With a total specific increment of less than 30 g and a maximum daily increment of about 250 mg, a retention of one-third of the allowance for pregnancy is implied, and that is in agreement with what might be expected with generous supplies of milk, as is usual in American diets, and an intake of 1500 mg. Absorption and retention will be much higher relatively where intake of calcium bears a closer relation to need.

FAO

In the 1957 report on Calorie Requirements FAO estimates the total extra requirement for a pregnancy of the reference woman of 55 kg, putting on 10 ±2 kg, as 80,000 kcal, but does not explain how the cost is distributed over the 9 months. In practice, it is argued, half the extra cost will be saved on activity, and only 40,000 kcal need be debited to the requirements of pregnancy. In the report in the same year of a different FAO committee on protein requirements the conclusion was that, for populations well supplied with protein, no extra provision is required; poor diets should be supplemented according to the non-pregnant woman's supply and the biological value of the protein of the habitual diet. The addition recommended, of 10 g above that of 'the unencumbered adult' is what we have reckoned to be needed in terms of food protein of only 40 biological value.

BRITISH MEDICAL ASSOCIATION

The British Medical Association allowances date from 1950 and have not been revised since. Their allowance for energy exceeds the value of consumption of the diets in Table 13.6 except for the artisan group in the English (1938) survey of McCance *et al.*, 1938 Dutch and German women after mid pregnancy, and one group of well-to-do Calcutta women in a questionnaire survey. For protein the British Medical Association allowance exceeds all present day allowances quoted. It is difficult to avoid the conclusion that both allowances are over-generous. There is no evidence to support them as applicable to the mean pregnant woman in any population.

GENERAL DISCUSSION

At one time it seemed as if targets for attainment in the supply of essential nutrients, and desirable foods, could not be fixed too high; as if it were axiomatic that we cannot have too much of a good thing, and as if all people were of the same build as the largest Americans to whose needs American allowances are tailored. In view of the effect of such targets on the morale of less well fed and smaller people, the alarm and despondency apt to be caused by, for instance, the implication that a Far East pregnant woman requires 1500 mg calcium daily when her normal supply is about 300 mg, it is good to see efforts being made to adjust proposals to present needs and to within reasonable distance of what Far East and other emergent populations have, or may hope to procure in the not too distant future. The American allowance of calcium is 1500 mg daily for the second half of pregnancy. The only justification for it may be found in the thought that, having built up large and well-calcified skeletons, and assuming the usual proportions of inert and exchangeable calcium in the skeleton, the maintenance of the large exchangeable store is important enough to warrant continuation of a high intake, even if the economy of utilization is extremely low.

FAO now suggests an allowance of 1.0 to 1.2 g, or less if there is a smaller child to produce and, presumably, less maternal skeleton to maintain. Even that allowance will be difficult to attain in some areas, at least if the whole is to be obtained from food. But we are apt to forget the lime that is rolled in betel leaves, or used to treat maize before tortillas are baked, or the bones of fish, or pig bones cooked in vinegar, or the crude salts, of which many contain calcium. We need a great deal more information.

There is only one estimate of what iron the pregnant woman needs, 15 mg daily, in the second half of pregnancy, which should be more than enough to supply the computed maximum increment of about 4 mg daily.

Of the other nutrients for which allowances are proposed only one, the allowance of the British Medical Association for vitamin C calls for comment. Allowances for other nutrients resemble each other so much as to suggest a common origin. The reason why the allowance proposed by the British Medical Association is as low as 40 mg is that the table was drawn up soon after the results became known of the Medical Research Council's experiment in production and cure of deficiency of vitamin C (Bartley, Krebs and O'Brien, 1953). In it, 10 mg ascorbic acid was sufficient to prevent and cure signs of scurvy in adult volunteers. The allowance of 40 mg provides a generous surplus over requirement to prevent scurvy. We still do not know whether the further rich excess provided by diets in the United Kingdom (Reports of the National Food Survey Committee, *passim*), connotes a proportionate, or any, benefit to health, but of all the debated nutrients and their allowances, vitamin C appears to be that least likely to be in deficit. The circumstances in which scurvy was once a common disorder fortunately have no parallel in modern life. Scurvy is still recorded on occasion in infants fed on boiled or otherwise heated milk, without any source of vitamin C, and in old bachelors too lazy, or too indifferent, to improve their diet habits. There is no excuse for either.

It is not without interest that Norwegian authorities use the NRC allowances as standards except for vitamin C, for which they prefer the BMA standard of 40 mg (Nicolaysen, 1961).

It would be far outside the scope of this book to comment in any detail on the present world picture of food supplies and needs. But, as regards pregnant women, we may say that if records are correct, it is astonishing on how little a woman can produce a viable child and feed it. Llewellyn-Jones (1962) says of the Malayan women: 'most of the women felt well and were able to do a full day's work, on less than 2000 kcal and less than the gram-per-kg-body-weight protein which the NRC allows'. We have shown that those intakes are not out of line with calculated requirements based on the small size of the women and their babies. What we do not know is to what extent the smallness is an ethnic difference and unchangeable, or would change with good feeding continued through growth and reproductive life over a number of generations.

CHAPTER 14

Childbearing under Adverse Conditions

This book has been concerned, so far, with the adaptation to pregnancy of normal healthy women living in normally comfortable conditions. We have been at pains to define normality of response, not in terms of any theoretical 'best' performance, but as that of a typical well-grown primigravida producing a well-grown infant at term. The response of such mothers includes the accumulation of reserves that would safeguard the pregnancy against at least short periods of deprivation, although, in the nature of things, the best fed and best grown are most sheltered from adversity.

Under adverse conditions are included both shortage of food and subsistence on diets which, though sufficient in quantity, are of poor quality; and, further, exposure to other hardships: poor housing, difficult climates, hard physical work and endemic disease, all of which tend to co-exist with poor and insufficient supplies of food.

There are three sorts of evidence to be examined. From sophisticated communities there are *ad hoc* studies of childbearing in small groups and general vital statistics which make possible comparisons between socio-economic classes. From the emergent countries there are vital statistics, usually patchy and incomplete, and small studies, almost all of hospital confinements and affording little information about the natural background of the mothers. And, third, there is information on the effects of sudden and severe deprivation in time of war.

CHILDBEARING IN 'SOPHISTICATED' COMMUNITIES

Even in countries such as Great Britain and the United States conditions are by no means uniformly favourable, and were much worse during the *laissez faire* economic conditions that existed up to 1939.

In industrial Britain during the 19th and early 20th centuries infection and rickets were the two greatest hazards to childbearing. A witness reporting to the Interdepartmental Committee on Physical Deterioration (Chalmers, 1904) said that 'during the seventies [of the 19th century] the surgeons began to perform the operation of osteotomy to counteract the injurious effects of rickets on bones—operations for contracted pelvis in childbed have increased in recent years'. Munro Kerr (1916) wrote that 'Taking the cases in the Glasgow Maternity Hospital for the last ten years, decided pelvic deformity has been found in fully 30 per cent of indoor patients. This high proportion is to be accounted for by the prevalence of rickets in the city'. In such circumstances the obstetricians of Glasgow became famous for their manipulative skill.

Active rickets was still common in young children in the larger industrial cities in the mid 30s and even now many mothers suffer from the effects on their physique. Baird (1945) showed that in Aberdeen, even with similar standards of medical care throughout pregnancy, women in the poorer socio-economic classes were at a disadvantage compared to the more affluent. The better off were, on the average, taller than the rest, a fact which Baird considered to be due to superior nutritional and other environmental circumstances during growth. In other words, short women were considered to include a high proportion of those whose growth had been stunted. Bernard (1952) produced confirmatory evidence of skeletal malformation by X-ray pelvimetry of 100 tall women and 100 short women. In the short group, but not in the tall, antero-posterior flattening of the pelvic brim was found to be common; the distortion was similar in kind to, but less marked than the serious pelvic deformity that may result from florid rickets.

The influence of maternal stature on reproductive efficiency has been discussed recently by Thomson (1959c), and Thomson and Bill-ewicz (1963). Whatever its origin it seems beyond doubt that short stature, in general, implies not only increased mechanical difficulty in childbearing, but also increased foetal mortality from all causes, which suggests a generally low foetal vitality.

The more general concept that maternal nutritional status has a bearing on reproductive efficiency was discussed by Mellanby in 1933, at a time when the 'newer knowledge of nutrition' was being used by many scientists to demonstrate the evil effects on health of the great economic depression. Mellanby thought that the high rates of mortality and morbidity in pregnancy could be much reduced by proper diet, but admitted that the scientific evidence was 'meagre', and that reproduction was often surprisingly good even when diet was seriously at fault. He instanced the osteomalacia of pregnancy in Indian and Chinese women with congenital rickets in their infants, theorized about anaemia in infants thought to be associated with deficiency of iron in maternal diet, and believed that both goitre and puerperal sepsis might be related to deficient diet in pregnancy.

Field surveys (e.g. McCance, Widdowson and Verdon-Roe, 1938, Table 13.6) confirmed that the diets of pregnant women, as of other groups in the population, showed a 'poverty gradient', the diets of the poor being much inferior to those of the well-to-do. About the same time, experiments in which extra food was provided for pregnant women, especially in the industrially depressed areas, suggested that improvement of diet reduced morbidity and mortality (e.g. Balfour, 1944; People's League of Health, 1946). The picture as a whole suggested strongly that many clinical abnormalities of pregnancy were caused by poor diet. The same was affirmed in the report of the Orr Committee (Department of Health for Scotland, 1943) which examined the position in Scotland before the 1939–45 war, and concluded that 'working-class mothers are often underfed and their diets are of poor quality, deficient in materials for bone and blood formation and in the vitamins needed for health. Such diets are important causes of poor physique and maternal ill-health, low vitality of the infant at birth and inability of the mother to suckle and care for her young'.

During the war years, the national nutritional scene was transformed by an enlightened food policy, which took care to improve the nutritive value of diets in general, and included pregnant and lactating women among the 'priority groups'. At the same time full employment abolished extremes of poverty. It is of great interest that the stillbirth rate in England and Wales fell from 38 per 1000 in 1940 to 28 in 1945, the steepest and most dramatic fall on record in this country. Duncan, Baird and Thomson (1952) considered that the most likely reason was the improvement of maternal nutrition.

Diet in pregnancy

Surveys and feeding experiments in North America during the war years strengthened the belief that the quality of the diet taken by the mother during pregnancy affects foetal growth and vitality (Ebbs, Tisdall and Scott, 1941; Burke *et al.* 1943). An interesting account of the encouraging position towards the end of the war may be found in two symposia of the Nutrition Society (1944a, b).

Nevertheless, caution and not enthusiasm is the keynote of many post-war reports. Garry and Wood (1945–46) introduced their review of dietary requirements for pregnancy and lactation by saying that 'In spite of the voluminous literature, the additions to scientific factual knowledge are somewhat meagre. There are signs of the development of a more critical attitude, even of disillusionment, and there is a tendency to discount the claims made by earlier workers. On the other hand, there has been a veritable spate of popular articles, reviews and books on nutrition, often with special reference to pregnancy and lactation. Many of these publications are, to say the least, not notable for a critical outlook. When to this intensive popularization of knowledge concerning nutrition there is added the by no means disinterested propaganda of manufacturers of "concentrates" and of vitamins, an atmosphere is created far from conducive to calm appraisal of known facts'.

A few of the post-war investigators (Jeans, Smith and Stearns, 1955; Woodhill *et al.* 1955) claimed to have found striking correlations between the reproductive histories and the diets of their subjects, and Dieckmann *et al.* (1951) and Berry and Wiehl (1952) reported benefits from giving protein supplements or advice on diet to pregnant women. In our opinion the data are not convincing. Other dietary and clinical surveys gave negative results even though some of the authors made the most of minor and inexplicable correlations, or argued that their technique must have been inadequate (Sontag and Wines, 1947; Hobson, 1948; Speert, Graff and Graff, 1951; Macy *et al.* 1954; McGanity *et al.* 1954; Thomson, 1959b). The extremely extensive study of the Vanderbilt team deserves special mention (McGanity *et al.* 1954).

Thomson (1958, 1959a, 1959b) took great care in the selection of the subjects (primigravidae) in his survey, and with the technique of collecting clinical and dietary information. He showed that there was an association between mean birth weight of the baby and the calorie value of the diets taken by their mothers during the later part of pregnancy; but the association disappeared when the data were adjusted statistically to allow for the fact that taller and

AA

heavier women took diets of higher calorie value and also had heavier babies than shorter and lighter women. 'The conclusion must be that, within the range of diets in this survey, the influence of diet on birth weight was small, indeed negligible'. The range of nutritive values of the diets in Thomson's sample was wide, and many were well below accepted 'recommended allowances' for pregnancy.

Women delivered by caesarean section had poorer diets than those who had normal deliveries, and they were also shorter. Thomson found no reason to think that diet during pregnancy itself had an effect on the incidence of difficult labour. This question will be raised again in Appendix A, which deals with attempts made many decades ago to prevent difficult delivery by restricting the maternal diet during pregnancy. It is sufficient to say here that a woman whose pelvis has been contracted and distorted by rickets in childhood cannot remedy the anatomical defect by taking a good diet during pregnancy.

The wartime national 'feeding experiment', which embraced the whole population and lasted 5 years, was associated with a reduction of stillbirth rate from 38 to 28 per 1000. It might be expected that an instantaneous sample of the population, showing a gradient in diet with social class, might show some association between quality or quantity of diet and perinatal mortality. Thomson found none in his sample of 489 women. There might be two reasons: first, to be reasonably sure of showing a change of the magnitude of the wartime reduction in a planned feeding trial, it would be necessary to use about 5000 fed subjects and the same number of controls. With a survey sample of less than 500 the negative result does not contradict the large-scale wartime result. Further, the dietary gradient in 1958 was probably less in important respects than that which existed at the beginning of the wartime experiment (Table 13.7).

Thomson (1959b) found a significant correlation (r = 0.3) between the calorie value of the maternal diet and the gain in weight during pregnancy; when the mother is allowed to eat to appetite weight gain appears not to be significantly correlated with maternal height or initial body weight (Thomson and Billewicz, 1957). Since high weight gain is associated with a raised incidence of pre-eclampsia, it might be expected that diets of high calorie value would be associated with an increased tendency to pre-eclampsia.

According to Thomson's data for women allowed to eat to appetite they are so correlated. McGanity *et al.* (1954), found their pre-eclamptic subjects to eat less than the average, but that was presumably because the obstetricians concerned attempted to limit the gain of weight.

Earlier in this section we said that small maternal stature has an adverse effect on reproductive performance. The study of body weight is less easy, since correction should be made for stature; the proper measure is weight-for-height. Thomson and Billewicz (1957; 1963) defined overweight women as the heaviest and underweight as the lightest 25 per cent for each height; in overweight women they found the incidence of pre-eclampsia and delivery by caesarean section to be above average, but that of prematurity to be relatively low. Conversely, underweight women had a high incidence of prematurity and a low incidence of pre-eclampsia.

To sum up, there seems to be little satisfactory evidence that under-feeding *during pregnancy itself* is of any great importance in a modern sophisticated community with a generally high standard of living. There is some evidence that over-feeding or under-exercise, through its effect on body weight and on the amount of weight gained during pregnancy, may be prejudicial, especially by pre-disposing to pre-eclampsia.

In such communities the state of the physique and health of the mothers, which is established before pregnancy, is the chief determinant of reproductive performance. In communities where the general standard of living is high, and where children grow to the full stature of which they are genetically capable, the reproductive results will generally be excellent. Where depressed standards result in poor growth, the girls will become relatively stunted mothers, and will be more liable to many kinds of reproductive disability. The main lesson is that to safeguard the mothers, we should look after the children. It is too late to seek dietetic remedies during pregnancy if damage has already been done.

Vital statistics

That having been said, we can look at some of the international, inter-regional and inter-class differences which appear in official statistics. While it is generally true that dietary practices are related to economic status, it has to be remembered that poor economic status implies a host of adverse conditions other than dietary, and statistical trends and associations must accordingly be interpreted with caution. Differences in the accuracy of registration, or in the definitions used, and also genetic differences, may complicate international comparisons.

Information for the United Kingdom may be obtained from annual and decennial reports of the Registrars General, and from the reports of numerous private investigations; international comparisons may be made with the aid of reports published by the United Nations and its agencies.

In Great Britain there is a steady increase of perinatal mortality as one moves from mothers in the best educated and most affluent occupational groups to those in the poorest groups. Rates tend to be relatively high in areas where industry is or has recently been depressed. The data of the Perinatal Mortality Survey of the National Birthday Trust (which, at the time of writing, are being prepared for publication in detail) show similar trends for most of the individual causes of perinatal death and for prematurity, and areas of high mortality and high prematurity are those in which high proportions of the mothers are of relatively short stature. Conversely, areas in which conditions are and have been generally prosperous have a larger proportion of tall mothers, who have relatively low rates of prematurity and perinatal mortality.

Stillbirths associated with congenital deformity of the central nervous system, anencephaly, hydrocephaly and spina bifida, are most common where social circumstances are least favourable (Anderson, Baird and Thomson 1958; Edwards, 1958; McDonald, 1961).

So far as international comparisons can be made, it appears that similar trends are present. Stillbirth and neonatal death rates are low in countries with a consistently high standard of living, such as the Netherlands, Scandinavia and New Zealand, and high in, for example, the Iberian peninsula. In the United States, rates are higher among negroes than among whites. There are some notable exceptions to such general trends. For example, the official stillbirth rate in Hong Kong is one of the lowest in the world. Thomson, Chun and Baird (1963) thought that the official rate might be about 30 per cent too low, but even then the reproductive efficiency of Chinese mothers in Hong Kong appears to be astonishingly great, and is not to be accounted for by a high standard of economic prosperity, or of maternal physique and health.

Ethnic differences may be responsible. There is evidence (Searle, 1958–59) that the incidence of congenital abnormalities of the central nervous system is less in the Chinese than in Indian and Western peoples. Similarly, genetic difference may explain at least in part the excess of congenital abnormalities of the central nervous system in the lower socio-economic groups of this country.

CHILDBEARING IN DEVELOPING COMMUNITIES

Theoretically, the effects of chronic dietary and other shortages should be seen more clearly in countries and areas where the benefits of modern methods of food production and distribution and the comforts of Western life are not generally available. But precise information about such countries and areas is understandably scarce. Where infective and parasitic diseases overwhelm the medical services, research and the collection of even elementary statistics are difficult. Official vital statistics are of doubtful accuracy. Most of the information collected by private investigators comes from selected groups, such as patients admitted to hospital, and the majority of mothers are usually not delivered in hospital.

Birth weight and prematurity

In Chapter 10 we concluded that the mean birth weight in most of Europe and North America (Caucasian ethnic stock) is about 3300 g. All other ethnic groups have means of the order of 3000 g with the exception of South Indian and Ceylonese, which have means about 2700, and African pygmies which are even smaller. The consistency of the reports for the major groups is impressive, and differences between groups are too big to be readily explained away as due to sampling errors. But the data available do not help us to decide whether, or how much of, the differences should be attributed to ethnic origin, genetic differences within ethnic groups, poor maternal diet and physique, adverse environment, or a mixture.

Estimates of the incidence of prematurity both confirm the reality of the mean differences and show how inappropriate to some populations is the international standard of 'maturity'. Thomson (unpublished data) extracted from records the birth weights of 341 babies born at home in two villages in the Gambia and weighed with tolerable accuracy by local midwives. The mean birth weight was 3016 g (SD 553 g). In the weighed series 17.3 per cent were less than 2500 g; if 13 unweighed babies that were stillborn or died soon after birth are taken as premature also, the rate is 20 per cent on the international standard. The perinatal mortality rate was 68 per 1000 births.

In his study of birth weights of the Wasukuma Bantu, the numerically most important tribe in Tanganyika, McLaren (1959) estimated the incidence of prematurity by applying the international criterion and by the use of unspecified clinical signs. The mean birth weights for over a thousand boys and girls are shown in Table 10.2. The incidence of prematurity is shown in Table 14.1.

De Silva, Fernando and Gunaratne (1962) by a more obscure argument came to the conclusion that the proper dividing line for prematurity in Colombo was 2100 g. The average birth weight of infants born in municipal maternity homes was 2500 g and of infants of higher economic class 2700 g.

We have seen in Chapter 10 that birth weight in the Caucasian ethnic group varies with the stature of the mother. The same is true in other ethnic groups. McLaren (1959) quotes his own earlier measurements in the hills of Orissa: for Oriya infants, male and female, weights of 2618 and 2627 g, and for Khond babies, 2596 and 2518 g, small even for Indians. Malnutrition in the area was uncommon, he says, and diet surveys showed a protein intake between 60 and 80 g daily. But then the mean heights and weights

TABLE 14.1. Prematurity in the Wasukuma
(McLaren, 1959)

Criterion of prematurity:	International standard	Clinical signs
	%	%
All parities	15.6	7.8
First births	30.8	12.1
Other birth orders	3.8 to 12.8	1.9 to 5.1
(No regular change with birth order after the first)		

of adults were: men 63.0" (160 cm) and 103 lb (47 kg), and women 58.1" (148 cm) and 88 lb (40 kg). Autret (1957) gives the birth weight of Basuku infants as 2400 g and their mothers' weight as 38–39 kg. He does not say whether the Basuku are ill nourished, but suggests that genetic differences are to be considered.

Part of the adverse environment in which infants in emergent countries are born is infective disease. Of particular importance in West Africa is malaria which not only affects general health but may injure the placenta. In the Gambian series described above and in another series with even smaller birth weights and a still poorer environment, it may be taken that all the mothers were malarious. Archibald (1958) sought to measure the direct effect of the disease. The mean birth weight of 62 infants where the placenta was malarious was 2778 g; that of 378 infants where the placenta was not infected, 3076 g.

The data assembled in Table 10.2 include several studies (Mukherjee and Biswas, 1959; Achar and Yankauer, 1962; Venkatachalam, 1962 in India; Jans, 1959; Hollingsworth, 1960 in Africa) which show the gradient with socio-economic status which is characteristic also of European and American peoples. The broad picture outlined by the data in Table 10.2 has been filled in and illuminated by a number of more intimate studies concerned particularly with the growth of infants and toddlers. Few of them give measurements of birth weights, but there is almost complete agreement that, even when the environment is bad, average birth weights are 'normal' or 'satisfactory'. The data for growth rates during the early months when the infants are fed entirely, or almost entirely, on breast milk, are more convincing than such vague pronouncements. Most of them show rates within the range of average samples of European or American children. Difficulty with the growth and health of children begins at any time after 4 months of age when the baby outgrows the supply of breast milk without satisfactory replacement, and inherited immunity to infection has waned. Some of the more important studies are those of Nicol (1949), Bruce Chwatt (1952), Matthews (1955), McGregor, Billewicz and Thomson (1961) and Frenk (1961).

From the evidence of *ad hoc* studies of birth weight and from that of growth during the first months of life we have to conclude that even where serious malnutrition in the weaned infant is believed to be common, in the form of kwashiorkor and marasmus, there is no

serious defect of birth weight, and capacity to lactate may be outstanding.

Fertility

It is well known that, at present, birth rates in emergent countries
exceed death rates by so wide a margin that the growing pressure
of population on limited, or poorly exploited, land is believed by
many authorities to be the most urgent problem in the world
today. *Prima facie* there is no reason to think that chronic under-
feeding impairs fertility and, manifestly, fertility is more than
adequate in the presence of such degrees of scarcity and privation
as exist today over large areas of the world. If the growth of population is to be controlled, we must look to 'sophistication' and improved standards of living.

Weight gain and its components

For obvious reasons there is not much information about the rate
at which pregnant women in underdeveloped countries gain
weight, or about the components of gain. Since such women are
presumed to be living at subsistence dietary levels and often have
to undertake hard physical work during pregnancy, exact information would be of great interest. There can be no exception to the
laws of thermodynamic equilibrium, and weight during pregnancy
must, in effect, reflect the balance between energy intake and
energy output.

Fragmentary, but interesting, data have been collected in a
Gambian village (Thomson, personal communication). Weights
during the last trimester of pregnancy in women doing hard
agricultural work show, on the average, a slight loss. Comparison
of weights about the end of the second trimester with those of the
same women before pregnancy suggests a gain during the earlier
part of pregnancy of about 13 lb (6 kg). Similar findings have been
reported from Nigeria (Hauck, 1963).

The most detailed studies available have been made by Gopalan
and his associates in South India (Venkatachalam, Shankar and
Gopalan, 1960). The average weight gain of these 'poor' Indians
was little more than half that of the average Aberdeen primigravida
(Chapter 9), about 7 kg (15 lb) and the shape of the curve is quite
different. Figure 14.1 shows the observed pattern and a tentative
analysis of the components.

The analysis has had to be made by interpolating figures from other sources and by making some assumptions. In the original series, only 15 out of 130 babies were weighed, and in these the mean birth weight was 3120 g. This is considerably higher than the averages reported elsewhere for poor-class South Indians, and we have chosen 2900 g as possibly more representative, although higher than the averages reported for South Indians of the poorest classes. The other components of weight gain have been scaled to a birth weight of 2900 g, using proportions derived from the Aberdeen data. It is known that placenta and liquor amnii are related to birth weight and so presumably is uterine growth. We have found the increase of maternal plasma volume to be related to foetal weight (Hytten and Paintin, 1963). Since women with oedema were excluded from the series reported by Venkatachalam *et al.*, no allowance has been made in Figure 14.1 for additional extracellular water. It can be seen from the figure that, on these

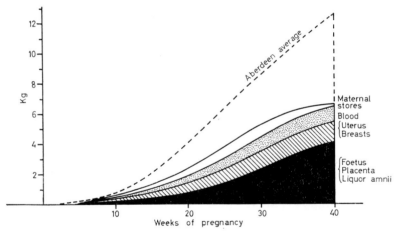

FIGURE 14.1. Possible components of weight gained by poor Indian women (Venkatachalam *et al.* 1960). Compare with Figure 11.3

assumptions, the Indian women were apparently able to store a little fat, perhaps 1 kg, during the earlier part of pregnancy, but most of it had been used by the end of pregnancy.

Whether or not the details are accurate, such a pattern makes physiological sense. As already suggested (Chapter 12) women lay down an energy reserve at a time when the direct needs of the foetus are still small, and the reserve can be used later when the foetus is growing at its fastest rate. If it were not so, foetal growth would be more susceptible of injury and maternal health more seriously impaired if shortage should occur.

Lactation makes much greater energy demands than pregnancy and one would expect that women who have been unable to store some fat during pregnancy would suffer a serious loss of tissue reserves during subsequent lactation. That this may happen is suggested by Venkatachalam (1962a) who showed a falling body weight with rising parity among the poorly-fed Chimbu women of New Guinea.

CHILDBEARING DURING WAR AND FAMINE

We have seen that the evidence from affluent and less affluent societies is by no means sufficiently clear-cut to show whether under-nutrition and malnutrition during pregnancy itself as distinct from the habitual dietary background of the mother can have a serious effect upon reproductive efficiency. An analysis of some of the reports on pregnancy during acute deprivation, the result of war and famine, may clarify the issue. Those for the first world war were assembled by systematic examination of many volumes of the two chief German journals of obstetrics. Those for the second world war are based on the statements of experts who visited occupied or war-devastated areas immediately after the armistice in order to report on the health conditions, especially of mothers and children.

The war of 1914–18

The blockade of Germany in the first world war was unexpected. No preparation to increase or modify home production of food had been made and agricultural work cannot be reorganized overnight, even in a country not already under arms. The effect of interruption or reduction of imports was soon felt and rationing was introduced. As much food as possible was procured from neighbouring countries by purchase or barter, grain from the Balkan countries and butter from Denmark for instance, in exchange for chemicals and manufactured goods. But as the blockade became more effective, neighbouring countries also were affected by being denied imports from America, and in Scandinavia as well as the whole of central

Europe food imports were shortest in the end of 1917 and 1918. According to the official report to the U.K. Government by Professor Starling (1919), the winter of 1916 to 1917 was the time of most acute deprivation in Germany. Those who had no priority for rations, he said, had just enough to keep alive; many did not have even that, for the civil death rate rose steadily to 9.5 per cent in 1915 and 37 per cent in 1918 above the pre-war level. By that time fulminating tuberculosis was a major cause of death, demonstrating the relation of good diet to resistance to that disease. Among the inmates of prisons and asylums hunger oedema was common. Starling says that some deaths were attributed to starvation and that these occurred when the loss of weight reached 30 per cent. A large part of the civil population was of 'low vitality'. The birth rate for the Reich as a whole in 1917 was about half the pre-war rate. Starling seems to have attributed the fall to reduction of fertility in both sexes, but part of it must, of course, have been due to absence of men on active service. There were certainly two or more components, of which, as will be described below, one was 'war amenorrhoea'.

That brief summary of conditions in Germany during the 1914–18 war makes it clear that there was, for a considerable proportion of the population not directly involved in the war effort, and even for some who were, a degree of food shortage far beyond any likely to be imposed in any ordinary physiological test. If food shortage does affect the outcome of pregnancy, it is almost inconceivable that clear evidence should not be found in the war records. Reports from Germany were reviewed by Murray in 1924 on behalf of the Medical Research Council, and since the German conclusions were accepted by Murray at their face value and since the issue is important, a reassessment of the position seems to be required.

What we find is a long series of reports from 1915 on into the post-war years to the effect that birth weights were equal to, or above, the pre-war averages, that there were more babies of high birth weight, and that the food shortage therefore was without effect. Where birth weights were above pre-war averages, the increase was attributed to welfare provisions (which included extra rations) for pregnant women, or to a reduction of the proportion of first births, or to a rise in the average age of pregnant women. The explanations in terms of rise of age or of parity were not related in the original accounts to the occurrence of 'war amenorrhoea' but there can be little doubt that there was an association, although that was, we believe, not the only reason for the apparent rise of birth weight.

Reports of 'war amenorrhoea' came from all over Germany, usually without discussion of aetiology. It occurred in all ranks of society, they said, but more often in women of the hospital class than in private practice. It was attributed to monotony of diet, to ergot poisoning from badly milled, ergot-infested rye in bread, to war neurosis; that it could be caused by shortage of food was even denied. Where the clinical signs and not merely incidence were discussed, atrophy of the uterus was consistently stated to have occurred. In at least two clinics biopsies of the ovary at operation for other reasons showed cystic changes with absence of corpora lutea and secondary changes in the uterus. The pathology of war amenorrhoea as there described is confirmed in a report from Leiden in the second world war. Holmer (1947) adds to the description that, even when menstruation occurred, the cycle was anovulatory. He says too that degeneration of the germinal epithelium occurred in men.

None of the German reports gives any indication of what effect war amenorrhoea might have had on the birth rate, but a report from Stockholm (Nilsson, 1920) is more informative. Before the war amenorrhoea occurred in less than 1 per cent of hospital patients, about 0.6 or 0.7 per cent. It rose steadily during the war to reach an incidence of 11 per cent. in the third quarter of 1918 The maximum incidence of amenorrhoea was followed, 9 months later, by a minimum for the birth rate. In January 1917 there were 600 births, followed by an almost continuous fall to 390 in May 1919, a fall of a third. It cannot of course be assumed that amenorrhoea was the sole cause in Sweden or elsewhere, but it looks as if it might account for a substantial part of the reduction of the birth rate. That view is supported by the age incidence of the disorder. In Stockholm it was most frequent in women of 20 to 30 years of age and almost all of the patients were nulliparae. In Germany also it was said to be most frequent between the ages of 20 and 30. In both descriptions therefore it occurred most frequently where it would reduce, and on the Swedish data reduce substantially, the proportion of first births. In Germany the rise of birth weight was attributed by some to deficit of first births.

A completely satisfying interpretation of the reports on weight is not possible because of the obvious differences in what is to be understood by 'birth weight'. Where a basis is stated at all, it may be simply 'mature' without any definition of maturity; or it may be all births over 2000 g weight or over 2500 g weight, with or without stillbirths; or a length criterion might be used, or a combination of length and weight. There is no guarantee that the earlier statistics with which comparison is made were on the same basis, and there is a general flavour of choosing a favourable basis for the calculation. An *ad hoc* analysis of Aberdeen data shows that, taking all single births less macerated foetuses and malformations as the standard, exclusion of all births of weight less than 2000 g would raise the mean by 50 g and exclusion of all births of weight less than 2500 g would raise it by 100 g. Hence increases of the order of 50 to 100 g need have no significance in the absence of a clear statement of the basis on which birth weight was computed at the dates compared.

There are other reasons for doubting the validity of the usual statement that war diet had not had any adverse effect on birth weight. The reports from Vienna and Budapest about birth weight, although they agree in general that there was no great change, at or after the end of the war admit reductions of from 100 to 200 g and, what is more important and more illuminating, they say that the patients had changed. Only the better fed were having babies at all. And finally there are one or two reports from Germany which offer a strong suspicion of general suppression of the truth in the interests of popular morale. Writing in 1916 Dr Mössmer said: 'The sensational statements of Kettner on the frequency at present of small, underdeveloped, fragile, very thin, new-born infants with a 'cerebral' tendency, if they reach the general public, are calculated to cause great anxiety because the alleged inferiority of the children would naturally be attributed to the food shortage.' Three years later, after the end of the war, Gessner (1919) wrote: 'Unfortunately we have no clinical investigations on the significance of bodily work and exercise during pregnancy for the course of birth and the size of the child and about the effect of different foods on the metabolism of the pregnant woman. These wide gaps in our knowledge have been filled in an empirical way by the mass experiment of the hunger blockade, in that it showed that, in pregnant women with plenty of exercise and work continued to delivery and at the same time restricted diet, deliveries are quicker and easier because the otherwise impeding layer of fat is absent and the children are smaller'. We can now summarise and interpret the position. First, the younger potential mothers did not conceive. Second, such babies as were produced were born to women in rural areas or with priority rations. That is to say that a reduction of birth weight would tend to be offset by the rise of maternal age, parity and maternal economic class. Third, there is a suggestion that even the children that were born *were not of normal vitality*. We shall see that such an interpretation is amply supported by events in the second world war.

The war of 1939–45

In Germany conditions were altogether different from what they were in the first world war. Food production and preservation were planned in advance to provide the maximum yield of energy and protein and the prelude to major war operations was the occupation of neighbouring countries so that, at need, they might be despoiled. The more significant reports come therefore not from Germany but from the invaded and occupied countries. In neither was there any reason for *suppressio veri*.

The siege of Leningrad began in August, 1941 and the city was relieved in August, 1943. Conditions in respect of food were worst between September 1941 and February 1942, before the air lift was organized. The picture of events at the State Pediatric Institute is shown in Table 14.2, in terms of birth weights of liveborn infants (Antonov, 1947).

TABLE 14.2. Infants Born at Term* in a Leningrad Clinic
1941–42 (Antonov, 1947)

	January to June				July to December			
	Boys		Girls		Boys		Girls	
	No.	Wt. g	No.	Wt. g	No.	Wt. g	No.	Wt. g
1941	933	3444	874	3302	503	3344	447	3222
1942	135	2815	120	2760	39	3199	32	2890
Difference		629		542		145		332

* Criterion a length at birth of 47 cm or more, irrespective of weight.

Amenorrhoea was common. Only 79 pregnancies were recorded for the second half of 1942, with 77 live births, 71 judged to be born at term. Of the 79 women pregnant, 73 were known not to have suffered from acute food shortage. They were professional or otherwise occupied women with priority rations.

Antonov says that the weight of infants born in other Leningrad clinics was, on the average, down by about 500 g for boys and 410 g for girls. It is clear from Antonov's description of Leningrad during the siege that conditions were much worse than any during the first world war. The city was bombed and shelled; there was no heating and no public transport, and the winter of 1941–42 was severe. On a diet scarcely sufficient to keep them alive, women had to queue for rations, chop wood, clear snow and ice, clean back yards and stand guard for air raids. They suffered hunger, vitamin deficiency, cold, excessive physical strain, lack of rest, constant nervous tension. Such children as were born in the first half of 1942 were described as of low vitality, inert, unable to maintain their temperature, easily chilled, sucking weakly and consequently suffering high mortality. The women produced little milk and the duration of lactation was short.

The position in blockaded Rotterdam during the famine period from October 1944 to May 1945, when details of the reports are brought together, was closely similar. Smith (1947) says that 50 per cent of urban women were amenorrhoeic and that the birth rate fell to about a third of normal. The numbers and weights of infants born were closely related to the acute food shortage. The number of infants born during February, March and April 1945 was normal but the average birth weight was less by about 240 g than the normal. Most women had gained no more than 2 kg during pregnancy and a large number lost weight. In contrast the number of infants born was at a minimum in October, November and December, 1945 (84, 87 and 89 from an average of about 220 for the same months in 1944) but the average weight was above pre-war level. Only the best fed women conceived during the severe shortage and, before the demands of the foetus were significant, the shortage was over. Even allowing for the fact that only the best fed women reproduced at all, it seems surprising that there was no evidence of reduced foetal vitality, in a high stillbirth rate. According to Holmer (1947), mortality in the first week was high, and reduction of foetal vitality may well have contributed to the rise.

Evidence from Austria and Germany itself, if less dramatic than that from the besieged cities, is to the same effect.

Reports from Vienna show conditions to have been more severe than in the first world war. There were fluctuations of average birth weight which improved with the home produce of summer and deteriorated during the winter, but rural areas and country towns showed no evidence of the shortage. Other areas reported changes, resembling those of the first world war with decreases of average weight of 100 or 200 g, without much critical examination of the circumstances. Lax (1947) in Leipzig, in addition to the fall in weight, reported also an increase of premature births from 10 per cent pre-war to 16 per cent in 1945–46 when there were less than half the total number of births. Giese and Kayser (1947) in Erfurt, including all births in their reckoning, not a selected sample such as most commentators used, found an average fall of over 200 g in mean birth weight between 1938–39 and 1945–46 and Umland (1948) confirmed that finding. Fink (1948) in Mannheim, taking a highly selected sample, still found a difference of 144 g between 1937 and 1946 and Budde (1948) in Bochum, with a sample of 10,000 infants over 2500 g in weight, reported a fall of 133 g in 1946–47 compared with the corresponding mean weight in 1936–39. Both Fink and Budde found a shift in the distribution of birth weights from the higher weights into the 2500 to 3000 class. These mean differences are not large, but since the infants were, in all likelihood, the best from the best fed mothers, they are probably real.

There are two other pieces of evidence pointing to an effect of the unfavourable environment on reproduction. First, it seems well established that, among the children that were born in Germany in the first two or three years after the war, while food supplies and other environmental conditions were still bad, the incidence of congenital malformations rose, especially malformations of the central nervous system (Pschyrembel, 1948; Gesenius, see Pschyrembel). Second, it has been shown that the incidence of dizygous twin births, which may be a measure of favourable conditions (p. 391) fell in occupied France, the Netherlands and Norway, but not in unoccupied France or in Denmark where there was no real shortage of food. Unfortunately, we have no information for Germany.

In summary we may say, notwithstanding any attempts that

were made in the interests of public morale to camouflage the position, that acute deprivation of food, in the quantitative and caloric sense, had the following effects in the two world wars:

(i) Amenorrhoea became common, especially in younger women, and the conception rate fell.

(ii) The women who did conceive were better fed than those who did not.

(iii) There were fewer first births and that, by itself, would minimize any reduction of mean birth weight.

(iv) There were fewer births to women of the poorer classes and that also would tend to minimize change in mean birth weight among the population as a whole.

Comparisons of wartime with pre-war birth weights were not made at the time by birth order and social class, and such comparisons cannot be made now from published accounts. But it is clear that, as a criterion of the effect of acute deprivation of food on reproductive performance, published mean birth weights give no true picture.

General interpretation

The most severe forms of deprivation, as in war and famine, are associated with widespread amenorrhoea and failure to conceive. Those women who do conceive are a selected group, biassed towards multiparae and the more privileged classes who are able to obtain more food than the others. This kind of selection minimizes the effects of famine on reproductive statistics, but the available evidence suggests that the babies born are undersized and of impaired vitality.

With chronic, but not critical degrees of deprivation, such as exist in many emergent countries, and also in the developed countries, there are socio-economic gradients in reproductive efficiency. In both types of country, the size and vitality of babies are lower in the poorer classes. Taken as a whole, the evidence does not suggest that there is much direct effect of deprivation during pregnancy itself on the 'efficiency' of pregnancy. It suggests, rather, that the general levels of feeding in different social strata, by their effects on the growth and vitality of children and on the physique and general health of adults, are of great significance. A well-fed population has well-grown and healthy mothers. The effects of

BB

generally depressed nutritional levels are complicated by the effects of disease and other adverse environmental conditions. As the evidence is at present, the possibility cannot be excluded that some genetic segregation may be contributing to the continued existence of socio-economic strata. If that is so, neither its extent nor its importance can be rightly judged until more progress has been made with the control of environment and the equitable distribution of food. Even then it may take generations of readaptation of mother and infant before we can be sure.

The Place of Prochownick in the History of Weight Control in Pregnancy

The idea of dieting the mother to control the size of her baby is usually attributed to the German physician Prochownick although reports of measures recommended by obstetricians to control birth weight go back to the 18th century, and those were probably not the first. Nor were they all based on restriction of diet. Periodic blood-letting and the use of purgatives were common, and indeed persisted into modern times. In the discussion following a paper in 1934, we read: (Dr Carl Henry Davis) 'Just as soon as I find a patient has gained too much during a week or ten-day period, an effort is made to increase elimination. If she has gained more than one or two pounds her diet is reduced and we give her Epsom salts before breakfast once or twice or three times a week, according to her condition.' Yet, as long ago as 1803 Professor Brünninghausen in Würzburg suggested that it was foolish to let pregnant women eat and then get rid of food and that it would be better for them to eat less. He experimented accordingly with a diet chiefly of thin soups, green vegetables and fruit. Legumes, potatoes and bread were forbidden. Only a few patients were treated and accounts of only two were published by Brünninghausen. One of the infants is described as 'very well nourished and fat', the other as 'not fat', but 'well nourished'. Both were said to have soft skulls with wide sutures, so that birth was easier. The diet was severely criticized by prominent obstetricians and presumably little used.

During the second half of the 19th century it became increasingly common to attempt to get live infants from women with contracted pelves by induction of labour, on the grounds that small premature infants would pass more easily through the small pelvis. Here is an extract from Cazeaux's *Theoretical and practical treatise on midwifery* published in 1871. 'It is really wonderful that the consequences of this operation [surgical induction of labour] have been so long dreaded; since, in two hundred and fifty cases collected by M. Lacour, in the commencement of 1844, more than one-half of the children survived, and scarcely one woman in sixteen died. Let any one compare these results with those furnished either by symphyseotomy or by the Caesarean operation.' Prochownick is nowadays credited with being the first person seriously to attempt control of birth weight by restriction of diet in pregnancy. Writing in 1889, he said of premature induction of labour that, although the prospects had improved slightly, the operation still had many opponents, especially among practising doctors whose main preoccupation was not with the improved prospects for the mother, but with the chance of survival of the child. In his second paper in 1901 he gave the mortality rates even in well-run hospitals in 1885 as between 45 and 50 per cent, in one as low as 42 per cent, and they were certainly not better in practice outside hospitals.

It was therefore in the hope of avoiding induction of labour that Prochownick took up the question of diet, for the first time since Brünninghausen. He published his first paper in 1889. It presented only three case reports but, Prochownick said, it was published in the hope that others would try his proposed diet. It introduced an entirely new idea. In modern terms it would be described as a high-protein, low-carbohydrate diet and it was said to be so restricted in energy value as to ensure that the woman would put on little or no weight beyond that of the foetus, and that neither mother nor child would put on much, or any, fat. Prochownick's second and main publication was in 1901 and because most of the subsequent experiments in control of birth weight are said to derive from it, we must consider in some detail just what Prochownick said and did. His paper begins with a general introduction which covers the effect on the pregnant woman of social conditions and employment in industry, and the benefit in terms of infant mortality of compulsory rest with payment before and after delivery. He says that among employees in the Dollfus factories in Mühlhausen infant mortality fell from 39 to 25 per cent when wages were paid to the women for 6 weeks before confinement, without the need to work. In the canton of Glarus infant mortality fell significantly when absence from work was enforced for only 6 weeks after delivery.[1]

---

[1] In den J. Dollfus' schen Fabriken (Mühlhausen i.E.) sank die Sterblichkeit der Kinder im ersten Lebensjahre von 39 auf 25 Proc., nachdem man den Arbeiterinnen 6 Wochen vor und nach der Niederkunft Lohn zahlte, ohne sie

Accepted views about physiological requirements in pregnancy were summarized, the main contention being that there was no question of 'eating for two', the needs of the foetus being met by metabolic economies on the part of the mother. On the other hand, Lahmann's view that weak, chlorotic, 'dysaemic' women produce cherubs (Posaunenengeln) was, he said, not supported by experience of obstetrics among the poor.

Prochownick's trials were of three types. First, he tried the effect of restricted diet on obese multiparae with pendulous abdomen and atrophic muscle. Patients of the second class for whom diets were prescribed were anaemic, chlorotic, exhausted women. For these a plentiful, substantial diet with iron was prescribed. His third class of patient, and that with which we are especially concerned, was a small and carefully selected group of women with a moderate degree of contracted pelvis, who had had at least one previous pregnancy, usually with a stillborn child.

The diet prescribed for the first and third groups was a high protein, low carbohydrate diet. The obese were allowed a little more food than the third group and their fluid was less severely restricted. The two diets are shown in Table A.1, side by side.

For both groups, fluid was restricted and the amount of fruit eaten *must not be sufficient to allay thirst* (... und vor Allem rohes Obst in beliebiger aber nicht zu grosser Menge und nicht viel auf einmal zur Durstbekämpfung erlaubt). The obese were allowed up to 500 or 600 cc in a day, those with contracted pelvis must never exceed 500 cc. The reason for restriction of fluid is stated to have been the belief that high fluid intake increased deposition of fat, restriction of fluid inhibited it. It is stated also, in reference to the patients with contracted pelvis, that the foetus during the last two months of pregnancy puts on weight rapidly, lays down fat in the skin, develops skin turgor and calcifies the skull bones. Hence the idea was, during that time, to make sure that the mother would be in nitrogen equilibrium but to prevent as far as possible the transfer of fat and water to the foetus. (Einen besonderen Nachdruck habe ich auf die möglichst geringe Flüssigkeitszufuhr gelegt).

The diet was calculated to provide 130 to 160 g protein, 80 to 130 g fat and 100 g carbohydrate, equivalent to from 1800 to 2000

zur Arbeit zu zwingen. Im Kanton Glarus sank dieselbe Sterblichkeit schon deutlich, als nur 6 Wochen gezwungene Arbeitsruhe nach der Niederkunft Einführung fand.

TABLE A.1

	Reducing diet	Diet in contracted pelvis
Morning	Coffee with milk, 125 cc Bread, 40 g with butter Egg, 1 or 2 A little fruit	Coffee, 100 cc Zwieback or bread and butter, 25 g
Forenoon	Fruit; 1 egg Bread and butter, 15 g	
Midday	Meat, vegetables (except turnip and peas), lettuce, fruit, cheese	Meat or egg or fish with little sauce, Green vegetables cooked in fat, lettuce, cheese
Afternoon	Coffee or tea, not more than 100 cc, bread and butter 15 g 1 egg if desired	
Evening	Egg or meat; Bread, 40–60 g butter, fruit, cheese; milk or tea 125–200 cc	As mid-day with bread 40–50 g and butter as desired Fruit or lettuce. Daily: 300–400 cc red or moselle wine. Forbidden: Water, soups, potatoes, cereal dishes (Mehlspeisen), sugar and beer.

kcal daily. It was later criticized on the basis that a pregnant woman requires 40 kcal per kg mean body weight, which, taken as 65 kg, gives a requirement of 2600. There is little or no evidence to suggest that the requirement is 2600 kcal, and recent findings would not class Prochownick's restricted diet as grossly insufficient in energy value.

So much for the actual composition of the diet. The points on which Prochownick laid special stress were as follows. Since we believe they are important if we are to understand why some who tried the diet subsequently did so without effect, we include quotations from the original.

In reference to his first, reducing diet, Prochownick says that he was not concerned with the weight of the child but 'ist in diesen sonst ja gesunded Frauen das Gewicht der Kinder mit der

Entfettung der Mutter deutlich heruntergegangen, obwohl es nach dem Alter der Mutter und der Geburtenzahl eher hätte steigen sollen. ... Auf die Länge der Kinder und Härte der Kopfknochen war ein sichtlichen Einfluss nicht vorhanden, hingegen war die Verschieblichkeit der Kopfhaut über die Kopfknocken und der geringere Turgor der Haut im Ansicht und am Rücken bei den Kinder mehrfach scharf ausgeprägt'. (... The weight of the children of these otherwise healthy women, with reduction of their mother's weight, was definitely reduced, although according to the age of the mothers and parity it might have been expected to rise. ... There was no obvious effect on the length of the children or hardness of the skull bones; on the other hand the mobility of the scalp over the skull bones, and the reduced turgor of the skin of the face and on the back were clearly to be seen.)

In the second part of his report of 1901, in which he deals chiefly with the selected women with contracted pelvis who took the more restricted diet, with more closely controlled fluid, Prochownick says the diet was well tolerated by all. The only complaints were of thirst (which is important) and of too much meat. He goes on to describe the children successfully delivered at term as follows.

'Bei einer grösseren Zahl der neugeborenen wird eine deutliche, mitunter ganz auffallende Magerkeit beschrieben; recht übereinstimmend lauten die Berichte über Faltung und Verschieblichkeit der fettarmen, wenig gespannten Kopfhaut und die ausgesprochene Verschieblichkeit der Kopfknochen.'

(In most of the newborn a definite and sometimes quite striking thinness is described; reports are in good agreement about wrinkling and mobility of the scalp which had little fat, and poor turgor, and the remarkable mobility of the skull bones.)

From these descriptions and a statement which Prochownick made more than once: 'Einen besonderen Nachdruck habe ich auf die möglichst geringe Flüssigkeitszufuhr gelegt' (I laid special emphasis on as small an intake of fluid as possible) we believe that the secret of his success lay, not so much in high protein or low carbohydrate or energy restriction as in restriction of fluid. Certainly, the high protein, low calorie diet in modern practice would pass muster as a slimming diet, but we know of no definite evidence to support the idea that restriction of fluid inhibits deposition of fat. The diet, Prochownick said, on account of the restriction of carbohydrate and water, had been described as a 'diabetic diet'. It did not deliberately follow the pattern of a diabetic diet, but it does resemble the restricted diet recommended by Naunyn, Prochownick's Austrian contemporary and authority on diabetes, in his (1906) textbook. Of water Naunyn says: 'It goes almost without saying that beverages should be controlled in quantity and kind, like foods. First the total fluid intake must be decided because if thirst is allowed to be the guide, harm may be done.'

We now know from experience of desert life and related experimental studies that the mode of induction of water loss by restriction of intake is important in relation to tolerance. If the onset is abrupt and loss is rapid, then desiccation of the blood is the first result and that is ill tolerated. If the onset is gradual and adjustment is by degrees, then the loss of water falls chiefly on muscle and skin, which normally carry a reserve, and they tolerate the loss of a considerable portion of their total water without obvious functional or structural damage. Prochownick says his treatment began slowly (alle langsam beginnend), with two or three weeks allowed for adjustment to the restricted diet and reduced fluid intake.

There is abundant evidence from animal experiments that restriction of the food intake in the last third or so of pregnancy will seriously affect the growth of the foetus and its chances of survival. For instance if the diet of ewes is so restricted that little or no weight is gained in the last third of pregnancy, there are few twins and all lambs are of less than normal weight. Twins are not only light but their vitality may be so impaired that they are unable to stand and so cannot reach the teats, or they may be too weak to suck, and so mortality is far above normal (Thomson and Thomson, 1949). We have shown in Chapter 14 that severe restriction of the diet of women also greatly prejudices the vitality of the infant, but, from Prochownick's description of the infants born to his restricted patients, there was no sign of loss or vigour. We have, so far, no data from animal experiment or clinical study to show beyond what limits of restricted fluid intake, and to what extend, dehydration of the mother is passed on to the child *in utero*. For that reason we have made the following calculation.

If we accept Laron's (1957) estimate that, when there is a significant loss of skin turgor in infants, they have lost at least 6 per cent of body weight as water, then, since the water content of the normal term infant is about 70 per cent, the loss represents between

8 and 9 per cent of total body water. Since mother and infant must be in approximate equilibrium in respect of water, the mother's loss is probably of the same order of magnitude, and an adult will tolerate such a loss without other disability than thirst. It appears therefore that the results that Prochownick claimed are possible, and to be attributed in large part to restriction of fluid.

Prochownick refers to a confirmatory report of the Dutch obstetrician Donath, which is translated in the Edinburgh Medical Journal of 1891. The patient is described as a 'little wee wifie' of 148 cm in height with a true conjugate of 11 cm. After four pregnancies with stillborn infants, she was put on the Prochownick diet and produced at term 'a boy of 2430 grammes . . . who from his meagreness looked like a miniature old mannie.'

There are some curious commentaries on Prochownick's work. Mussey in his review (1949) says: 'As a result of sheer persistence and assertive publications, Prochownick extended the use of the diet, which I previously mentioned as having been rejected by Cazeaux in 1850, until it became known as the Prochownick diet.' Yet the sum total of Prochownick's publications were the short paper in the Centralblatt für Gynäkologie in 1889 in which he described three cases and invited others to test the diet; the detailed paper in Therapeutische Monatshefte in two parts in 1901 (of which at least one reviewer had read only the first part), and a paper in Zentralblatt für Gynäkologie in 1917, which so far seems to have escaped the attention of reviewers.

In the last of these papers Prochownick, invited to comment on the effect on birth weight of the restricted wartime diet in Germany, conceded that, up to 1915, with a low protein, low fat diet made up with carbohydrate, there had been no effect, but like the cautious clinician he appears to have been, he thought a final judgment must await the statistics for 1916–17.

About his own work and criticisms of it he had to say: 'In our age it is commonly required that an empirically established fact is proved by animal experiment, and then, if the animal experiment agrees, the objection is raised that such a result cannot be transferred to man. But, if the experiment does not give the same result, the empirical finding is still not accepted; . . . .' The acid proof of whether his diet did what he claimed lay, he said, in those cases described in which there was a difficult first birth, then with the prescribed diet, an easy second birth, and with unrestricted diet in the third pregnancy a difficult labour and death of the child, and, in three cases since 1901, a fourth easy labour on the diet. To make his own attitude to the whole procedure plain he said further: 'My aim was not and is not *eo ipso* to produce small babies but to avoid premature induction in medium degrees of contracted pelvis, and translated into modern obstetrical language, to avoid surgical interference at term. If women with normal pelves wish to bring small babies into the world and are encouraged by doctors, such treatment should not be associated with my name. Usually it is not taken seriously and not conscientiously carried through.' Certainly the impression we get of Prochownick is not that of a self-assertive person at all, but of a modest, careful, clinically observant doctor who took considerable pains to know what physiologists said of diet in pregnancy, but, in our interpretation, missed the full significance of the restriction of water, on which he was so mercilessly insistent. His commentators sometimes remark on the restriction of fluid, sometimes ignore it, but do not attribute any special importance to it. Indeed most comments are inaccurate in that or other details of the diet or procedure, and questions about it are not consistently answered in the same way even in the same medical periodical. (See Journal of the American Medical Association 1911, 1913 and 1918).

APPENDIX B

The Sex Ratio

The proportion of male to female infants at birth is relevant in this book because it may be influenced by events and circumstances in pregnancy. Nevertheless we will attempt only a quick outline of the many complexities of the subject.

It seems quite certain that many more males than females are conceived and the sex-ratio at conception, the primary sex ratio, is probably about 120; i.e. 120 males for every 100 females (Parkes, 1925–26). Throughout life, including foetal life, the male has a greater mortality until at the age of 95 or more only about 25 males remain for every 100 females. Figure B.1 shows the changing sex ratio from conception to old age; the post-natal figures are from the 1951 Census of England and Wales (Registrar-General, 1956a).

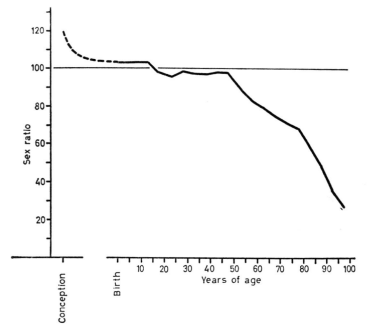

FIGURE B.1. Changing sex ratio from conception to old age

383

From the biological point of view it is important only that the sex ratio should be about 100 at the age of mating, since equality ensures the smallest amount of inbreeding (Kalmus and Smith, 1960).

The secondary sex ratio has been extensively studied and huge amounts of data are available from national birth statistics. It can be altered by changing the primary sex ratio, the proportion of males conceived, and by changing the differential of mortality between conception and birth; but so little is known, or can be known at present about the primary sex ratio that it is not possible to say at what point most of the known influences act.

The male determining sperm (containing the Y chromosome) has a smaller head than the female-determining sperm (containing the X chromosome), moves more rapidly and is present in greater numbers (Shettles, 1961), which may explain the high sex ratio at conception. Shettles suggests that the characteristics of the endo-cervical mucus at the time of ovulation favour the migration of the male-determining sperm, but that the female-determining sperm may be better able to tolerate a less favourable environment. That would explain the great excess of males which had been repeatedly recorded when conception is deliberately effected at the time of ovulation.

If influences such as the proximity of conception to ovulation affect the sex ratio, they will also seriously reduce the value of the Weinberg formula for the calculation of uniovular twinning rates from national statistics. The formula (see p. 390) assumes that the chances of conception of a male or a female are equal, so that for binovular twins the numbers of pairs of like sex will be approximately equal to the number of pairs of unlike sex. But if the maternal environment, or other influence at the time of conception, favours males or females then there will be a preponderance of twins of like sex in binovular pregnancies.

The evidence for the greater mortality of males during foetal life is overwhelming. For example, Table B.1, taken from Ciocco (1938a) shows the sex ratio in foetal deaths occurring between 1925 and 1934 in seven States of the U.S.A. where reliable information was available. Even if we ignore early abortions, where the recognition of sex is difficult if not impossible without histological examination, there is a striking excess of males at three and four months of gestation. The sex ratio falls until seven months and then rises again

TABLE B.1. Sex Ratio of Abortions and Stillbirths in Seven States
of the U.S.A., 1925–34 (from Ciocco, 1938a)

Period of gestation (months)	Sex ratio males/100 females	Sex recognized in No.	%
Under 2	228	82	10.1
2	431	563	27.8
3	361	2388	63.2
4	201	6401	89.5
5	140	12541	97.4
6	123	17857	99.0
7	112	23109	99.4
8	125	28903	99.6
9	135	68932	99.8
10 and over	133	2667	99.6

towards term. It is difficult to interpret the trend without more knowledge of the causes of foetal death. Ciocco (1938b) has given details also of the sex ratio for stillbirths by stated cause. Males preponderated for all causes except malformation where there was a clear excess of females, particulatly in spina bifida. The highest sex ratio was, as might have been expected, when death was due to 'difficult labour'.

More recent evidence of the high sex ratio of aborted foetuses has been given by Tricomi, Serr and Solish (1960) who studied the sex chromatin pattern in placental cells. In 242 abortions before the 24th week of pregnancy, 149 were male, a sex ratio of about 160.

Some of the influences affecting the sex ratio appear to be genetically determined. There is a considerable body of evidence to suggest that differences of sex ratio are associated with different blood groups. For example, babies of group AB mothers have a significantly higher sex ratio than those born to mothers with other blood groups and group O babies have a higher sex ratio than babies of other groups (Allan, 1959). Renkonen, Mäkelä and Lehtovaara (1961) in a study of 158,000 families suggest that some families have a tendency to produce children of one sex and

Renkonen and Lehtovaara (1962) present evidence which suggests the possibility that women who have borne boys may develop some sort of reaction to male infants which reduces their chances of producing a subsequent male child. It is not possible to make a final judgement about the possibility of familial tendency to produce children of a single sex. Data are not easy to acquire, and interpretation of the data is far from straightforward. The statistical pitfalls have been pointed out by Edwards (1958–59).

Schull and Neel (1958) in a study of Japanese who survived the atomic bombing, found an excess of male infants born to parents where the father had been irradiated and a reduced sex ratio where the mother had been irradiated, changes which would be expected if exposure to radiation had induced sex-linked lethal mutations.

It has long been recognized that the sex ratio declines with

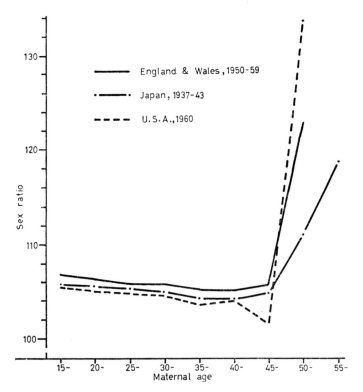

FIGURE B.2. Sex ratio in relation to maternal age

maternal age and Figure B.2 shows the remarkable similarity of the rate of change in three countries: Japan (Takahashi, 1954), U.S.A. (U.S. Department of Health, Education and Welfare, 1962) and England and Wales (Registrar General 1953-56, 57, 57a, 59-60a). A curious reversal of the trend in the upper age groups with extremely high ratios for women over 50 occurred in each set of data, and although it was necessarily based on small numbers, it was too consistent to be dismissed. Apart from the late effect, for which no explanation can be offered, the effect of maternal age is spurious. It has been convincingly demonstrated by Novitski and Kimball (1958) that the downward trend with age is due very largely to the effect of birth order with some contribution from paternal age; maternal age, as such, has no effect on sex ratio Calculations based on Takahashi's data support the view that birth order and not maternal age is the important influence.

It has been accepted for a long time that more males are born in wartime but the data are often contradictory. The evidence was reviewed by Panunzio (1943) who concluded that there was some support for the view.

There may also be ethnic differences in sex ratio. Ciocco (1938a) showed that both U.S. negroes and migrant Italians had low secondary sex ratios, too low to be explained by a higher rate of foetal loss, and that there were relatively more males born to parents of mixed race, 'hybrids', than to parents of the same racial stock. Kang and Cho (1962) have shown that Koreans have a particularly high secondary sex ratio; it was about 115 in 11,131 births.

Other influences on sex ratio have been demonstrated. The sex ratio for infants of mothers who smoked cigarettes during pregnancy was below 100 in two series where it was examined (Frazier *et al.* 1961; Heriott, Billewicz and Hytten, 1962).

Air-force personnel who fly high-performance military aircraft have infants with a dramatically low sex ratio compared to their colleagues who fly transport aircraft or who do not fly (Snyder, 1961).

It should be evident from this very brief, and far from comprehensive review, that the sex ratio offers considerable opportunities for further research.

Multiple Births

The product of conception usually, and in the sense in which the term is used in this book, contains only one child, but multiple births do occur and account must be taken of them. From the physiological point of view we should like to know how many human pregnancies begin with the embedding of more than one ovum and how many with the splitting of one zygote and the subsequent embedding of the two or more parts.

The human ovary contains about half a million oocytes at birth. No more than about 500 will be shed during 30 years of reproductive life; the other 99.9 per cent degenerate, or undergo 'atresia'. The phenomenon of atresia is discussed by Ingram (1962); little is known about it. It seems remarkable that hundreds of oocytes should be started on the way to ovulation in each sexual cycle, presumably by some hormonal, probably pituitary, stimulus and yet only one should finally become a fertilizable egg. Viewed from that angle dizygotic twin births might be regarded as due to a failure of some mechanism, at present unknown, to limit ovulation to one of the many possible oocyte candidates available at each cycle.

That disturbance of an endocrine pattern may be responsible is suggested by the dramatic results of injecting human pituitary follicle stimulating hormone (HPFSH) and human chorionic gonadotrophin into women (Gemzell, 1963). Gemzell induced ovulation in women who had long standing amenorrhoea by giving HPFSH for 10 days followed by HCG for 3 days. When the report was made, four of these women had completed full term pregnancies and three of them had dizygous twins; two others aborted at 5 and 6 months, one dizygous twins, the other 4-egg quadruplets.

There is no reliable evidence to show how many fertilized ova perish at early stages of development and, because the stillbirth rate in multiple pregnancy is higher than that in single pregnancy (Karn, 1951–52; Anderson, 1956), it seems likely that the embryonic wastage also may be higher when more than one ovum is shed at one time, or an ovum divides into independent parts at some early cleavage. Guttmacher (1939) claimed that one abortion in 37 was of twins, which would make the abortion rate for twins much higher than for a single conceptus, but his information came from hospital records and his estimate is therefore probably an overestimate. We can compare only birth rates, remembering that, when the statistics available are based on live births or births in which at least one twin survived, the error of underestimation will be greater than it is for single births.

There are two other sources of error. Because of the known hazards of multiple pregnancy a higher proportion of the mothers are confined in hospital and so the incidence is inflated in hospital statistics in comparison with that in the general population. The magnitude of the difference varies. Anderson's (1956) data for the maternity hospital in Aberdeen with a twinning incidence of 15 per 1000 total maternities was only one point ahead of the estimate of the Registrar General (Scotland) of 14 per 1000. But Karn's (1951–52) analysis of University College Hospital (London) records from 1927 to 1948 gave an incidence of 16.7 per 1000 while the incidence in England and Wales from the Registrar General's returns was only 11.4 (Bulmer, 1957–58). That makes it the more difficult to interpret the hospital data given by Bulmer (1960b) for Africa, and discussed further below.

Triplets and multiple births of higher order are rare. Estimates for the United States from 1951–57 are shown in Table C.1; they refer to multiple births where at least one infant survived and so underestimate the actual incidence. Per million confinements there were 10,539 twins, 93 triplets and 1.1 quadruplet; the rates were higher in non-whites than in whites (Statistical Bulletin of the

TABLE C.1. The Incidence of Twins, Triplets and Quadruplets in the U.S.A. 1951–57. (Statistical Bulletin of the Metropolitan Life Insurance Co., 1960)

Colour	No. of confinements	Plural births per million confinements			
		Twins	Triplets	Quadruplets	Total
White	23,751,611	10,059	85	1.0	10,145
Non-white	3,946,146	13,423	141	1.8	13,576
Total	27,697,757	10,539	93	1.1	10,634

CC

Metropolitan Life Insurance Co, 1960). So little is known of the statistical relations of triplet and quadruplet infants in respect of sex or of the number of ova concerned, that we shall deal only with twins. Everyone knows that there are two kinds of twin, identical and non-identical and, with the help of Weinberg's (1909) simple device, the incidence of the two types may be studied separately wherever the sex of the twins is recorded. Weinberg says the number of dizygous (non-identical) twin pairs is twice the number of unlike-sexed twin pairs, on the assumption that the chances of one male and one female in a pair is twice the chance of two males or two females, and so half the total number of dizygous pairs. Identical twins are then counted as the total number of twin pairs less the number of dizygous. Weinberg's assumption is almost certainly inaccurate, since there is a greater likelihood of like-sexed twins than unlike-sexed twins (see p. 384, Appendix B) but failure to take this into account will not seriously affect the trends we describe below.

Table C.2 summarizes recent data. Some remarkable suggestions arise at once from it. Most obvious, there appear to be considerable ethnic differences in the tendency to multiple birth, but, because most of the African and Far East data come from hospitals, the true magnitude of the differences cannot be assessed. It seems likely that the African negro has a high dizygous twinning rate but some of the West African groups, possibly of different ethnic origin, have rates about the upper limit of European populations. When allowance for small numbers and the hospital bias is made, there is no evidence that the monozygous rate is above the European. On the other hand, in Japan (Komai and Fukuoka, 1936) the dizygous rate seems to be well below that in Europe; and in 'poor Chinese' in Singapore (Millis, 1958–59b) the dizygous rate is low but the monozygous rate, which does not rise above an average of 4 per 1000 in Europe, is 6.7. At Trivandrum, on the south tip of peninsular India, the monozygous rate is still higher, 8.3 per 1000 (Namboodiri and Balakrishnan, 1958–59b). A small sample from Arctic Russia (Kandror, 1961) suggests a low twinning rate, in the range of the Far Eastern rather than European rates.

Within Europe itself Bulmer (1960b) records lowest twinning rates in Spain and Portugal (1951–56) and highest (with the exception of Rumania) in the Baltic countries (1935–38). Dizygous are not distinguished where the total rates are highest. The identical twin rates, where recorded, vary only between 2.9 and 3.8 per 1000. American (United States) rates for the white population correspond with central Europe and the United Kingdom; for the negro population the rates, like some of the west African, are about the upper limit of the European.

The evidence certainly suggests that the incidence of twinning and its type might yield interesting pointers for the ethnographer. It may be of interest also to the sociologist, with special emphasis on the rates of dizygous twinning. It is common knowledge for polytocous farm animals that the number of ova shed at one oestrus depends on the state of nutrition of the animal. For instance, in a well-fed flock of ewes twins and triplets are the rule; in an ill-fed flock, with little or no shelter, there may be far less than one lamb per ewe. It would be rash to argue from that to human populations even if Spain and Portugal are less well fed, on the average, than the Baltic countries; and the 'poor Chinese' in Singapore, and hospital women in Trivandrum are still less well-off; but, nevertheless, Bulmer (1959a) holds that the dizygotic twinning rate fell significantly in occupied France, Holland and Norway during the last world war, but not in Denmark, Sweden or North-west France where there was no severe restriction of diet during that time. In the light of these figures we have re-examined the twinning rates recorded by Morton (1955) in Hiroshima and Nagasaki. With 60,000 single births he records only 260 pairs of twins, a total rate of only 4.3 per 1000. Of those, there were 40 pairs of unlike sex, which means 80 dizygous pairs and leaves 180 pairs of identical twins. The corresponding rates are: monozygous 3, which is not abnormal, and dizygous 1.3 per thousand, which is half the apparently normal Japanese rate and the lowest so far recorded.

The Registrar-General (1958) has reviewed returns for England and Wales from 1938 to 1956, and we have examined the collected data in search of a possible upward trend associated with the great improvement in the diet of the population in general over those years. The dizygous rate shows a continuous rise from 8.54 in 1938–45 to 9.04 in 1951–56. It is difficult to imagine any reason other than better feeding to account for the difference.

One further point of interest. In his study of twinning in Aberdeen women Anderson (1956) compared the total twinning rate in three height groups: small, less than 5′ 1″, medium, 5′ 1″ to 5′ 3¾″, and tall, 5′ 4″ and over. The rates were roughly 9, 12 and 15 per

TABLE C.2. Rates of Twin

Author	Date of Investigation	Place EUROPE
Bulmer (1960b)	1951–53	Spain
	1955–56	Portugal
	1946–51	France
	1950	Belgium
	1952–56	Austria
	1901–53	Luxembourg
	1950–55	West Germany
	1930–32	Lithuania
	1935–41	Hungary
	1931–32	Poland
	1946–55	Sweden
	1943–48	Switzerland
	1946–55	Holland
	1935–39	Bulgaria
	1946–54	Norway
	1949–55	Italy
	1950–55	East Germany
	1955	Jugoslavia
	1931–33	Czechoslovakia
	1931–38	Greece
	1946–55	Denmark
	1935–37	Finland
	1935–37	Estonia
	1936–38	Roumania
	1935–38	Latvia
Registrar-General (1958)	1938–56	England and Wa
Karn (1951–52)	1927–48	London
Anderson (1956)	1938–52	Aberdeen
	1939–52	Scotland
Bulmer (1957–58)	1938	UNITED STAT U.S.

ffferent Populations

ulation	Incidence of twins/1000 births			Other information
	Total	Dizygous	Mono-zygous	
onal birth statistics	9.1	5.9	3.2	Standardised for
,, ,, ,,	10.1	6.5	3.6	maternal age
,, ,, ,,	10.8	7.1	3.7	
,, ,, ,,	10.9	7.3	3.6	
,, ,, ,,	10.9	7.5	3.4	
,, ,, ,,	11.4	7.9	3.5	
,, ,, ,,	11.5	8.2	3.3	
,, ,, ,,	11.5	—	—	
,, ,, ,,	11.6	—	—	
,, ,, ,,	11.7	—	—	
,, ,, ,,	11.7	8.6	3.2	
,, ,, ,,	11.7	8.1	3.6	
,, ,, ,,	11.9	8.1	3.7	
,, ,, ,,	11.9	—	—	
,, ,, ,,	12.1	8.3	3.8	
,, ,, ,,	12.3	8.6	3.7	
,, ,, ,,	12.4	9.1	3.3	
,, ,, ,,	12.6	—	—	
,, ,, ,,	13.2	9.8	3.4	
,, ,, ,,	13.8	10.9	2.9	
,, ,, ,,	14.2	—	—	
,, ,, ,,	14.6	—	—	
,, ,, ,,	15.1	—	—	
,, ,, ,,	15.6	—	—	
,, ,, ,,	16.3	—	—	
onal birth statistics	12.3	8.8	3.5	
versity College pital	16.6	10.9	5.7	
ernity Hospital	15.2	—	—	Stillbirths before the 28th
onal birth statistics	13.9	—	—	week of pregnancy excluded
te Population Statistics	11.3	7.1	4.2	Figures adjusted from those published by
ro	15.8	11.1	4.7	Enders and Stern (1948)

TABLE

Author	Date of Investigation	Place
Statistical Bulletin of the Metropolitan Life Insurance Co. (1960)	1951–57	U.S.
Bulmer (1960b)	1954–58 No date No date No date	AFRICA Gambia Nigeria S. Rhodesia Congo
Bulmer (1960b)	1857–1951 No date	WEST INDIES Antigua Jamaica
Namboodiri and Balakrishnan (1958–59b)	1956–58	FAR EAST India
Millis (1958–59b)	1950–53	Singapore
Komai and Fukuoka (1936)	1926–31	Japan
Morton (1955)	post-1945 no detail	Japan
Kandror (1961)	1944–46 1946–50	U.S.S.R.

thousand total births in these groups. Identical and non-identical twins were not distinguished, and the numbers are too small to give confidence. More analyses of this sort, to give larger numbers and with types distinguished, would clarify the question whether the dizygous twinning rate is, or is not, a sensitive index of well-being, nutritional or genetic.

inued)

| | Incidence of twins/1000 births | | | |
ılation	Total	Dizygous	Mono-zygous	Other information
te Population Statistics	10.1	—	—	At least one twin surviving
ro	13.4	—	—	
urst, birth statistics	16.6	9.9	6.7	Based on only 57 twins
an, hospital statistics	44.9	39.9	5.0	603 twins
bury, ,, ,,	28.9	26.6	2.3	100 twins
oldville ,,	21.8	18.7	3.1	500 twins
bethville ,,	16.9	13.3	3.6	270 twins
onal statistics	15.4	11.5	3.9	2253 twins
ital ,,	17.2	13.4	3.8	95 twins
andrum, hospital stics	16.8	8.5	8.3	
Chinese in hospital	10.9	4.2	6.7	
wives' records from				
ca	5.6	2.7	2.9	Authors say data from
shu	6.8	2.9	3.9	Korea and Formosa
shu	7.1	2.6	4.5	similar
asaki and Hiroshima; birth statistics	4.3	1.3	3.0	
ic region	7.7	—	—	9 sets of twins in 1181 births

Several important studies have been made of twinning in relation to age and parity of the mother (Bulmer, 1959b Registrar General (England and Wales), 1958). Figures for Denmark (1944–55) were provided by Dr H. F. Helweg-Larsen (personal communication). These are in almost perfect agreement, and the nature of the relation to age is shown in Figure C.1 for

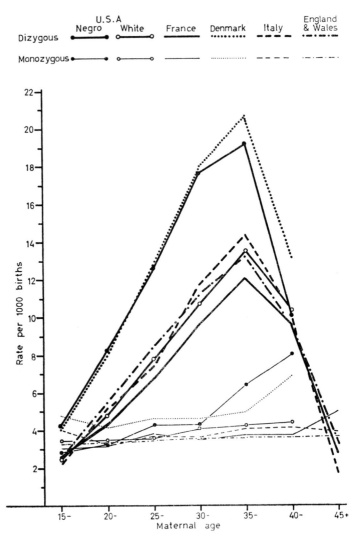

FIGURE C.1. Incidence of monozygous and dizygous twins in relation to maternal age

Italy, England and Wales, United States, France and Denmark. Monozygous twins are slightly more frequent at higher ages of the mother, but the big change is in dizygous twinning. The dizygous rate in the youngest age group lies between 2 and 3 per thousand; it rises steeply to five, or more than five, times that rate in the age group 35–39 and then falls even more steeply to the original level or less; the agreement in this pattern for different ethnic groups in five countries is remarkable. Assuming that there is no change in the chances of fertilization and successful embedding, that implies that the frequency with which the ovary discharges two ova during one cycle is five times at age 35–39 what it is before twenty years of age. Perhaps this represents an increasing incidence of failure of the mechanism which normally limits the discharge of ova to one per cycle. The steep fall after 40 is no doubt due to exhaustion of Graafian follicles and the approaching menopause. There is no evidence to show whether the vitality of the late-born twins is equal to that of the earlier-born.

Within each age group the twinning rate rises with birth order, sometimes throughout the range, sometimes with a decline at the highest orders. The combined effect of high age and high parity is to give rates up to 20 per thousand.

Bulmer (1959b) presents an analysis of United States twin pregnancies which shows for a given maternal age, a rise in incidence of twinning with age of father. But the rise with parity in each maternal age group is more striking than the rise with age of father and the apparent effect of father's age seems to be merely a reflection of the association of maternal parity with paternal age.

A popular belief is that twinning 'runs in families'. Bulmer's (1960a) analysis of family histories suggests some excess in the mother's line, in that 4 per cent of mothers of twins were themselves twins but only 1.7 per cent of fathers.

Twins together weigh more than single infants, but not twice as much; they also tend to be born before term. For example Karn (1951–52) showed the mean length of gestation in a hospital series to be about 257 days and the mean birth weight to be about 2300 g. At a mean gestation of 280 days twins in that series weighed about 2700 g. compared with 3250 g for single births in the same hospital (Karn and Penrose, 1951–52).

It is not easy to decide how multiple births should be regarded in terms of physiological performance. In sheep, for example, twins are more 'normal' than a single lamb and the best ewe has twins more often than not. In women also the healthiest have more twins than the less healthy and the twin rate is higher in a population when feeding is adequate than when it is not, suggesting that at least a certain incidence of twins is a desirable physiological target. And yet twin pregnancy, even in women of the best physique, is a load which taxes the mother to, and often beyond safe limits and is associated with a considerable increase in perinatal deaths and such complications as pre-eclampsia and anaemia.

References

ABBAS T.M. and TOVEY J.E. (1960) Proteins of the liquor amnii. *Brit. med. J.* i, 476

ABDUL-KARIM R. and ASSALI N.S. (1961) Renal function in human pregnancy. V. Effects of oxytocin on renal hemodynamics and water and electrolyte excretion. *J. Lab. clin. Med.* **57**, 522

ABOLINS J.A. (1961) The weight and length of newborn infants in relation to parental age. *Acta obstet. gynec. scand.* **40**, 339

ABRAMSON D.I., FLACHS K. and FIERST S.M. (1943) Peripheral blood flow during gestation. *Amer. J. Obstet. Gynec.* **45**, 666

ACHAR S.T. and YANKAUER A. (1962) Studies on the birth weight of South Indian infants. *Indian J. Child Hlth.* **11**, 157

ADAMS J.Q. (1954) Cardiovascular physiology in normal pregnancy: studies with the dye dilution technique. *Amer. J. Obstet. Gynec.* **67**, 741

ALBERT A. and BERKSON J. (1951) A clinical bio-assay for chorionic gonadotropin. *J. clin. Endocr.* **11**, 805

ALBERT A. and DERNER I. (1960) Studies on the biologic characterization of human gonadotropin. VI. Nature and number of gonadotropins in human pregnancy urine. *J. clin. Endocr.* **20**, 1225

ALLAN T.M. (1953) ABO blood groups and human fertility. *Brit. J. prev. soc. Med.* **7**, 220

ALLAN T.M. (1959) ABO blood groups and sex ratio at birth. *Brit. med. J.* i, 553

ALLEN D.W., WYMAN J. Jr. and SMITH C.A. (1953) The oxygen equilibrium of fetal and adult human hemoglobin. *J. biol. Chem.* **203**, 81

ALLEN T.H. (1951) Extraction of T-1824 in the presence of gross haemolysis and lipaemia. *Proc. Soc. exp. Biol.* **76**, 145

ALLISON J.B. (1961) The ideal aminogram. *Fed. Proc.* **20**, 66

ALVAREZ H. and CALDEYRO-BARCIA R. (1954) *Fisiopatologia de la contraccion uterina y sus aplicaciones en la clinica obstetrica.* [Physiopathology of contraction of the uterus and its bearing on clinical obstetrics]. Facultad. de Medicina de Montevideo, Uruguay

DE ALVAREZ R.R. (1958) Renal glomerulo-tubular mechanisms during normal pregnancy. 1. Glomerular filtration rate, renal plasma flow and creatinine clearance. *Amer. J. Obstet. Gynec.* **75**, 931

DE ALVAREZ R.R., AFONSO J.F. and SHERRARD D.J. (1961) Serum protein fractionation in normal pregnancy. *Amer. J. Obstet. Gynec.* **82**, 1096

DE ALVAREZ R.R., GAISER D.F., SIMKINS D.M., SMITH E.K. and BRATVOLD G.E. (1959) Serial studies of serum lipids in normal human pregnancy. *Amer. J. Obstet. Gynec.* **77**, 743

ALWARD H.C. (1930) Observations on the vital capacity during the last month of pregnancy and the puerperium. *Amer. J. Obstet. Gynec.* **20**, 373

AMOROSO E.C. (1958) in *Marshall's Physiology of Reproduction*. A. S. Parkes Ed. Vol. 2. Longmans, Green & Co, London

AMOROSO E.C. (1961) Histology of the placenta. *Brit. med. Bull.* **17**, 81

ANDERSON N.A., BROWN E.W. and LYON R.A. (1943) Causes of prematurity. III. Influence of race and sex on duration of gestation and weight at birth. *Amer. J. Dis. Child* **65**, 523

ANDERSON R.K., ROBINSON W.D., CALVO J. and PAYNE G.C. (1946) Nutritional status during pregnancy and after delivery of a group of women in Mexico City. *J. Amer. diet. Ass.* **22**, 588

ANDERSON W.J.R. (1956) Stillbirth and neonatal mortality in twin pregnancy. *J. Obstet. Gynaec. Brit. Emp.* **63**, 205

ANDERSON W.J.R., BAIRD D. and THOMSON A.M. (1958) Epidemiology of stillbirths and infant deaths due to congenital malformation. *Lancet* **i**, 1304

ANDREWS W.C. and BONSNES R.W. (1951) The leucocytes during pregnancy. *Amer. J. Obstet. Gynec.* **61**, 1129

ANDROS G.J. (1945) Blood pressure in normal pregnancy. *Amer. J. Obstet. Gynec.* **50**, 300

ANGELINO P.F., ACTIS-DATO A., LEVI V., SILIQUINI P.N. and REVELLI E. (1954) Nuovi concetti di emodinamica in gravidanza da indagini con cateterismo angiocardiaco. [New views on haemodynamics in pregnancy based on observations with catheterisation of cardiac vessels]. *Minerva ginec.* **6**, 517

ANTONOV A.N. (1947) Children born during the siege of Leningrad in 1942. *J. Pediat.* **30**, 250

ARCHIBALD H.M. (1958) Influence of maternal malaria on newborn infants. *Brit. med. J.* **ii**, 1512

ARNOLD L.E. (1940) An attempt to control fetal weight. *Amer. J. Obstet. Gynec.* **39**, 99

ASSALI N.S., DIGNAM W.J. and DASGUPTA K. (1959) Renal function in human pregnancy. II. Effects of venous pooling on renal hemodynamics and water, electrolyte and aldosterone excretion during normal gestation. *J. Lab. clin. Med.* **54**, 394

ASSALI N.S., DIGNAM W.J. and LONGO L. (1960) Renal function in human pregnancy. III. Effects of antidiuretic hormone (ADH) on renal hemodynamics and water and electrolyte excretion near term and post-partum. *J. clin. Endocr.* **20**, 58

ASSALI N.S., DOUGLASS R.A. Jr., BAIRD W.W., NICHOLSON D.B. and SUYEMOTO R. (1953a) Measurement of uterine blood flow and uterine metabolism. II. The techniques of catheterization and cannulation of the uterine veins and sampling of arterial and venous blood in pregnant women. *Amer. J. Obstet. Gynec.* **66**, 11

ASSALI N.S., DOUGLASS R.A. Jr., BAIRD W.W., NICHOLSON D.B. and SUYEMOTO R. (1953b) Measurement of uterine blood flow and uterine metabolism. IV. Results in normal pregnancy. *Amer. J. Obstet. Gynec.* **66**, 248

ASSALI N.S., HERZIG D. and SINGH B. P. (1954–55) Renal response to ammonium chloride acidosis in normal and toxemic pregnancies. *J. appl. Physiol.* **7**, 367

REFERENCES   401

ASSALI N.S., RAURAMO L. and PELTONEN T. (1960) Measurement of uterine blood flow and uterine metabolism. VIII. Uterine and fetal blood flow and oxygen consumption in early human pregnancy. *Amer. J. Obstet. Gynec.* **79**, 86

ASSALI N.S., VERGON J.M., TADA Y. and GARBER S.T. (1952) Studies on autonomic blockade. VI. The mechanisms regulating the hemodynamic changes in the pregnant woman and their relation to the hypertension of toxemia of pregnancy. *Amer. J. Obstet. Gynec.* **63**, 978

AUTRET M. (1957) in *Human protein requirements and their fulfilment in practice.* Proceedings of a conference sponsored jointly by F.A.O., W.H.O. and the Josiah Macy, Jr. Foundation. Eds. J. C. Waterlow and J. M. L. Stephen.

BADER R.A., BADER M.E. and ROSE D.J. (1959) The oxygen cost of breathing in dyspnoeic subjects as studied in normal pregnant women. *Clin. Sci.* **18**, 223

BADER R.A., BADER, M.E., ROSE D.J. and BRAUNWALD E. (1955) Hemodynamics at rest and during exercise in normal pregnancy as studied by cardiac catheterization. *J. clin. Invest.* **34**, 1524

BAGCHI K. and BOSE A.K. (1962) Effect of low nutrient intake during pregnancy on obstetrical performance and offspring. *Amer. J. clin. Nutr.* **11**, 586

BAINES A.H.J., HOLLINGSWORTH D.F. and LEITCH I. (1963) Diets of working-class families with children before and after the second world war, with a section on height and weight of children. *Nutr. Abstr. Rev.* **33**, 653

BAIRD D. (1935) The upper urinary tract in pregnancy and puerperium, with special reference to pyelitis of pregnancy. *J. Obstet. Gynaec. Brit. Emp.* **42**, 733

BAIRD D. (1945) The influence of social and economic factors on stillbirths and neonatal deaths. *J. Obstet. Gynaec. Brit. Emp.* **52**, 217

BAIRD D. (1960) The evolution of modern obstetrics. *Lancet* **ii**, 557

BAIRD D. (1963) The contribution of operative obstetrics to the prevention of perinatal death. *J. Obstet. Gynaec. Brit. Commonw.* **70**, 204

BAIRD D., HYTTEN F.E. and THOMSON A.M. (1958) Age and human reproduction. *J. Obstet. Gynaec. Brit. Emp.* **65**, 865

BAIRD D., THOMSON A.M. and BILLEWICZ W.Z. (1957) Birth weights and placental weights in pre-eclampsia. *J. Obstet. Gynaec. Brit. Emp.* **64**, 370

BAIRD J.D. and FARQUHAR J.W. (1962) Insulin-secreting capacity in newborn infants of normal and diabetic women. *Lancet* **i**, 71

BALAKRISHNAN V. and NAMBOODIRI N.K. (1960) Data on the gestation period of Indian mothers. *Ann. hum. Genet.* **24**, 5

BALFOUR M.I. (1944) Supplementary feeding in pregnancy: the National Birthday Trust Fund experiment. *Proc. Nutr. Soc.* **2**, 27

BARCROFT H. and EDHOLM O.G. (1945) Temperature and blood flow in the human forearm. *J. Physiol. (Lond.)* **104**, 366.

BARCROFT J. (1936) Fetal circulation and respiration. *Physiol. Rev.* **16**, 103

BARCROFT J. (1944) Nutritional functions of the placenta. *Proc. Nutr. Soc.* **2**, 14

BARCROFT J. (1946) *Researches on pre-natal life.* Blackwell Scientific Publications, Oxford

BARDAWIL W.A., MITCHELL G.W., McKEOGH R.D. and MARCHANT D.J. (1962) Behavior of skin homografts in human pregnancy. I. Habitual abortion. *Amer. J. Obstet. Gynec.* **84**, 1283

BARNES A.C., KUMAR D. and GOODNO J.A. (1962) Studies in human myometrium during pregnancy. V. Myometrial tissue progesterone analyses by gas-liquid phase chromatography. *Amer. J. Obstet. Gynec.* **84**, 1207

BARRON D.H. (1959) in *Oxygen supply to the human foetus*. Eds. J. Walker and A. C. Turnbull. Blackwell Scientific Publications, Oxford

BARRON D.H. (1960) The placenta as the fetal lung, in *The placenta and fetal membranes*. Ed. C. A. Villee. The Williams and Wilkins Co, Baltimore.

BASCH K. (1910) Ueber experimentelle Milchauslösung und über das Verhalten der Milchabsonderung bei den zusammengewachsenen Schwestern Blažek. [Experimental induction of lactation and the occurrence of lactation in the Blažek Siamese twins]. *Dtsch. med. Wschr.* **36**, 987

BARTELS H. (1959) in *Oxygen supply to the human foetus*. Eds. J. Walker and A. C. Turnbull. Blackwell Scientific Publications, Oxford

BARTELS H., MOLL W. and METCALFE J. (1962) Physiology of gas exchange in the human placenta. *Amer. J. Obstet. Gynec.* **84**, 1714

BARTLEY W., KREBS H.A. and O'BRIEN J.R.P. (1953) Vitamin C requirements of human adults. A report of the vitamin C subcommittee of the Accessory Food Factors Committee M.R.C. Spec. Rept. Ser., No. 280. H.M.S.O., London.

BATTAGLIA F., PRYSTOWSKY H., SMISSON C., HELLEGERS A. and BRUNS P. (1959) Fetal blood studies. XVI. On the changes in total osmotic pressure and sodium and potassium concentrations of amniotic fluid during the course of human gestation. *Surg. Gynec. Obstet.* **109**, 509

BAYLISS R.I.S., BROWNE J.C.M., ROUND B.P. and STEINBECK A.W. (1955) Plasma 17-hydroxycortiosteroids in pregnancy. *Lancet* **i**, 62

BEAN W.B., DEXTER M.W. and COGSWELL R.C. (1947) Vascular spiders and palmer erythema in pregnancy. *J. clin. Invest.* **26**, 1173

BEARDSLEY G.S. (1941) Implications of weight gain during pregnancy. *West. J. Surg.* **49**, 350.

BEATON G.H., BEARE J., RYU M.H. and McHENRY E.W. (1954) Protein metabolism of the pregnant rat. *J. Nutr.* **54**, 291

BEILLY J.S. and KURLAND I.I. (1945) Relationship of maternal weight gain and weight of newborn infant. *Amer. J. Obstet. Gynec.* **50**, 202

BENGTSSON L.P. (1962) Endocrine factors in labour. *Acta obstet. gynec. scand.* **41**, Suppl. 1, 87

BENNHOLD H., PETERS H. and ROTH E. (1954) Über einen Fall von kompletter Analbuminaemie ohne wesentliche klinische Krankheitszeichen. [A case of total absence of blood albumin without significant clinical signs]. *Verh. dtsch. Ges. inn. Med.* **60**, Kongr. p. 630

BENSON G.K., COWIE A.T., FOLLEY S.J. and TINDAL J.S. (1959) Recent developments in endocrine studies on mammary growth and lactation, in *Recent Progress in the Endocrinology of Reproduction*. Ed. C. W. Lloyd. Academic Press, New York

BENSTEAD N. and THEOBALD G.W. (1952) Iron and the 'physiological' anaemia of pregnancy. *Brit. med. J.* **i**, 407

BENZIE D., BOYNE A.W., DALGARNO A.C., DUCKWORTH J., HILL R. and WALKER D.M. (1955) Studies of the skeleton of the sheep. 1. The effect of different levels of dietary calcium during pregnancy and lactation on individual bones. *J. agric. Sci.* **46**, 425

BERLIN N.I., GOETSCH, C., HYDE G.M. and PARSONS R.J. (1953) The blood volume in pregnancy as determined by P[32] labelled red blood cells. *Surg. Gynec. Obstet.* **97**, 173

BERNARD R.M. (1952) The shape and size of the female pelvis. *Edinb. med. J.* **59**, *Proc. Edinb. obstet. Soc.* p. 1

BERRY K. and WIEHL D.G. (1952) An experiment in diet education during pregnancy. *Milbank mem. Fd. quart. Bull.* **30**, 119

BEST C.H. and TAYLOR N.B. (1961) *The physiological basis of medical practice*, 7th edition. Bailliere, Tindall and Cox Ltd, London.

DE BETTENCOURT J.M. and FRAGOSO J.C.B. (1952) L'electrocardiogramme de la femme enciente. [The electro cardiogram of the pregnant woman]. *Acta cardiol. (Brux.)* **7**, 123

BICKERS W. (1942) The placenta: a modified arterio-venous fistula. *Sth. med. J.* **35**, 593

BIEZENSKI J.J. (1960) Antifibrinolytic activity in normal pregnancy. *J. clin. Path.* **13**, 220

BIEZENSKI J.J. and MOORE H.C. (1958) Fibrinolysis in normal pregnancy. *J. clin. Path.* **11**, 306

BINGHAM A.W. (1932) The prevention of obstetric complications by diet and exercise. *Amer. J. Obstet. Gynec.* **23**, 38

BIRKE G., GEMZELL C.A., PLANTIN L.O. and ROBBE H. (1958) Plasma levels of 17-hydroxycorticosteroids and urinary excretion pattern of keto-steroids in normal pregnancy. *Acta endocr. (Kbh.)* **27**, 389

BLAIKLEY J., CLARKE S., MACKEITH R. and OGDEN K.M. (1953) Breast-feeding: factors affecting success. *J. Obstet. Gynaec. Brit. Emp.* **60**, 657

BLOCK R.J. and MITCHELL H.H. (1946) The correlation of the amino-acid composition of proteins with their nutritive value. *Nutr. Abstr. Rev.* **16**, 249

BOCCI A. and DAVITTI L. (1956) L'importanza dell'igiene alimentare in gravidanza. (Contributo clinico e statistico). [Importance of diet in pregnancy. Clinical and statistical study]. *Quad. Nutr.* **16**, 145

BONSNES R.W. and Lange W.A. (1950) Inulin clearance during pregnancy. *Fed. Proc.* **9**, 154

BORDLEY J. III, CONNOR C.A.R., HAMILTON W.F., KERR W.J. and WIGGERS C.J. (1951) Recommendations for human blood pressure determinations by sphygmomanometer. *Circulation* **4**, 503

BORGLIN N.E. (1959) Effect of oestriol on the female genital tract. *Acta obstet. gynec. scand.* **38**, 157

BOUTERLINE-YOUNG H. and BOUTERLINE-YOUNG E. (1956) Alveolar carbon-dioxide levels in pregnant, parturient and lactating subjects. *J. Obstet. Gynaec. Brit. Emp.* **63**, 509

BOYDEN E.A. and RIGLER L.G. (1944) Initial emptying time of stomach in primigravidae as related to evacuation of biliary tract. *Proc. Soc. exp. Biol.* **56**, 200

BRAITENBERG H.V. (1942) Zur Frage der Entwicklungsbeschleunigung der Neugeborenen. [The question of accelerated development of the new-born]. *Arch. Gynäk.* **174**, 193

Brambell F.W.R. and Hemmings W.A. (1960) in *The Placenta and Fetal Membranes* Ed. C. A. Villee. Williams and Wilkens Company, Baltimore.

Brandstetter F. and Schüller E. (1956) Die Clearanceuntersuchung in der Gravidität. Ein Beitrag zur Physiopathologie der Niere und Leber in der Schwangershaft. [Investigation of renal clearance in pregnancy. Contribution to the physiology and pathology of kidney and liver in pregnancy]. *Fortschr. Geburtsh. Gynäk.* No. 14

Bray P.N. (1938) Weight changes in pregnancy. *Amer. J. Obstet. Gynec.* **35**, 802

Brehm H. and Kindling E. (1955) Der Kreislauf während Schwangerschaft und Wochenbett. [The circulation in pregnancy and the puerperium]. *Arch. Gynäk.* **185**, 696

Breyere E.J. and Barrett M.K. (1960) Prolonged survival of skin homografts in parous female mice. *J. nat. Cancer Inst.* **25**, 1405

British Association (1879) Report of the Anthropometric Committee. *Report of the 49th meeting of the British Association for the Advancement of Science.* p. 175. John Murray, London

British Association (1884) Report of the Anthropometric Committee 1882–83. *Report of the 53rd meeting of the British Association for the Advancement of Science*, 1883. John Murray, London

British Medical Association (1950) Report of the Committee on Nutrition. British Medical Association, London

Bro-Rasmussen F. (1958) The riboflavin requirement of animals and man and associated metabolic relations. Part I. Technique of estimating requirement and modifying circumstances. Part II. Relation of requirement to the metabolism of protein and energy. *Nutr. Abstr. Rev.* **28**, 1; 369

Bro-Rasmussen F., Buus O., Lundwall F. and Trolle D. (1962) Variations in plasma cortisol during pregnancy, delivery and the puerperium. *Acta endocr. (Kbh.)* **40**, 571

Brown E.S. (1963) Foetal erythrocytes in the maternal circulation. *Brit. med. J.* **i**, 1000

Brown J.B. (1956) Urinary excretion of oestrogens during pregnancy, lactation and the re-establishment of menstruation. *Lancet* **i**, 704

Brown J.B. (1959) The metabolism of oestrogens and the measurement of the excretory products in the urine. *J. Obstet. Gynaec. Brit. Emp.* **66**, 795

Brown W.E. and Bradbury J.T. (1947) A study of the physiologic action of human chorionic hormone. The production of pseudo-pregnancy in women by chorionic hormone. *Amer. J. Obstet. Gynec.* **53**, 749

Browne J.C.M. (1959) The measurement and significance of utero-placental and uterine muscle flow, in *Oxygen supply to the human foetus.* Eds. J. Walker and A. C. Turnbull. Blackwell Scientific Publications, Oxford

Bruce-Chwatt L.J. (1952) Malaria in African infants and children in Southern Nigeria. *Ann. trop. Med. Parasit.* **46**, 173

Bruner J.A. (1951) Distribution of chorionic gonadotropin in mother and fetus at various stages of pregnancy. *J. clin. Endocr.* **11**, 360

Brzezinski A., Bercovici B. and Gedalia J. (1960) Fluorine in the human fetus. *Obstet. and Gynec.* **15**, 329

Bucht H. (1951) Studies on renal function in man with special reference to glomerular filtration and renal plasma flow in pregnancy. *Scand. J. clin. Lab. Invest.* **3**, Suppl. 3.

BUDDE S. (1948) Hat die Mangelernährung einen Einfluss auf die intrauterine Fruchtentwicklung. [Has insufficient diet an effect on intrauterine development of the foetus]. *Zbl. Gynäk.* **70**, 487

BUHS A. (1959) Caries, saliva and pregnancy. I. Clinical. II. Physiological Chemistry. *Sammlung. Meusser* **42**, 1, 96

BULMER M.G. (1957–58) The numbers of human multiple births. *Ann. hum. Genet.* **22**, 158

BULMER M.G. (1959a) Twinning rate in Europe during the war. *Brit. med. J.* **i**, 29

BULMER M.G. (1959b) The effect of parental age, parity and duration of marriage on the twinning rate. *Ann. hum. Genet.* **23**, 454

BULMER M.G. (1960a) The familial incidence of twinning. *Ann. hum. Genet.* **24**, 1

BULMER M.G. (1960b) The twinning rate in Europe and Africa. *Ann. hum. Genet.* **24**, 121

BURGEN A.S.V. and EMMELIN N.G. (1961) *Physiology of the salivary glands.* Edward Arnold Ltd, London

BURKE B.S., BEAL V.A., KIRKWOOD S.B. and STUART H.C. (1943) The influence of nutrition during pregnancy upon the condition of the infant at birth. *J. Nutr.* **26**, 569

BURROWS H. (1949) *Biological actions of sex hormones.* 2nd Ed. Cambridge University Press, London

BURT C.C. (1949) Peripheral skin temperature in normal pregnancy. *Lancet* **ii**, 787

BURT C.C. (1950) The peripheral circulation in pregnancy. *Edinb. med. J.* **57**, Trans. 18

BURT R.L. (1954) Peripheral utilization of glucose in pregnancy and the puerperium. *Obstet. and Gynec.* **4**, 58

BURT R.L. (1960) Carbohydrate metabolism in pregnancy, in *Clinical Obstetrics and Gynaecology*, Vol. 3. Paul B. Hoeber, Inc, N.Y.

BURT R.L. and PULLIAM R.P. (1959) Carbohydrate metabolism in pregnancy. Lactic acid production following insulin administration. *Obstet. and Gynec.* **14**, 518

BURWELL C.S. (1938) The placenta as a modified arterio-venous fistula considered in relation to the circulatory adjustments to pregnancy. *Amer. J. med. Sci.* **195**, 1

BURWELL C.S. and METCALFE J. (1958) *Heart Disease in Pregnancy. Physiology and management.* J. and A. Churchill, London

BURWELL C.S., STRAYHORN W.D., FLICKINGER D., CORLETTE M.B., BOWERMAN E.P. and KENNEDY J.A. (1938) Circulation during pregnancy. *Arch. intern. Med.* **62**, 979

BUTTERMANN K. (1958) Clearance-Untersuchungen in der normalen und pathologischen Schwangerschaft. Zugleich eine kritische Beurteilung des Verfahrens. [Renal clearance in normal and pathological pregnancy. Critical examination of the technique]. *Arch. Gynäk.* **190**, 448

BUXTON C.L. and ATKINSON W.B. (1948) Hormonal factors involved in the regulation of basal body temperature during the menstrual cycle and pregnancy. *J. clin. Endocr.* **8**, 544

DD

CAMERON C.S. and GRAHAM S. (1944) Antenatal diet and its influence on stillbirths and prematurity. *Glasgow med. J.* **24,** 1

CAMPBELL E.J.M. and HOWELL J.B.L. (1963) The sensation of breathlessness. *Brit. med. Bull.* **19,** 36

CAMPBELL E.J.M., WESTLAKE E.K. and CHERNIACK R.M. (1959) The oxygen consumption and efficiency of the respiratory muscles of young male subjects. *Clin. Sci.* **18,** 55

CANADIAN COUNCIL ON NUTRITION (1950) A dietary standard for Canada approved by the Canadian Council on Nutrition, the Department of National Health and Welfare Ottawa, December 7, 1948. *Canad. Bull. Nutr.* **2,** No. 1

CARDELL B.S. (1953) The infants of diabetic mothers: a morphological study. *J. Obstet. Gynaec. Brit. Emp.* **60,** 834

CARPENTER T.M. and MURLIN J.R. (1911) The energy metabolism of mother and child just before and just after birth. *Arch. intern. Med.* **7,** 184

CARTWRIGHT G.E., HUGULEY C.M. Jr., ASHENBRUCKER H., FAY J. and WINTROBE M.M. (1948) Studies on free erythrocyte protoporphyrin, plasma iron and plasma copper in normal and anemic subjects. *Blood* **3,** 501

CASSANO F. and TARANTINO C. (1959) Il metabolismo glicidico della gravida studiato per mezzo del glucagone. [Carbohydrate metabolism in pregnancy studied with glucagon]. *Folia endocr. (Pisa)* **12,** 417

CASSMER O. (1959) Hormone production of the isolated human placenta. *Acta endocr. (Kbh.)* **32,** Suppl. 45

CATON W.L., ROBY C.C., REID D.E., CASWELL R., MALETSKOS C.J., FLUHARTY R.G. and GIBSON J.G. (1951) The circulating red cell volume and body hematocrit in normal pregnancy and the puerperium. *Amer. J. Obstet. Gynec.* **61,** 1207

CATON W.L., ROBY C.C., REID D.E. and GIBSON J.G. (1949) Plasma volume and extravascular fluid volume during pregnancy and the puerperium. *Amer. J. Obstet. Gynec.* **57,** 471

CAZEAUX P. (1871) *A theoretical and practical treatise on midwifery.* 5th American from the 7th French Edition. H. K. Lewis, London

CHALMERS A.K. (1904) (Rickets and contracted pelvis). Rept. of the Inter-departmental Committee on Physical Deterioration, Vol. 2, p. 239. Cd. 2210. H.M.S.O., London

CHANARIN I., MACGIBBON B.M., O'SULLIVAN W.J. and MOLLIN D.L. (1959) Folic acid deficiency in pregnancy. The pathogenesis of megaloblastic anaemia of pregnancy. *Lancet* **ii,** 634

CHAPLIN H. Jr., MOLLISON P.L. and VETTER H. (1953) The body/venous hematocrit ratio: its constancy over a wide hematocrit range. *J. clin. Invest.* **32,** 1309

CHESLEY L.C. (1943) A study of extracellular water changes in pregnancy. *Surg. Gynec. Obstet.* **76,** 589

CHESLEY L.C. (1944) Weight changes and water balance in normal and toxic pregnancy. *Amer. J. Obstet. Gynec.* **48,** 565

CHESLEY L.C. (1960) Renal functional changes in normal pregnancy, in *Clinical Obstetrics and Gynacology.* Vol. 3, No. 2. Paul B. Hoeber, Inc, N.Y.

CHESLEY L.C. and CHESLEY E.R. (1939) The diodrast clearance and renal blood flow in normal pregnant and non-pregnant women. *Amer. J. Physiol.* **127**, 731

CHESLEY L.C., VALENTI C. and REIN H. (1958) Excretion of sodium loads by non-pregnant and pregnant normal, hypertensive and pre-eclamptic women. *Metabolism* **7**, 575

CHEYNE G.A. and HYTTEN, F.E. (1963) Iron loss during menstruation. *Proc. nutr. Soc.* **22**, xix

CHRISTENSEN H.N. and STREICHER J.A. (1948) Association between rapid growth and elevated cell concentrations of amino acids. I. In fetal tissues. *J. biol. Chem.* **175**, 95

CHRISTENSEN P.J. (1958) Tubular reabsorption of glucose during pregnancy. *Scand. J. clin. Lab. Invest.* **10**, 364

CHRISTENSEN P.J., DATE J.W., SCHØNHEYDER F. and VOLQVARTZ K. (1957) Amino acids in blood plasma and urine during pregnancy. *Scand. J. clin. Lab. Invest.* **9**, 54

CIOCCO A. (1938a) Variation in the sex ratio at birth in the United States. *Hum. Biol.* **10**, 36

CIOCCO A. (1938b) The masculinity of stillbirths and abortions in relation to the duration of uterogestation and to the stated causes of fetal mortality. *Hum. Biol.* **10**, 235

CLARKE D.H. (1953) Peptic ulcer in women. *Brit. med. J.* i, 1254

CLAVERO J.A. and BOTELLA LLUSIÁ J. (1963) Measurement of the villus surface in normal and pathologic placentae. *Amer. J. Obstet. Gynec.* **86**, 234

COHEN M.E. and THOMSON K.J. (1936) Studies on the circulation in pregnancy. I. The velocity of blood flow and related aspects of the circulation in normal pregnant women. *J. clin. Invest.* **15**, 607

COMMISSIE VOEDINGSNORMEN VAN DE VOEDINGSRAAD (1961) Aanbevolen hoeveelheden voedingsstoffen. [Recommended amounts of nutrients]. *Voeding* **22**, 210

COMROE J.H., FORSTER R.E., DUBOIS A.B., BRISCOE W.A. and Carlsen E. (1955) *The Lung: clinical physiology and pulmonary function tests.* The Year Book Publishers, Chicago

CONE T.E. (1961) De pondere infantum recens natorum. The history of weighing the newborn infant. *Pediatrics* **28**, 490

CONNOR A., BENNETT C.G. and LOUIS L.S.K. (1957) Birth weight patterns by race in Hawaii. *Hawaii med. J.* **16**, 626

COONS C.M. (1933–34) Dietary habits during pregnancy. *J. Amer. diet. Ass.* **9**, 95

COONS C.M. and BLUNT K. (1930) The retention of nitrogen, calcium, phosphorus and magnesium by pregnant women. *J. biol. Chem.* **86**, 1

COONS C.M. and COONS R.R. (1935) Some effects of cod liver oil and wheat germ on the retention of iron, nitrogen, phosphorus, calcium and magnesium during human pregnancy. *J. Nutr.* **10**, 289

COPE C.L. and BLACK E. (1959) The hydrocortisone production in late pregnancy. *J. Obstet. Gynaec. Brit. Emp.* **66**, 404

COPE I. (1958) Plasma and blood volume changes in late and prolonged pregnancy. *J. Obstet. Gynaec. Brit. Emp.* **65**, 877

COURNAND A.F. (1945) Symposium on cardiac output. *Fed. Proc.* **4**, 183

COURRIER R. (1950) Interactions between estrogens and progesterone. *Vitam. and Horm.* **8**, 179

COYLE M.G. and BROWN J.B. (1963) Urinary excretion of oestriol during pregnancy. II. Results in normal and abnormal pregnancies. *J. Obstet. Gynaec. Brit. Commonw.* **70**, 225

CRAWFORD J.M. (1959) A study of human placental growth with observations on the placenta in erythroblastosis foetalis. *J. Obstet. Gynaec. Brit. Emp.* **66**, 885

CRAWFORD J.M. (1962) Vascular anatomy of the human placenta. *Amer. J. Obstet. Gynec.* **84**, 1543

CROOKE A.C. and BUTT W.R. (1959) The excretion of follicle stimulating hormone by pregnant women. *J. Obstet. Gynaec. Brit. Emp.* **66**, 297

CROOKS J., ABOUL-KHAIR S.A., TURNBULL A.C. and HYTTEN F.E. (1964) The incidence and causes of thyroid enlargement during pregnancy. To be published.

CROSS K.W., HOOPER J.M.D. and OPPÉ T.E. (1953) The effect of carbon dioxide on the respiration of the full term and premature infant. *J. Physiol. (Lond.)* **119**, 11 P.

CRUMP E.P., HORTON C.P., MASUOKA J. and RYAN D. (1957) Growth and development. I. Relation of birth weight in negro infants to sex, maternal age, parity, prenatal care, and socioeconomic status. *J. Pediat.* **51**, 678

CSAPO A. (1961) The *in vivo* and *in vitro* effects of estrogen and progesterone on the myometrium, in *Mechanisms of action of Steroid Hormones.* Eds. C. A. Villee and L. L. Engel. Pergamon Press, Oxford

CUGELL D.W., FRANK N.R., GAENSLER E.A. and BADGER T.L. (1953) Pulmonary function in pregnancy. I. Serial observations in normal women. *Amer. Rev. Tuberc.* **67**, 568

CUMMINGS H.H. (1934) An interpretation of weight changes during pregnancy. *Amer. J. Obstet. Gynec.* **27**, 808

CUSWORTH D.C. and DENT C.E. (1960) Renal clearances and amino acids in normal adults and in patients with aminoaciduria. *Biochem. J.* **74**, 550

DAHL S. (1948) Serum iron in normal women. *Brit. med. J.* **i**, 731

DAHLSTRÖM H. and IHRMAN K. (1960) A clinical and physiological study of pregnancy in a material from northern Sweden. V. The results of work tests during and after pregnancy. *Acta Soc. Med. upsalien.* **65**, 305

DAISER K.W. (1949) Bemerkungen zu H. Hosemann: Schwangerschaftsdauer und Neugeborenengewicht, Neugeborenengrösse. [Remarks on the publication of Hosemann: Duration of pregnancy and the weight of the newborn and length of the newborn]. *Arch. Gynäk.* **176**, 582

DANCIS J. (1959) The placenta. *J. Pediat.* **55**, 85

DANCIS J., BRENNER M.A. and MONEY W.L. (1962) Some factors affecting the permeability of the guinea pig placenta. *Amer. J. Obstet. Gynec.* **84**, 570

DANCIS J., SAMUELS B.D. and DOUGLAS G.W. (1962) Immunological competence of placenta. *Science* **136**, 382

DARBY W.J., McGANITY W.J., MARTIN M.B., BRIGFORTH E., DENSON P.M., KASER M.M., OGLE P.J., NEWBILL J.A., STOCKELL A., FERGUSON M.E., TOUSTER O., McLELLAN G.S., WILLIAMS C. and CANNON R.O. (1953) The Vanderbilt Co-operative Study of maternal and infant nutrition. IV.

Dietary, laboratory and physical findings in 2129 delivered pregnancies. *J. Nutr.* **51**, 565

DARLING R.C., SMITH C.A., ASMUSSEN E. and COHEN F.M. (1941) Some properties of human fetal and maternal blood. *J. clin. Invest.* **20**, 739

DAVEY D.A., O'SULLIVAN W.J. and BROWNE J.C.M. (1961) Total exchangeable sodium in normal pregnancy and in pre-eclampsia. *Lancet* **i**, 519

DAVIDSON W.M. and JENNISON R.F. (1952) The relationship between iron storage and anaemia. *J. clin. Path.* **5**, 281

DAVIS C.H. (1923) Weight in pregnancy: its value as a routine test. *Amer. J. Obstet. Gynec.* **6**, 575

DAVIS C.H. (1934) *Amer. J. Obstet. Gynec.* **27**, 808

DAVIS L.R. and JENNISON R.F. (1954) Response of the 'physiological anaemia' of pregnancy to iron therapy. *J. Obstet. Gynaec. Brit. Emp.* **61**, 103

DAVIS M.E. (1946) The clinical use of oral basal temperatures. *J. Amer. med. Ass.* **130**, 929

DAVIS M.E. and PLOTZ E.J. (1958) Hormones in human reproduction. Part II. Further investigations of steroid metabolism in human pregnancy. *Amer. J. Obstet. Gynec.* **76**, 939

DEAKINS M. and LOOBY J. (1943) Effect of pregnancy on the mineral content of dentin of human teeth. *Amer. J. Obstet. Gynec.* **46**, 265

DEANE H.W. and SELIGMAN A.M. (1953) Evaluation of procedures for the cytological localization of ketosteroids. *Vitam. and Horm.* **11**, 173

DEN HARTOG C., POSTHUMA J.H. and DE HASS J.H. (1953) Onderzoek naar de voeding van de zwangere op het platteland. [Study of the diet of pregnant women in rural areas]. *Voeding* **14**, 1

DEPARTMENT OF HEALTH FOR SCOTLAND (1943) Sub-committee of the Scientific Advisory Council (Orr Committee). Infant Mortality in Scotland. H.M.S.O. Edinburgh

DERRINGTON M.M. and SOOTHILL J.F. (1961) An immunochemical study of the proteins of amniotic fluid and of maternal and foetal serum. *J. Obstet. Gynaec. Brit. Commonw.* **68**, 755

DE SILVA C.C., FERNANDO P.V.D. and GUNARATNE C.D.H. (1962) The search for a prematurity level in Colombo, Ceylon. *J. trop. Pediat.* **8**, 29

DICKER S.E. (1956) in *Modern Views on the Secretion of urine.* Ed. F. R. Winton. J. & A. Churchill Ltd., London

DICZFALUSY E. (1953) Chorionic gonadotrophin and oestrogens in the human placenta. *Acta endocr. (Kbh.) Suppl.* **12**, 1

DICZFALUSY E. and BORELL U. (1961) Influence of oophorectomy on steroid excretion in early pregnancy. *J. clin. Endocr.* **21**, 1119

DICZFALUSY E., CASSMER O., ALONSO C. and DE MIGUEL M. (1961) Estrogen metabolism in the human fetus and newborn, in *Recent Progress in Hormone Research.* Academic Press, New York

DICZFALUSY E. and LAURITZEN C. (1961) *Oestrogene beim Menschen.* [Oestrogens in man]. Springer, Berlin

DICZFALUSY E., NILSSON L. and WESTMAN A. (1958) Chorionic gonadotrophin in hydatidiform moles. *Acta endocr. (Kbh.)* **28**, 137

DICZFALUSY E. and TROEN P. (1961) Endocrine functions of the human placenta. *Vitam. and Horm.* **19**, 229

DIECKMANN W.J. (1952) *The Toxaemias of Pregnancy*. 2nd Ed. Henry Kimpton, London

DIECKMANN W.J., TURNER D.F., MEILLER E.J., SAVAGE L.J., HILL A.J., STRAUBE M.T., POTTINGER R.E. and RYNKIEWICZ L.M. (1951) Observations on protein intake and the health of the mother and baby. 1. Clinical and laboratory findings. 2. Food intake. *J. Amer. diet. Ass.* **27**, 1046

DIECKMANN W.J. and WEGNER C.R. (1934) The blood in normal pregnancy. I. Blood and plasma volumes. *Arch. intern. Med.* **53**, 71

DIGNAM W.J., TITUS P. and ASSALI N.S. (1958) Renal function in human pregnancy. I. Changes in glomerular filtration rate and renal plasma flow. *Proc. Soc. exp. Biol.* **97**, 512

DIGNAM W.S., VOSKIAN J. and ASSALI N.S. (1956) Effects of estrogens on renal hemodynamics and excretion of electrolytes in human subjects. *J. clin. Endocr.* **16**, 1032

DILL L.V., ISENHOUR C.E., CADDEN J.F. and SCHAFFER N.K. (1942) Glomerular filtration and renal blood flow in the toxemias of pregnancy. *Amer. J. Obstet. Gynec.* **43**, 32

DOCUMENTA GEIGY. *Scientific Tables* (1956) J. R. Geigy, S.A., Basle

DOE R.P., ZINNEMAN H.H., FLINK E.B. and ULSTROM R.A. (1960) Significance of the concentration of non-protein-bound plasma cortisol in normal subjects, Cushing's syndrome, pregnancy and during estrogen therapy. *J. clin. Endocr.* **20**, 1484

DONALD H.P. (1938–39) Sources of variation in human birth weights. *Proc. roy. Soc. Edinb.* **59**, 91

DOUGLAS G.W., THOMAS L., CARR M., CULLEN N.M. and MORRIS R. (1959) Trophoblast in the circulating blood during pregnancy. *Amer. J. Obstet. Gynec.* **78**, 960

DOWLING J.T., FREINKEL N. and INGBAR S.H. (1956) Thyroxine-binding by sera of pregnant women. *J. clin. Endocr.* **16**, 280

DOWLING J.T., FREINKEL N. and INGBAR S.H. (1960) The effect of estrogens upon the peripheral metabolism of thyroxine. *J. clin. Invest.* **39**, 1119

DRAGIFF D.A. and KARSHAN M. (1943) Effect of pregnancy on the chemical composition of human dentin. *J. dent. Res.* **22**, 261

DUNCAN D.L. (1964) The balance study and its limitations. In preparation.

DUNCAN E.H.L., BAIRD D. and THOMSON A.M. (1952) The causes and prevention of stillbirths and first week deaths. Part 1. The evidence of vital statistics. *J. Obstet. Gynaec. Brit. Emp.* **59**, 183

DUNCAN J.M. (1864–65) On the weight and length of the newly-born child in relation to the mother's age. *Edinb. med. J.* **10**, 497

DUNPHY D. (1962) Observations on cord blood oxygen values. *Amer. J. Obstet. Gynec.* **84**, 1320

DUPIN H., MASSÉ L. and CORRÉA P. (1962) Contribution à l'étude des poids de naissance à la maternité Africaine de Dakar. Evolution au cours des années. Variations saisonnières. [Contribution to the study of birth weight in the African maternity hospital at Dakar. Secular change. Seasonal variation]. *Courrier* **12**, 1

EBBS J.H., TISDALL F.F. and SCOTT W.A. (1941) The influence of prenatal diet on the mother and child. *J. Nutr.* **22**, 515

REFERENCES 411

EDGAR W. and RICE H.M. (1956) Administration of iron in antenatal clinics. *Lancet* **i**, 599

EDGREN R.A., ELTON R.L. and CALHOUN D.W. (1961) Studies on the interaction of oestriol and progesterone. *J. Reprod. Fertil.* **2**, 98

EDWARDS A.W.F. (1958–59) An analysis of Geissler's data on the human sex ratio. *Ann hum. Genet.* **23**, 6

EDWARDS D.A.W. (1950) Observations on the distribution of subcutaneous fat. *Clin. Sci.* **9**, 259

EDWARDS E.A. and DUNTLEY S.Q. (1949) Cutaneous vascular changes in women in reference to the menstrual cycle and ovariectomy. *Amer. J. Obstet. Gynec.* **57**, 501

EDWARDS J.H. (1958) Congenital malformations of the central nervous system in Scotland. *Brit. J. prev. soc. Med.* **12**, 115

EJARQUE P.M. and BENGTSSON L.P. (1962) Production rate of progesterone in human mid-pregnancy. *Acta endocr. (Kbh.)* **41**, 521

ELKINGTON J.R. and TAFFEL M. (1942) Prolonged water deprivation in dog. *J. clin. Invest.* **21**, 787

ELLIOTT G.A. (1944) Anaemia of pregnancy—report on the haematological study of 48 cases of pregnancy with review to the literature. *J. Obstet. Gynaec. Brit. Emp.* **51**, 198

ELLIOTT P.M. and INMAN W.H.W. (1961) Volume of liquor amnii in normal and abnormal pregnancy. *Lancet* **ii**, 835

ENGEL S. (1941) Anatomy of the lactating breast. *Brit. J. Child Dis.* **38**, 14

ENGEL S. (1947) Discussion on some recent developments in knowledge of the physiology of the breast. *Proc. roy. Soc. Med.* **40**, 899

ENGLE R.L. Jr. and WOODS K.R. (1960) in *The Plasma Proteins*, Vol. 2. Academic Press, New York and London

ENTENMAN C., GOLDWATER W.H., AYRES N.S. and BEHNKE A.R. Jr. (1958) Analysis of adipose tissue in relation to body weight loss in man. *J. appl. Physiol.* **13**, 129

ETON B. and SHORT R.V. (1960) Blood progesterone levels in abnormal pregnancies. *J. Obstet. Gynaec. Brit. Emp.* **67**, 785

FABRICANT N.D. (1960) Sexual functions and the nose. *Amer. J. med. Sci.* **239**, 498

FALLER I.L., PETTY D., LAST J.H., PASCALE L.R. and BOND E.E. (1955) A comparison of the deuterium oxide and antipyrine dilution methods for measuring total body water in normal and hydropic human subjects. *J. Lab. clin. Med.* **45**, 748

FAO (1957a) *Protein Requirements.* FAO Nutritional Studies No. 16. Food and Agriculture Organization of the United Nations, Rome

FAO (1957b) *Calorie Requirements.* FAO Nutritional Studies No. 15. Food and Agriculture Organization of the United Nations, Rome

FAO/WHO EXPERT GROUP (1962) *Calcium Requirements.* FAO Nutrition Meetings Report Series No. 30. Food and Agriculture Organization of the United Nations, Rome

FARQUHAR J.W. (1962) Maternal hyperglycaemia and foetal hyperinsulinism in diabetic pregnancy. *Postgrad. med. J.* **38**, 612

FAY J., CARTWRIGHT G.E. and WINTROBE M.M. (1949) Studies on free erythrocyte protoporphyrin, serum iron, serum iron-binding capacity and plasma copper during normal pregnancy. *J. clin. Invest.* **28**, 487

FEHLING H. (1877) Beiträge zur Physiologie des placentaren Stoffverkehrs. [Contributions to the physiology of placental exchange]. *Arch. Gynäk.* **11**, 523

FELLERS F.X., BARNETT H.L., HARE K. and McNAMARA H. (1949) Change in thiocyanate and sodium[24] spaces during growth. *Pediatrics* **3**, 622

FERRIS E.B. and WILKINS R.W. (1937) The clinical value of comparative measurements of the pressure in the femoral and cubital veins. *Amer. Heart J.* **13**, 431

FINCH S.C. and FINCH C.A. (1955) Idiopathic hemochromatosis, and iron storage disease. A. Iron metabolism in hemochromatosis. *Medicine (Baltimore)* **34**, 381

FINK H. (1948) Geburtsgewicht und physiologischer Geburtsverlust der Neugeborenen in ihrer Beziehung zum Ernährungszustand der Mutter. [Birth weight and physiological loss of weight by the newborn in relation to the nutritional state of the mother]. *Zbl. Gynäk.* **70**, 481

FISHER M. and BIGGS R. (1955) Iron deficiency in pregnancy. *Brit. med. J.* **i**, 385

FISHMAN J. (1963) Role of 2-hydroxyestrone in estrogen metabolism. *J. clin. Endocr.* **23**, 207

FISHMAN J., BROWN J.B., HELLMAN L., ZUMOFF B. and GALLAGHER T.F. (1962) Estrogen metabolism in normal and pregnant women. *J. biol. Chem.* **237**, 1489

FITZGERALD M.G., MALINS J.M., O'SULLIVAN D.J. (1961a) Prevalence of diabetes in woman thirteen years after bearing a big baby. *Lancet* **i**, 1260

FITZGERALD M.G., MALINS J.M., O'SULLIVAN D.J. and WALL M. (1961b) The effect of sex and parity on the incidence of diabetes mellitus. *Quart. J. Med.* **54**, 57

FLEXNER L.B., COWIE D.B., HELLMAN L.M., WILDE W.S. and VOSBURGH G. J. (1948) The permeability of the human placenta to sodium in normal and abnormal pregnancies and the supply of sodium to the human fetus as determined with radioactive sodium. *Amer. J. Obstet. Gynec.* **55**, 469

FLYNN F.V., HARPER C. and DE MAYO P. (1953) Lactosuria and glycosuria in pregnancy and the puerperium. *Lancet* **ii**, 698

FORBES G.B., GALLUP J. and HURSH J.B. (1961) Estimation of total body fat from potassium[40] content. *Science* **133**, 101

FORSHAW J.W.B., JONES A.T., CHISHOLM W.N. and McGINLEY W.K. (1957) Megaloblastic anaemia of pregnancy and the puerperium. *J. Obstet. Gynaec. Brit. Emp.* **64**, 255

FOURMAN J. and MOFFAT D.B. (1961) The effect of intra-arterial cushions on plasma skimming in small arteries. *J. Physiol.* **158**, 374

FOWLER W.M. and BARER A.P. (1941) Some effect of iron on hemoglobin formation. *Amer. J. med. Sci.* **201**, 642

FOWLER W.M. and BARER A.P. (1952) Plasma iron: normal values; response following medication. *Amer. J. med. Sci.* **223**, 633

FRACCARO M. (1955–56) A contribution to the study of birth weight based on an Italian sample. *Ann. hum. Genet.* **20**, 282

FRACCARO M. (1958) Data for quantitative genetics in man. Birth weight in official statistics. *Hum. Biol.* **30**, 142

FRANDSEN V.A. and STAKEMANN G. (1961) The site of production of oestrogenic hormones in human pregnancy. *Acta endocr. (Kbh.)* **38**, 383

FRAZIER T.M., DAVIS G.H., GOLDSTEIN H. and GOLDBERG I.D. (1961) Cigarette smoking and prematurity: a prospective study. *Amer. J. Obstet. Gynec.* **81**, 988

FREDA V.J. (1962) Placental transfer of antibodies in man. *Amer. J. Obstet. Gynec.* **84**, 1756

FREEDBERG I.M., HAMOLSKY M.W. and FREEDBERG A.S. (1957) The thyroid gland in pregnancy. *New Engl. J. Med.* **256**, 505

FREINKEL N. and GOODNER C.J. (1960) Carbohydrate metabolism in pregnancy. I. The metabolism of insulin by human placental tissue. *J. clin. Invest*, **39**, 116

FREIS E.D. and KENNY J.F. (1948) Plasma volume, total circulating protein and 'available fluid' abnormalities in pre-eclampsia and eclampsia. *J. clin. Invest.* **27**, 283

FRENK S. (1961) Some aspects of protein malnutrition in childhood. *Fed. Proc.* **20**, 96

FREUDENBERG K. (1950) Zur Kritik extremer Schwangerschaftsdauern. [Doubts about extremely long gestations]. *Arch. Gynäk.* **177**, 736

FRIED P.H. and RAKOFF A.E. (1951) The effects of chorionic gonadotropin and luteotropin on the maintenance of corpus luteum function. *J. clin. Endocr.* **11**, 768

FRIEDEN E.H., STONE N.R. and LAYMAN N.W. (1960) Non-steroid ovarian hormones. III. The properties of relaxin preparations purified by countercurrent distribution. *J. biol. Chem.* **235**, 2267

FRIEDLANDER M., LASKEY N. and SILBERT S. (1935) Studies in thromboangiitis obliterans (Buerger). X. Reduction in blood volume following bilateral oophorectomy. *Endocrinology* **19**, 461

FRIEDLANDER M., LASKEY N. and SILBERT S. (1936) Effect of estrogenic substance on blood volume. *Endocrinology* **20**, 329

FRIEDMAN E.A., LITTLE W.A. and SACHTLEBEN M.R. (1962) Placental oxygen consumption in vitro. 2. Total uptake as an index of placental function. *Amer. J. Obstet. Gynec.* **84**, 561

FRIEDMAN M.M., GOODFRIEND M.J., BERLIN P.F. and GOLDSTEIN T. (1951) Extracellular fluid in normal pregnancy. *Amer. J. Obstet. Gynec.* **61**, 609

FUCHS F. (1957) Studies on the passage of phosphate between mother and foetus in the guinea pig. Thesis, Ejnar Munksgaard, Copenhagen

FUCHS F. (1962) Endocrine factors in the maintenance of pregnancy. *Acta obstet. gynec. scand.* **41**, Suppl. 1, 7

FUCHS F., SPACKMAN T. and ASSALI N.S. (1963) Complexity and nonhomogeneity of the intervillous space. *Amer. J. Obstet. Gynec.* **86**, 226

FULLERTON H.W. (1937) The iron deficiency anaemia of late infancy. *Arch. Dis. Childh.* **12**, 91

FURUHJELM U. (1956) Maternal and cord blood. A comparative investigation with reference to blood sugar, serum proteins, erythrocyte sedimentation rate and total serum lipids. *Ann. Paediat. Fenn.* **2**, Suppl. 5, 1

GALLETTI F. and KLOPPER A. (1962) Influenza della somministrazione di progesterone sulla quantita e sulla distribuzione del grasso corporeo nel ratto feminina. [Effect of administration of progesterone on the quantity and distribution of body fat in the female rat]. Excerpta Medica, International Congress Series No. 51, 253

GAMONDI P. and SANTOS REIS C. (1960) Contribuição para o estudo dos pesos dos recém-nascidos de Sawah Lunto (Sumatra). [Contribution to the study of birth weight in Sawah Lunto, Sumatra]. An. Inst. Med. trop. (Lisbon) 17, 705

GARDNER D.E., SMITH F.A., HODGE H.C., OVERTON D.E. and FELTMAN R. (1952) The fluoride content of placental tissue as related to the fluoride content of drinking water. Science 115, 208

GARRY R.C. and STIVEN D. (1935-6) Review of recent work on dietary requirements in pregnancy and lactation with attempt to assess human requirements. Nutr. Abstr. Rev. 5, 855

GARRY R.C. and WOOD H.O. (1945-46) Dietary requirements in human pregnancy and lactation. A review of recent work. Nutr. Abstr. Rev. 15, 591

GARRY R.C., SLOAN A.W., WEIR J.B. de V. and WISHART M. (1954) The concentration of haemoglobin in the blood of young adult men and women: the effect of administering small doses of iron for prolonged periods. Brit. J. Nutr. 8, 253

GEMZELL C.A. (1963) in Modern Trends in Gynaecology. Ed. R. J. Kellar. Butterworths & Co Ltd, London

GEMZELL C.A., ROBBE H. and SJÖSTRAND T. (1954) Blood volume and total amount of haemoglobin in normal pregnancy and the puerperium. Acta obstet. gynec. scand. 33, 289

GEMZELL C.A., ROBBE H. and STRÖM G. (1957) Total amount of haemoglobin and physical working capacity in normal pregnancy and puerperium (with iron medication). Acta obstet. gynec. scand. 36, 93

GERDES M.M. and BOYDEN E.A. (1938) The rate of emptying of the human gall-bladder in pregnancy. Surg. Gynec. Obstet. 66, 145

GERRITSEN T. and WALKER A.R.P. (1954) The effect of habitually high iron intake on certain blood values in pregnant Bantu women. J. clin. Invest. 33, 23

GESSNER W. (1919) Eklampsie und Weltkrieg im Lichte einer amtlichen Landesstatistik. [Eclampsia and World War in the light of regional departmental statistics]. Zbl. Gynäk. 43, 1033

GIACOMETTI L. and MONTAGNA W. (1962) The nipple and the areola of the human female breast. Anat. Rec. 144, 191

GIESE R. and KAYSER K. (1947) Die Beeinflussung des Geburtsgewichts durch schlechte Ernährungs verhältnisse wahrend des Krieges und der Nachkriegsjahre von 1938-1946. [Effect on birth weight of bad nutritional conditions during the war and the post-war years 1938-46]. Zbl. Gynäk. 69, 583

GILBERT R., EPIFANO L. and AUCHINCLOSS J.H. Jr. (1962) Dyspnea of pregnancy. J. Amer. med. Ass. 182, 1073

GILES C. and SHUTTLEWORTH E.M. (1958) Megaloblastic anaemia of pregnancy and the puerperium. Lancet ii, 1341

GILLESPIE E.C. (1950) Principles of uterine growth in pregnancy. *Amer. J. Obstet. Gynec.* **59**, 949

GILLMAN T., NAIDOO S.S. and HATHORN M. (1959) Plasma fibrinolytic activity in pregnancy. *Lancet* ii, 70

GOLDECK H., REMY D. and LABHARD H. (1954) Eisenmangel und Schwangerschaft. [Iron deficiency and pregnancy]. *Dtsch. med. Wschr.* **79**, 211

GOODALL J.R. and GOTTLIEB R. (1936) The association of pregnancy, hypochromic anemia and achlorhydria. *Canad. med. Ass. J.* **35**, 50

GOODLAND R.L. and POMMERENKE W.T. (1952) Cyclic fluctuations of the alveolar carbon dioxide tension during the normal menstrual cycle. *Fertil. and Steril.* **3**, 394

GOODLAND R.L., REYNOLDS J.G., McCOORD A.B. and POMMERENKE W.T. (1953) Respiratory and electrolyte effects induced by estrogen and progesterone. *Fertil. and Steril.* **4**, 300

GOUDSMIT A. and LOUIS L. (1942) Extracellular fluid volume in man. Its measurement and relation to season. *Amer. J. med. Sci.* **203**, 914

GRÄFE H.K. (1961) Aktuelle Beitrag zur Schwangeren-Ernährung. 1. Bericht über die Ernährungsbefunde von 89 Frauen im 5. Monat der Schwangerschaft. 2. Bericht über die Ernährungsbefunde von 89 Frauen im 8. Monat der Schwangerschaft. [Recent contribution to nutrition in pregnancy. 1. Diet findings in 89 women in the 5th month of pregnancy. 2. Diet findings in 89 women in the 8th month of pregnancy. *Dtsch. Gesundh.-Wes.* **16**, 461, 509, 813, 845

GRANGER G.B. (1941) The significance of weight changes during pregnancy. *Med. Tms.* (*N.Y.*) **69**, 68

GRAY M.J. and PLENTL A.A. (1954) The variations of the sodium space and the total exchangeable sodium during pregnancy. *J. clin. Invest.* **33**, 347

GREENSTEIN N.M. and CLAHR J. (1937) Circulation time studies in pregnant women. *Amer. J. Obstet. Gynec.* **33**, 414

GREGERSEN M.I. and RAWSON R.A. (1959) Blood volume. *Physiol. Rev.* **39**, 307

GREGORY R.A. (1962) *Secretory mechanisms of the gastro-intestinal tract.* Edward Arnold Ltd, London

GREIG M., COYLE M.G., COOPER W. and WALKER J. (1962) Plasma progesterone in mother and foetus in the second half of human pregnancy. *J. Obstet. Gynaec. Brit. Commonw.* **69**, 772

GRUMBACH M.M. and WERNER S.C. (1956) Transfer of thyroid hormone across the human placenta at term. *J. clin. Endocr.* **16**, 1392

GRYBOSKI W.A. and SPIRO H.M. (1956) The effect of pregnancy on gastric secretion. *New Engl. J. Med.* **255**, 1131

GUTHMANN H. and MAY W. (1930) Gibt es eine intrauterine Nierensekretion? [Is there an intrauterine renal section?] *Arch. Gynäk.* **141**, 450

GUTTMACHER A.F. (1939) An analysis of 573 cases of twin pregnancy. II. The hazards of pregnancy itself. *Amer. J. Obstet. Gynec.* **38**, 277

GYLLING T. (1961) Renal haemodynamics and heart volume in normal pregnancy. *Acta obstet. gynec. scand.* **40**, Suppl. 5

HADDON W., NESBITT R.E.L. and GARCIA R. (1961) Smoking and pregnancy: carbon monoxide in blood during gestation and at term. *Obstet. and Gynec.* **18**, 262

HAGERMAN D.D. and VILLEE C.A. (1961) A mechanism of action for estrogenic steroid hormones, in *Mechanism of Action of Steroid Hormones*. Eds. C. A· Villee and L. L. Engel. Pergamon Press, Oxford

HAHN P.F., CAROTHERS E.L., DARBY W.J., MARTIN M., SHEPPARD C.W., CANNON R.O., BEAM A.S., DENSEN P.M., PETERSON J.C. and McCLELLAN G.S. (1951) Iron metabolism in human pregnancy as studied with the radioactive isotope Fe⁵⁹. *Amer. J. Obstet. Gynec.* **61**, 477

HALEY H.B. and WOODBURY J.W. (1956) Body composition and body water metabolism in normal pregnancy. *Surg. Gynec. Obstet.* **103**, 227

HALL K. (1960) Relaxin. *J. Reprod. Fertil.* **1**, 368

HALNAN K.E. (1958) The radioiodine uptake of the human thyroid in pregnancy. *Clin. Sci.* **17**, 281

HAMILTON B. and MORIARTY M. (1929) The composition of growth in infancy. *Amer. J. Dis. Child.* **37**, 1169

HAMILTON H.F.H. (1949) The cardiac output in normal pregnancy. As determined by the Cournand right heart catheterization technique. *J. Obstet. Gynaec. Brit. Emp.* **56**, 548

HAMILTON H.F.H. (1950) Blood viscosity in pregnancy. *J. Obstet. Gynaec. Brit. Emp.* **57**, 530

HAMILTON W.F., RILEY R.L., ATTYAH A.M., COURNAND A., FOWELL D.M., HIMMELSTEIN A., NOBLE R.P., REMINGTON J.W., RICHARDS D.W. Jr., WHEELER N.C. and WITHAM A.C. (1948) Comparison of the Fick and dye injection methods of measuring the cardiac output in man. *Amer. J. Physiol.* **153**, 309

HAMILTON W.J. and BOYD J.D. (1951) Observations on the human placenta. *Proc. roy. Soc. Med.* **44**, 489

HAMILTON W.J., BOYD J.D. and MOSSMAN H.W. (1956) *Human Embryology. Prenatal development of form and function*. 2nd Ed. (1st Ed. 1945). W. Heffer and Sons Ltd, Cambridge

HANNAH C.R. (1925) Weight during pregnancy with observations and statistics. *Amer. J. Obstet. Gynec.* **9**, 854

HANON F. (1957) Liquide amniotique et système amniotique. [Amniotic fluid and the amniotic system]. *Rev. franç. Gynéc.* **52**, 57

HANSEN H.A. and KLEWESAHL-PALM H.V. (1963) Blood folic acid levels and clearance rate of injected folic acid in normal pregnancy and puerperium. *Scand. J. clin. Lab. Invest.* **15**, Suppl. 69, 78

HANSEN R. and LANGER W. (1935) Über Geschmacksveränderungen in der Schwangerschaft. [Changes of taste in pregnancy]. *Klin. Wschr.* **14**, 1173

HANSEN R. (1937) Zur Physiologie des Magens in der Schwangershaft. [Physiology of the stomach in pregnancy]. *Zbl. Gynäk.* **61**, 2306

HARDINGE M.G. and STARE F.J. (1954) Nutritional studies of vegetarians. 1. Nutritional, physical and laboratory studies. *Amer. J. clin. Nutr.* **2**, 73

HARE D.C. and KARN M.N. (1929) An investigation of blood pressure, pulse rate and the response to exercise during normal pregnancy, and some observations after confinement. *Quart. J. Med.* **22**, 381

HARKNESS M.L.R. and HARKNESS R.D. (1959) Changes in the physical properties of the uterine cervix of the rat during pregnancy. *J. Physiol.* **148**, 524

HARRIES J.M. and HUGHES T.F. (1957) An enumeration of the 'cravings' of some pregnant women. *Proc. Nutr. Soc.* **16**, xx

HARRIS E.A. (1958) Exercise-tolerance tests. *Lancet* ii, 409

HARRISON H.E., DARROW D.C. and YANNET H. (1936) Total electrolyte content of animals and its probable relation to distribution of body water. *J. biol. Chem.* **113**, 515

HASKINS A.L. and TAUBERT H.D. (1963) Progesterone transportation in blood. *Obstet. and Gynec.* **21**, 395

HAUCK H.M. (1963) Weight changes during pregnancy. Awo Omamma, Nigeria, 1960. *Brit. J. Obstet. Gynaec. Brit. Commonw.* **70**, 885

HAUROWITZ F. (1961) in *Function of the blood.* Eds. R. G. MacFarlane and A. H. T. Robb-Smith. Blackwell Scientific Publications, Oxford

HAWKER R.W. (1956) Inactivation of antidiuretic hormone and oxytocin during pregnancy. *Quart. J. exp. Physiol.* **41**, 301

HAWKINS D.F. and NIXON W.C.W. (1958) The electrolyte composition of the human uterus in normal pregnancy and labour and in prolonged labour. *J. Obstet. Gynaec. Brit. Emp.* **65**, 895

HAYASHI T. (1956) Uric acid and endogenous creatinine clearance studies in normal pregnancy and toxemias of pregnancy. *Amer. J. Obstet. Gynec.* **71**, 859

HECKEL G.P. and TOBIN C.E. (1956) Arteriovenous shunts in the myometrium. *Amer. J. Obstet. Gynec.* **71**, 199

HELLEGERS A., OKUDA K., NESBIT R.E.L., SMITH D.W. and CHOW B.F. (1957) Vitamin B_{12} absorption in pregnancy and in the newborn. *Amer. J. clin. Nutr.* **5**, 327

HELLEGERS A., METCALFE J., HUCKABEE W., MESCHIA G., PRYSTOWSKY H. and BARRON D. (1959) The alveolar pCO_2 and pO_2 in pregnant and non-pregnant women at altitude. *J. clin. Invest.* **38**, 1010

HELLER L. (1955) Stickstoffbilanzen in den letzhen drei Schwangershaftsmonaten. [Nitrogen balances in the last three months of pregnancy]. *Arch. Gynäk.* **185**, 566

HELLMAN L.M., TRICOMI V. and GUPTA O. (1957) Pressures in the human amniotic fluid and intervillous space. *Amer. J. Obstet. Gynec.* **74**, 1018

HENDRICKS C.H. (1954) The neurohypophysis in pregnancy. *Obstet. gynec. Surv.* **9**, 323

HENDRICKS C.H. (1958) The hemodynamics of a uterine contraction. *Amer. J. Obstet. Gynec.* **76**, 969

HENRY J.S. (1936) The effect of pregnancy upon the blood pressure. *J. Obstet. Gynaec. Brit. Emp.* **43**, 908

HERBERT C.M., BANNER E.A. and WAKIM K.G. (1958) Variations in the peripheral circulation during pregnancy. *Amer. J. Obstet. Gynec.* **76**, 742

HERRIOT A., BILLEWICZ W.Z. and HYTTEN F.E. (1962) Cigarette smoking in pregnancy. *Lancet* i, 771

HILLMAN R.W. (1960) Fingernail growth in pregnancy. Relations to some common parameters of the reproductive process. *Hum. Biol.* **32**, 119

HOBSON W. (1948) A dietary and clinical survey of pregnant women with particular reference to toxaemia of pregnancy. *J, Hyg. (Lond.)* **46**, 198

HODGE H.C. and SMITH F.A. (1954) in *Fluoridation as a public health measure.* Ed.

418   THE PHYSIOLOGY OF HUMAN PREGNANCY

J. H. Shaw. American Association for the Advancement of Science, Washington, D.C.

HOFFSTRÖM K.A. (1910) Eine Stoffwechseluntersuchung während der Schwangerschaft. [Study of metabolism during pregnancy]. *Skand. Arch. Physiol.* **23**, 326

HOLLANDER A.G. and CRAWFORD J.H. (1943) Roentgenologic and electrocardiographic changes in the normal heart during pregnancy. *Amer. Heart J.* **26**, 364

HOLLINGSWORTH M.G. (1960) The birth weights of African and European babies born in Ghana. *W. African med. J.* **9**, 256

HOLMER A.J.M. (1947) in *Medische Ervaringen in Nederland tijdens de Bezetting, 1940–45.* [Medical observations in the Netherlands during the occupation, 1940–45]. Ed. I. Boerema. J. B. Wolters, Groningen

HOOVER C.R. and TURNER C.W. (1954) *In vitro* metabolism of the rat mammary gland. *Missouri Agric. Exp. Stat. Res. Bull. No.* 563

HOSEMANN H.A. (1949a) Schwangerschaftsdauer und Neugeborenengewicht. [Duration of pregnancy and birth weight]. *Arch. Gynäk.* **176**, 109

HOSEMANN H. (1949b) Schwangerschaftsdauer und Gewicht der Placenta. [Duration of pregnancy and weight of the placenta]. *Arch. Gynäk.* **176**, 453

HOWARD B.K., GOODSON J.H. and MENGERT W.F. (1953) Supine hypotensive syndrome in late pregnancy. *Obstet. and Gynec.* **1**, 371

HOWARD R.B. (1953) Diurnal rhythm of the serum iron level: effect of diet and of environmental temperature. *J. Lab. clin. Med.* **42**, 817

HUCKABEE W.E. (1962) Uterine blood flow. *Amer. J. Obstet. Gynec.* **84**, 1623

HUCKABEE W.E., METCALFE J., PRYSTOWSKY, H. and BARRON D.H. (1962) Insufficiency of O_2 supply to pregnant uterus. *Amer. J. Physiol.* **202**, 198

HUGGINS R.R., HARDEN B. and GRIER G.W. (1935) A study of the relationship of pregnancy to disease of the gall bladder. *Surg. Gynec. Obstet.* **61**, 471

HULKA J.F., HSU K.C. and BEISER S.M. (1961) Antibodies to trophoblasts during the post-partum period. *Nature* **191**, 510

HUMMEL F.C., STERNBERGER H.R., HUNSCHER H.A. and MACY I.G. (1936) Metabolism of women during the reproductive cycle. VII. Utilization of inorganic elements (a continuous case study of a multipara). *J. Nutr.* **11**, 235

HUMMEL F.C., HUNSCHER H.A., BATES M.F., BONNER P. and MACY I.G. (1937) A consideration of the nutritive state in the metabolism of women during pregnancy. *J. Nutr.* **13**, 263

HUMOLLER F.L., MOCKLER M.P., HOLTHAUS J.M. and MAHLER D.J. (1960) Enzymatic properties of coeruloplasmin. *J. Lab. clin. Med.* **56**, 222

HUMPHREYS R.C. (1954) An analysis of the maternal and foetal weight factors in normal pregnancy. *J. Obstet. Gynaec. Brit. Emp.* **61**, 764

HUNSCHER H.A., HUMMEL F.C., ERICKSON B.N. and MACY I.G. (1935) Metabolism of women during the reproductive cycle. VI. A case study of the continuous nitrogen utilization of a multipara during pregnancy, parturition, puerperium and lactation. *J. Nutr.* **10**, 579

HUNT J.N. and MURRAY F.A. (1958) Gastric function in pregnancy. *J. Obstet. Gynaec. Brit. Emp.* **65**, 78

HUTCHISON D.L., HUNTER C.B., NESLEN E.D. and PLENTL A.A. (1955) The

REFERENCES 419

exchange of water and electrolytes in the mechanism of amniotic fluid formation and the relationship to hydramnios. *Surg. Gynec. Obstet.* **100**, 391

HUTCHINSON D.L., PLENTL A.A. and TAYLOR H.C. Jr. (1954) The total body water and the water turnover in pregnancy studied with deuterium oxide as isotopic tracer. *J. clin. Invest.* **33**, 235

HYTTEN F.E. (1954a) Clinical and chemical studies in human lactation. IV. Trends in milk composition during course of lactation. *Brit. med. J.* **i**, 249

HYTTEN F.E. (1954b) Clinical and chemical studies in human lactation. VI. The functional capacity of the breast. *Brit. med. J.* **i**, 912

HYTTEN F.E. (1964) Measurement of total body fat in man with [85]Kypton. *Proc. nutr. Soc.* **23** in press.

HYTTEN F.E. and BAIRD D. (1958) The development of the nipple in pregnancy. *Lancet* **ii**, 1201

HYTTEN F.E. and CHEYNE G.A. (1962) The distribution of thiocyanate in the product of conception. *Clin. Sci.* **23**, 125

HYTTEN F.E. and DUNCAN D.L. (1956) Iron-deficiency anaemia in the pregnant woman and its relation to normal physiological changes. *Nutr. Abstr. Rev.* **26**, 855

HYTTEN F.E. and KLOPPER A.I. (1963) Response to a water load in pregnancy. *J. Obstet. Gynaec. Brit. Commonw.* **70**, 811

HYTTEN F.E. and PAINTIN D.B. (1963) Increase in plasma volume during normal pregnancy. *J. Obstet. Gynaec. Brit. Commonw.* **70**, 402

HYTTEN F.E., PAINTIN D.B., STEWART A.M. and PALMER J.H. (1963) The relation of maternal heart size, blood volume and stature to the birth weight of the baby. *J. Obstet. Gynaec. Brit. Commonw.* **70**, 817

HYTTEN F.E., TAGGART N., BILLEWICZ W.Z. and JASON A.C. (1962) The estimation of small concentrations of deuterium oxide in water by the falling drop method. *Phys. in Med. Biol.* **6**, 415

HYTTEN F.E. and THOMSON A.M. (1961) in *Milk: the Mammary Gland and its Secretion.* Eds. S. K. Kon and A. T. Cowie. Vol. II. Academic Press, New York and London

IHRMAN K. (1960a) A clinical and physiological study of pregnancy in a material from Northern Sweden. *Acta Soc. Med. upsalien.* **65**, 137

IHRMAN K. (1960b) A clinical and physiological study of pregnancy in a material from Northern Sweden. III. Vital capacity and maximal breathing capacity during and after pregnancy. *Acta Soc. Med. upsalien.* **65**, 147

IHRMAN K. (1960c) A clinical and physiological study of pregnancy in a material from Northern Sweden. VI. The arterial blood pressure at rest and in orthostatic test during and after pregnancy. *Acta Soc. Med. upsalien.* **65**, 315

IHRMAN K. (1960d) A clinical and physiological study of pregnancy in a material from Northern Sweden. VII. The heart volume during and after pregnancy. *Acta Soc. Med. upsalien.* **65**, 326

INGLEBY H. (1949) Changes in breast volume in a group of normal young women. *Bull. int. Ass. med. Mus.* **29**, 87

INGELMAN-SUNDBERG A. (1958) The value of antenatal massage of nipples and expression of colostrum. *J. Obstet. Gynaec. Brit. Emp.* **65**, 448

420 THE PHYSIOLOGY OF HUMAN PREGNANCY

INGRAM D.L. (1962) in *The Ovary*. Vol. I. Ed. S. Zuckerman. Academic Press, New York

INKLEY S.R., BROOKS L. and KRIEGER H. (1955) A study of methods for the prediction of plasma volume. *J. Lab. clin. Med.* **45**, 841

IOB V. and SWANSON W.W. (1934) Mineral growth of the human fetus. *Amer. J. Dis. Child*, **47**, 302

ISRAEL S.L., STROUP P.E., SELIGSON H.T. and SELIGSON D. (1959) Epinephrine and *nor*-epinephrine in pregnancy and labor. *Obstet. and Gynec.* **14**, 68

JACKSON C.M. (1909) On the prenatal growth of the human body and the relative growth of the various organs and parts. *Amer. J. Anat.* **9**, 119

JACKSON W.P.U. (1952) Studies in pre-diabetes. *Brit. med. J.* **2**, 690

JACKSON W.P.U. (1955) A concept of diabetes. *Lancet* **ii**, 625

JACKSON W.P.U. (1961a) Is pregnancy diabetogenic? *Lancet* **ii**, 1369

JACKSON W.P.U. (1961b) The cortisone-glucose tolerance test with special reference to the prediction of diabetes. *Diabetes* **10**, 33

JACOT B. (1951) Influence du jeûne sur les oscillations nycthémérales du fer sérique. [Effect of fasting on the daily fluctuations of serum iron]. *Experientia (Basel)*, **7**, 33

JAMES A.H. (1957) *The physiology of gastric digestion*. Edward Arnold Ltd, London

JAMES J.D. (1941) Dental caries in pregnancy. *J. Amer. dent. Ass.* **28**, 1857

JAMES L.S., WEISBROT I.M., PRINCE C.E., HOLADAY D.A. and APGAR V. (1958) The acid-base status of human infants in relation to birth asphyxia and the onset of respiration. *J. Pediat.* **52**, 379

JAMES S. and BURNARD E. (1961) Biochemical changes occurring during asphyxia at birth and some effects on the heart, in *Ciba Foundation Symposium on Somatic Stability in the newly born*. J. and A. Churchill, London

JANNEY J.C. and WALKER E.W. (1932) Kidney function in pregnancy. I. Water diuresis in normal pregnancy. *J. Amer. med. Ass.* **99**, 2078

JANS C. (1959) La croissance ponderale du nourrisson pygmée (Bambuti-Ituri). [Growth in weight of pygmy infants (Bambuti-Ituri)]. *Ann. Soc. Belge de Med. Trop.* **39**, 851

JANZ G.J., FERREIRA A.P., SANTOS REIS C. and PORTELA R. (1959) O peso do recém-nascido Africano da Guiné-Portuguesa. [Birth weight of African infants in Portuguese Guinea]. *An. Inst. Med. trop. (Lisbon)* **16**, 73

JARUSOVA N.S. (1961) O novyh sutocnyh normah potrebnosti celoveka v vitaminah. [New standards for daily vitamin requirements in man]. *Vop. Pitan.* **20**, No. 3, 3

JÄRVINEN P.A. and ÖSTERLUND K. (1963) Effect of smoking during pregnancy on the fetus, placenta and delivery. *Ann. Paediat. Fenn.* **9**, 18

JEANS P.C., SMITH M.B. and STEARNS G. (1952) Dietary habits of pregnant women of low income in a rural state. *J. Amer. diet. Ass.* **28**, 27

JEANS P.C., SMITH M.B. and STEARNS G. (1955) Incidence of prematurity in relation to maternal nutrition. *J. Amer. diet. Ass.* **31**, 576

JENSEN E.V. and JACOBSON H.I. (1962) Basic guides to the mechanism of estrogen action, in *Recent Progress in hormone research*. Ed. G. Pincus. Academic Press, New York

JOHNSON N.C. (1961) Studies of copper and zinc metabolism during pregnancy.

Proc. Soc. exp. Biol. (N.Y.) **108**, 518

JONES K.M., LLOYD-JONES R., RIONDEL A., TAIT J.F., TAIT S.A.S., BULBROOK R.D. and GREENWOOD F.C. (1959) Aldosterone secretion and metabolism in normal men and women and in pregnancy. *Acta endocr. (Kbh.)* **30**, 321

JOUBERT D.M. and HAMMOND J. (1954) Maternal effect on birth weight in South Devon x Dexter cattle crosses. *Nature, Lond.* **174**, 647

KAISER R. (1955) Oestrogene und Progesteronstoffwechsel. [Oestrogens and progesterone metabolism]. *Klin. Wschr.* **33**, 15

KALMUS H. and SMITH C.A.B. (1960) Evolutionary origin of sexual differentiation and the sex ratio. *Nature (Lond.)*, **186**, 1004

KALTREIDER N.L. and MENEELY G.R. (1940) The effect of exercise on the volume of the blood. *J. clin. Invest.* **19**, 627

KALTREIDER N.L., MENEELY G.R., ALLEN J.R. and BALE W.F. (1941) Determination of volume of extracellular fluid of body with radioactive sodium. *J. exp. Med.* **74**, 569

KANDROR I.S. (1961) Fizičeskoe razvitie novoroždennyh i detej v vozraste do 3 let, rodivšihsja v Arktike. [Physical development of newborn infants and children up to 3 years, born in the Arctic]. *Pediatrija* **40**, 41

KANG Y.S. and CHO W.K. (1962) The sex ratio at birth and other attributes of the newborn from maternity hospitals in Korea. *Hum. Biol.* **34**, 38

KAPLAN A. and CHAIKOFF I. L. (1936) The relation of glycogen, fat and protein to water storage in the liver, *J. biol. Chem.* **116**, 663

KAPLAN N.M. (1961) Successful pregnancy following hypophysectomy during the twelfth week of gestation. *J. clin. Endocr.* **21**, 1139

KAPPAS A., PALMER R.H. and GLICKMAN P.B. (1961) Steroid fever. *Amer. J. Med.* **31**, 167

KARN M.N. (1947–49) Length of human gestation with special reference to prematurity. *Ann Eugen. (Lond.)* **14**, 44

KARN M.N. (1951–52) Birth weight and length of gestation of twins, together with maternal age, parity and survival rate. *Ann. Eugen. (Lond.)* **16**, 365

KARN M.N. (1957–58) Considerations arising from weight and some other variables recorded in the survey of women's measurements (1957). *Ann. hum. Genet.* **22**, 385

KARN M.N. and PENROSE L.S. (1951–52) Birth weight and gestation time in relation to maternal age, parity and infant survival. *Ann. Eugen. (Lond.)* **16**, 147

KELLAR R.S. (1957) in *Combined Textbook of Obstetrics and Gynaecology.* Ed. D. Baird. 6th Ed. E. and S. Livingstone Ltd, Edinburgh

KELLY H.J., SLOAN R.E., HOFFMAN W. and SAUNDERS C. (1951) Accumulation of nitrogen and six minerals in the human fetus during gestation. *Hum. Biol.* **23**, 61

KEMSLEY W.F.F., BILLEWICZ W.Z. and THOMSON A.M. (1962) A new weight-for-height standard based on British anthropometric data. *Brit. J. prev. soc. Med.* **16**, 189

KERR A. Jr. (1943) Weight gain in pregnancy and its relation to weight of infants and to length of labor. *Amer. J. Obstet. Gynec.* **45**, 950

KERR D.N.S. and DAVIDSON S. (1958) The prophylaxis of iron deficiency

EE

422   THE PHYSIOLOGY OF HUMAN PREGNANCY

anaemia in pregnancy. *Lancet* ii, 483

KERR J.M.M. (1916) *Operative Midwifery.* Ballière, Tindall and Cox, London

KERWIN W. (1926) Weight estimates during pregnancy and the puerperium. *Amer. J. Obstet. Gynec.* 11, 473

KETY S.S. (1948) Quantitative determination of cerebral blood flow in man. *Methods in Medical Research I*, 204. Year Book Publishers, Chicago

KEYS A., ANDERSON J.T. and BROZEK J. (1955) Weight gain from simple overeating. 1. Character of the tissue gained. *Metabolism* 4, 427

KILLANDER A. (1957) The serum vitamin B_{12} levels at various ages. *Acta paediat. (Uppsala)* 46, 585

KING A.G. (1949) Free-feeding pregnant women. *Amer. J. Obstet. Gynec.* 58, 299

KJELLBERG S.R., LONROTH H., RUDHE U. and SJÖSTRAND T. (1950) Blood volume and heart volume during pregnancy and the puerperium. *Acta med. scand.* 138, 421

KLAFTEN E. and PALUGYAY J. (1926) Zur Physiologie der Atmung in der Schwangerschaft. [Physiology of respiration in pregnancy]. *Arch. Gynäk.* 129, 414

KLAFTEN E. and PALUGYAY J. (1927) Vergleichende Untersuchungen über Lage und Ausdehnung von Herz und Lunge in her Schwangerschaft und im Wochenbett. [Comparative studies of the position and size of heart and lungs in pregnancy and the puerperium]. *Arch. Gynäk.* 131, 347

KLEIBER M. (1961) *The fire of life. An introduction to animal energetics.* John Wiley & Sons, Inc., New York

KLEIN J. (1946) The relationship of maternal weight gain to the weight of the newborn infant. *Amer. J. Obstet. Gynec.* 52, 574

KLOPPER A. (1953) The use of oestrogens, in *Modern Trends in Obstetrics.* Ed. R. Kellar. Butterworths, London

KLOPPER A. and BILLEWICZ W. (1963) Urinary excretion of oestriol and pregnanediol during normal pregnancy. *J. Obstet. Gynaec. Brit. Commonw.* 70, 1024.

KLOPPER A.I. and DENNIS K.J. (1962) Effect of oestrogens on myometrial contractions. *Brit. med. J.* ii, 1157

KLOPPER A.I. and MACNAUGHTON M.C. (1959) The identification of pregnanediol in liquor amnii, bile and faeces. *J. Endocr.* 18, 319

KLOPPER A. and MICHIE E.A. (1956) The excretion of urinary pregnanediol after the administration of progesterone. *J. Endocr.* 13, 360

KLOPPER A.I., MICHIE E.A. and BROWN J.B. (1955) A method for the determination of urinary pregnanediol. *J. Endocr.* 12, 209

KOMAI T. and FUKUOKA G. (1936) Frequency of multiple births among the Japanese and related people. *Amer. J. phys. Anthropol.* 21, 433

KOSTERLITZ H.W. and CAMPBELL R. M. (1957) Nutrition and gestation. *Ann. Nutr. (Paris)* 11, A85

KREIGER D.T., GABRILOVE J.L. and SOFFER L.J. (1960) Adrenal function in a pregnant bilaterally adrenalectomized woman. *J. clin. Endocr.* 20, 1493

KRUKENBERG H. (1932) Arbeitsphysiologische Studien |an Graviden. 2. Der Einfluss der Körperarbeit auf Herz und Kreislauf. [Work physiology in pregnant women. 2. Effect of bodily work on heart and circulation]. *Arch. Gynäk.* 149, 663

KUMAR D. (1962) *In vitro* inhibitory effect of progesterone on extrauterine human smooth muscle. *Amer. J. Obstet. Gynec.* **84**, 1300

KUO C.C. (1941) Weight gain in normal pregnancy in Chinese pateints. *Chin. med. J.* **59**, 278

LAGERLÖF H., WERKÖ L., BUCHT H. and HOLMGREN A. (1949) Separate determination of the blood volume of the right and left heart and the lungs in man with the aid of the dye injection method. *Scand. J. clin. Lab. Invest.* **1**, 114

LAHEY M.E., GUBLER C.J., CARTWRIGHT G.E. and WINTROBE M.M. (1953) Studies on copper metabolism. 7. Blood copper in pregnancy and various pathologic states. *J. clin. Invest.* **32**, 329

LAHMANN H. quoted by Prochownick (1901)

LAIDLER K.J. and KRUPKA R.M. (1961) Enzyme mechanisms in relation to the mode of action of steroid hormones, in *Mechanism of action of steroid hormones*. Eds. C. A. Villee and L. L. Engel. Pergamon Press, Oxford

LAMBIOTTE C., BLANCHARD J. and GRAFF S. (1950) Thiosulphate clearance in pregnancy. *J. clin. Invest.* **29**, 1207

LANDAU R.L. and LUGIBIHL K. (1961) The catabolic and natruretic effects of progesterone in man, in *Recent Progress in hormone research*. Ed. G. Pincus. Academic Press, New York

LANDAU R.L., PLOTZ E.J. and LUGIBIHL K. (1960) Effect of pregnancy on the metabolic influence of administered progesterone. *J. clin. Endocr.* **20**, 1561

LANDT H. and BENJAMIN J.E. (1936) Cardiodynamic and electrocardiographic changes in normal pregnancy. *Amer. Heart J.* **12**, 592

LANZ R. and HOCHULI E. (1955) Über die Nierenclearance in der normalen Schwangerschaft und bei hypertensiven Spättoxikosen. Ihre Beeinflüssung durch hypotensive Medikamenta. [Renal clearance in normal pregnancy and in late hypertensive toxicoses. Effect of hypotensive drugs]. *Schweiz. med. Wschr.* **85**, 395

LARGE A.M., JOHNSTON C.G., KATSUKI T. and FACHNIE H.L. (1960) Gallstones and pregnancy: the composition of gall-bladder bile in the pregnant woman at term. *Amer. J. med. Sci.* **239**, 713

LARON Z. (1957) Skin turgor as a quantitative index of dehydration in children. *Pediatrics* **19**, 816

LAURELL C.B. (1947) Studies on the transportation and metabolism of iron in the body, with special reference to the iron-binding component in human plasma. *Acta physiol. scand.* **14**, Suppl. 46

LAWSON H.W. (1934) Weight curve and Benedict test during pregnancy. *Med. Ann. D. C.* **III**, 6

LAX H. (1947) Die Auswirkung der veränderten Ernährungslage in der Klinik. [The effect of the changed nutritional position in the clinic]. *Zbl. Gynäk.* **69**, 310

LEE C.-C. (1948) Birth weights of full term infants in West China. *Chin. med. J.* **66**, 153

LECK I. (1963) Incidence of malformations following influenza epidemics. *Brit. J. prev. soc. Med.* **17**, 70

LEITCH I. (1964) in *Nutrition: A comprehensive treatise*. Ed. G. A. Beaton. Academic Press, New York and London.

LEITCH I. and AITKEN F.C. (1959) The estimation of calcium requirement: a re-examination. *Nutr. Abstr. Rev.* **29**, 393

LEITCH I., HYTTEN F.E. and BILLEWICZ W.Z. (1959) The maternal and neonatal weights of some mammalia. *Proc. zool. Soc. Lond.* **133**, 11.

LERNER A.B., SHIZUME K. and BUNDING I. (1954) The mechanism of endocrine control of melanin pigmentation. *J. clin. Endocr.* **14**, 1463

LEVIANT S.M. (1960) Leningrad infants. *Pediatriya* **7**, 27

LI C.H. (1962) Synthesis and biological properties of ACTH peptides, in *Recent Progress in Hormone Research.* Ed. G. Pincus. Academic Press, New York

LITTLE B., SMITH O.W., JESSIMAN A.G., SELENKOW H.A., VAN'T HOFF W., EGLIN J.M. and MOORE F.D. (1958) Hypophysectomy during pregnancy in a patient with cancer of the breast: case report with hormone studies. *J. clin. Endocr.* **18**, 425

LLEWELLYN-JONES D. (1955) Premature babies in the tropics. *J. Obstet. Gynaec. Brit. Emp.* **62**, 275

LLEWELLYN-JONES D. (1962) Nutritional supplements in pregnancy (with special reference to the developing countries) *Med. J. Malaya*, **16**, 260

LONGO L.D. and ASSALI N.S. (1960) Renal function in human pregnancy. IV. The Urinary tract 'dead-space' during normal gestation. *Amer. J. Obstet. Gynec.* **80**, 495

LORAINE J.A. (1961) Human chorionic gonadotrophin (HCG), in *Hormones in blood.* Eds. C. H. Gray and A. L. Bacharach. Academic Press, New York

LOWE C.R. (1959) Effect of mothers' smoking habits on birth weight of their children. *Brit. med. J.* **ii**, 673

LOWENSTEIN L., PICK C.A. and PHILPOTT N.W. (1950) Correlation of blood loss with blood volume and other hematological studies before, during and after childbirth. *Amer. J. Obstet. Gynec.* **60**, 1206

LUND C.J. (1951) Studies on the iron-deficiency anemia of pregnancy, including plasma volume, total hemoglobin, erythrocyte protoporphyrin in treated and untreated normal and anemic patients. *Amer. J. Obstet. Gynec.* **62**, 947

LUNDSTRÖM P. (1950) Studies on erythroid elements and serum iron in normal pregnancy. *Acta Soc. Med. upsalien.* **55**, 1

LYSGAARD H. (1962) Kvindens vaegtøgning under graviditeten i relation til barnets fødselsstørrelse. [Weight increase in pregnant women in relation to the birth weight of their infants]. *Nord. Med.* **67**, 539

MCCALL M.L. (1949) Cerebral blood flow and metabolism in toxemias of pregnancy. *Surg. Gynec. Obstet.* **89**, 715

MCCANCE R.A., WIDDOWSON E.M. and VERDON-ROE C.M. (1938) A study of English diets by the individual method. III. Pregnant women at different economic levels. *J. Hyg. (Lond.)* **38**, 596

MCCARTNEY C.P., POTTINGER R.E. and HARROD J.P. (1959) Alterations in body composition during pregnancy. *Am. J. Obstet. Gynec.* **77**, 1038

MCCAUSLAND A.M., HYMAN C., WINSOR T. and TROTTER A.D. (1961) Venous distensibility during pregnancy. *Amer. J. Obstet. Gynec.* **81**, 472

MCCLURE J.H. and JAMES J.M. (1960) Oxygen administration to the mother and its relation to blood oxygen in the newborn infant. *Amer. J. Obstet. Gynec.* **80**, 554

McCoy B.A., Bleiler R.E. and Ohlson M.A. (1961) Iron content of intact placentas and cords. *Amer. J. clin. Nutr.* **9**, 613

McDonald A.D. (1961) Maternal health in early pregnancy and congenital defect. *Brit. J. prev. soc. Med.* **15**, 154

MacFarlane R.G. (1943) The error of haemoglobin estimation by the Haldane-Gowers method, in *Haemoglobin levels in Great Britain in 1943.* M.R.C. spec. rep. ser. No. 252. H.M.S.O., London

MacFarlane R.G. (1961) in *Functions of the Blood.* Eds. R. G. MacFarlane and A. H. T. Robb-Smith. Blackwell Scientific Publications, Oxford

McGanity W.J., Cannon R.O., Bridgforth E.B., Martin M.P., Densen P.M., Newbill J.A., McClellan G.S., Christie A., Peterson J.C. and Darby W.J. (1954) The Vanderbilt cooperative study of maternal and infant nutrition. VI. Relationship of obstetric performance to nutrition *Amer. J. Obstet. Gynec.* **67**, 501

MacGillivray I. (1961) Hypertension in pregnancy and its consequences. *J. Obstet. Gynaec. Brit. Commonw.* **68**, 557

MacGillivray I. and Buchanan T.J. (1958) Total exchangeable sodium and potassium in non-pregnant women and in normal and pre-eclamptic pregnancy. *Lancet* **ii**, 1090

MacGillivray I. and Tovey J.E. (1957) A study of the serum protein changes in pregnancy and toxaemia, using paper strip electrophoresis. *J. Obstet. Gynaec. Brit. Emp.* **64**, 361

McGinty A.P. (1938) The comparative effects of pregnancy and phrenic nerve interruption on the diaphragm and their relation to pulmonary tuberculosis. *Amer. J. Obstet. Gynec.* **35**, 237

McGregor I.A., Billewicz W.Z. and Thomson A.M. (1961) Growth and mortality in children in an African village. *Brit. med. J.* **ii**, 1661

McGuinness B.W. (1961) Skin pigmentation and the menstrual cycle. *Brit. med. J.* **2**, 563

McKay D.G., Hertig A.T., Adams E.C. and Richardson M.V. (1958) Histochemical observations on the human placenta. *Obstet. and Gynec.* **12**, 1

MacKay R.B. (1957) Observations on the oxygenation of the foetus in normal and abnormal pregnancy. *J. Obstet. Gynaec. Brit. Emp.* **64**, 185

Mackenzie A. and Tindle J. (1959) Determination of plasma volume using intravenous iron dextran. *Lancet* **i**, 333

McKenzie C.H. and Swain F.M. (1955) Diabetes insipidus and pregnancy. *Minn. Med.* **38**, 809

McKeown T. and Gibson J.R. (1951) Observations on all births (23970) in Birmingham, 1947. *Brit. J. soc. Med.* **5**, 98

McKeown T. and Record R.G. (1953) The influence of placental size on foetal growth according to sex and order of birth. *J. Endocr.* **10**, 73

McKeown T. and Record R.G. (1954) Influence of pre-natal environment on correlation between birth weight and parental height. *Amer. J. hum. genet.* **6**, 457

McLaren D.S. (1955) Health and disease in the Khond Hills, India. A contribution to global epidemiology. M.D. Thesis, Edinburgh

McLaren D.S. (1959) Records of birth weight and prematurity in the Wasukuma of Lake Province, Tanganyika. *Tr. roy. Soc. trop. Med. Hyg.* **53**, 173

426 THE PHYSIOLOGY OF HUMAN PREGNANCY

McLennan C.E. (1943) Antecubital and femoral venous pressure in normal and toxemic pregnancy. *Amer. J. Obstet. Gynec.* **45**, 568

McLennan C.E. and Corey D.L. (1950) Plasma volume in late pregnancy. *Amer. J. Obstet. Gynec,* **59**, 662

McLennan C.E. and Thouin L.G. (1948) Blood volume in pregnancy. A critical review and preliminary report of results with a new technique. *Amer. J. Obstet. Gynec.* **55**, 189

McManus M.A., Riley G.A. and Janney J.C. (1934) Kidney function in pregnancy. III. Water diuresis in the toxemias of pregnancy. *Amer. J. Obstet. Gynec.* **28**, 524

McSwiney R.R. and De Wardener H.E. (1950) Renal tract delay time and dead space. *Lancet* **ii**, 845

Macy I.G. (1958) Metabolic and biochemical changes in normal pregnancy. *J. Amer. med. Ass.* **168**, 2265

Macy I.G., Hunscher H.A., Nims B. and McCosh S.S. (1930) Metabolism of women during the reproductive cycle. I. Calcium and phosphorus utilization in pregnancy. *J. biol. Chem.* **86**, 17

Macy I.G. and Hunscher H.A. (1934) An evaluation of maternal nitrogen and mineral needs during embryonic and infant development. *Amer. J. Obstet. Gynec.* **27**, 878

Macy I.G., Moyer E.Z., Kelly H.J., Mack H.C., Di Loretto P.C. and Pratt J.P. (1954) Physiological adaptation and nutritional status during and after pregnancy. *J. Nutr.* **52**, Suppl. 1.

Magee H.E. and Milligan E.H.M. (1951) Haemoglobin levels before and after labour. *Brit. med. J.* **ii**, 1307

Mall F.P. (1918) On the age of human embryos. *Amer. J. Anat.* **23**, 397

Man E.B., Heinemann M., Johnson C.E., Leary D.C. and Peters J.P. (1951) The precipitable iodine of serum in normal pregnancy and its relation to abortions. *J. clin. Invest.* **30**, 137

Manchester B. and Loube S.D. (1946) The velocity of blood flow in normal pregnant women. *Amer. Heart J.* **32**, 215

Manery J.F. (1954) Water and electrolyte metabolism. *Physiol. Rev,* **34**, 334

Marañón G. (1947) Diabetes insipidus and uterine atony. *Brit. med. J.* **2**, 769

Marks I.N., Komarov S.A. and Shay H. (1960) Maximal acid secretory response to histamine and its relation to parietal mass in the dog. *Amer. J. Physiol.* **199**, 579

Martin J.D. and Mills I.H. (1956) Aldosterone excretion in normal and toxaemic pregnancies. *Brit. med. J.* **2**, 571

Martin J.D. and Mills I.H. (1958) The effects of pregnancy on adrenal steroid metabolism. *Clin. Sci.* **17**, 137

Martland H.S. and Martland H.S. Jr. (1950) Placental barrier in carbon monoxide, barbiturate and radium poisoning. *Amer. J. Surg.* **80**, 270

Masters M. and Clayton S.G. (1940) Calcification of the human placenta. *J. Obstet. Gynaec. Brit. Emp.* **47**, 437

Matsunaga E. and Itoh S. (1957–58) Blood groups and fertility in a Japanese population, with special reference to intrauterine selection due to maternal fetal incompatibility. *Ann. hum. Genet.* **22**, 111

MATTHEWS D.S. (1955) The ethnological and medical significance of breast feeding: with special reference to the Yorubas of Nigeria. *J. trop. Pediat.* **1**, 9

MAUKS K. Jr. (1939) Die Bedeutung der Körpergewichtsmessung für die Früherkennung der Schwangerschaftstoxikosen. [Significance of measurement of body weight for the early diagnosis of pregnancy toxicosis]. *Zbl. Gynäk,* **63**, 1409

MEDAWAR P.B. (1953) Some immunological and endocrinological problems raised by the evolution of viviparity in vertebrates, in *Symposia of the Society for experimental biology.* No. 7. Cambridge University Press, London

MEDICAL RESEARCH COUNCIL (1945) *Haemoglobin levels in Great Britain in 1943.* Spec. Rep. Ser. No. 252. H.M.S.O., London

MELBARD S.M. (1938) Valeur diagnostique de la capillaroscopie dans la grossesse et dans la sepsie puerpérale. [Diagnostic value of capillaroscopy in pregnancy and puerperal sepsis]. *Gynéc. et Obstét.* **37**, 200

MELLANBY E. (1933) Nutrition and child-bearing. *Lancet* ii, 1131

MELLBIN T. (1962) The children of Swedish nomad Lapps. A study of their health, growth and development. *Acta paediat. (Uppsala)* **51**, Suppl. 131

MEREDITH H.V. (1952) North American negro infants: size at birth and growth during the first postnatal year. *Hum. Biol.* **24**, 290

MERIVALE W.H.H. and RICHARDSON G.O. (1950) Changes in size of red cells during normal pregnancy. *Brit. med. J.* i, 463

METCALFE J. (1959) in *Oxygen Supply to the Human Foetus.* Eds. J. Walker and A. C. Turnbull. Blackwell Scientific Publications, Oxford

METCALFE J., ROMNEY S.L., RAMSEY L.H., REID D.E. and BURWELL C.S. (1955) Estimation of uterine blood flow in normal human pregnancy at term. *J. clin. Invest.* **34**, 1632

MICHIE A.J. and MICHIE C.R. (1951) Attainment of equilibrium between plasma and urine with reference to the measurement of renal clearances. *J. Urol. (Baltimore)* **66**, 518

MIGEON C.J., BERTRAND J. and GEMZELL C.A. (1962) The transplacental passage of 4, ^{14}C-cortisol in mid-pregnancy, in *The Human Adrenal Cortex.* Eds. A. R. Currie, T. Symington and J. K. Grant. E. and S. Livingstone, Edinburgh

MILES B.E. and DE WARDENER H.E. (1953) Effect of emotion on renal function in normotensive and hypertensive women. *Lancet* ii, 539

MILLER J.R., KEITH N.M. and ROWNTREE L.G. (1915) Plasma and blood volume in pregnancy. *J. Amer. med. Ass.* **65**, 779

MILLIS J. (1958-59a) Distribution of birth weights of Chinese and Indian infants born in Singapore: birth weight as an index of maturity. *Ann. hum. Genet.* **23**, 164

MILLIS J. (1958-59b) The frequency of twinning in poor Chinese in the maternity hospital, Singapore. *Ann. hum. Genet,* **23**, 171

MILLIS J. and YOU POH SENG (1954-55) The effect of age and parity of the mother on birth weight of the offspring. *Ann. hum. Genet.* **19**, 58

MILLS I.H., SCHEDL H.P., CHEN P.S. and BARTTER F.C. (1960) The effect of estrogen administration on the metabolism and protein binding of hydrocortisone. *J. clin. Endocr.* **20**, 515

MINISTRY OF HEALTH (1944) *Report on the breast feeding of infants*. Rep. publ. Hlth. med. Subj. No. 91. H.M.S.O., London

MINISTRY OF HEALTH (1959) *Standards of normal weight in infancy*. Rep. publ. Hlth. med. Subj. No. 99. H.M.S.O., London

MISCHEL W. (1957–58a) Die anorganischen Bestandteile der Placenta. 1. Der Wassergehalt, die Trockensubstanz und der Aschegehalt der reifen und unreifen, normalen und pathologischen menschlichen Placenta. [The inorganic components of the placenta. 1. The water content, dry matter and ash content of the mature and immature, normal and pathological human placenta]. *Arch. Gynäk.* **190**, 8

MISCHEL W. (1957–58b) Die anorganischen Bestandteile der Placenta. 2. Die Natriumgehalt der reifen und unreifen, normalen und pathologischen menschlichen Placenta. [The inorganic components of the placenta. 2. The sodium content of the mature and immature, normal and pathological human placenta]. *Arch. Gynäk.* **190**, 111

MISCHEL W. (1957–58c) Die anorganischen. Bestandteile der Placenta. 4. Der Calciumgehalt der reifen und unreifen, normalen und pathologischen menschlichen Placenta. [The inorganic components of the placenta. 4. The calcium content of the mature and immature, normal and pathological human placenta]. *Arch. Gynäk.* **190**, 228

MISCHEL W. (1957–58d) Die anorganischen Bestandteile der Placenta. 6. Der Gesamt- und Gewebseisengehalt der reifen und unreifen, normalen und pathologischen menschlichen Placenta. [The inorganic components of the placenta. 6. Total and tissue iron content of the mature and immature, normal and pathological human placenta]. *Arch. Gynäk.* **190**, 638

MISHELL D.R. Jr., WIDE L. and GEMZELL C.A. (1963) Immunologic determination of human chorionic gonadotrophin in serum. *J. clin. Endocr.* **23**, 125

MOISTER F.C. and FREIS E.D. (1949) The metabolism of thiocyanate after prolonged administration in man. *Amer. J. med. Sci.* **218**, 549

MÖLLER E., McINTOSH J.F. and VAN SLYKE D.D. (1929) Studies of urea excretion. II. Relationship between urine volume and the rate of urea excretion by normal adults. *J. clin. Invest.* **6**, 427

MOLLER M.S.G. (1961) Custom, pregnancy and child rearing in Tanganyika. *J. trop. Pediat.* **7**, 66

MONIE I.W. (1953) The volume of the amniotic fluid in the early months of pregnancy. *Amer. J. Obstet. Gynec.* **66**, 616

MONTGOMERY T.L. and PINCUS I.J. (1955) A nutritional problem in pregnancy resulting from extensive resection of the small bowel. *Amer. J. Obstet. Gynec.* **69**, 865

MOR A., YANG W., SCHWARZ A. and JONES W.C. (1960) Platelet counts in pregnancy and labor. A comparative study. *Obstet. and Gynec.* **16**, 338

MORGAN E.H. (1961) Plasma-iron and haemoglobin levels in pregnancy. The effect of oral iron. *Lancet* **i**, 9

MORRIS I.G. (1963) Interference with the uptake of guinea-pig agglutinins in mice due to fractions of papain hydrolyzed rabbit γ-globulin. *Proc. roy. Soc. B* **157**, 160

MORRISON S.D., RUSSELL F.C. and STEVENSON J. (1949) Estimating food intake by questioning and weighing: a one-day survey of eight subjects. *Brit. J. Nutr.* **3**, V

MORTON N.E. (1955) The inheritance of human birth weight. *Ann. hum. Genet.* **20**, 125

MOSES A.M., LOBOTSKY J. and LLOYD C.W. (1959) The occurrence of pre-eclampsia in a bilaterally adrenolectomized woman. *J. clin. Endocr.* **19**, 987

MÖSSMER (Dr) (1916) Über 'Kriegsneugeborene'. ['War babies']. *Zbl. Gynäk.* **40**, (ii) 684

MOYA F. and THORNDIKE V. (1962) Passage of drugs across the placenta. *Amer. J. Obstet. Gynec.* **84**, 1778

MUELLER G.C., HERRANEN A.M. and JERVELL K.F. (1958) Studies on the mechanism of action of estrogens. in *Recent Progress in Hormone Research.* Ed. G. Pincus. Academic Press, New York

MUKHERJEE C. and MUKHERJEE S.K. (1953) Studies in iron metabolism in anaemias in pregnancy. 1. Serum iron. *J. Indian med. Ass.* **22**, 345

MUKHERJEE S. and BISWAS S. (1959) Birth weight and its relationship to gestation period, sex, maternal age, parity and socio-economic status. *J. Indian med. Ass.* **32**, 389

MUNNELL E.W. and TAYLOR H.C. Jr. (1947) Liver blood flow in pregnancy—hepatic vein catheterization. *J. clin. Invest.* **26**, 952

MURRAY F.A., ERSKINE J.P. and FIELDING J. (1957) Gastric secretion in pregnancy. *J. Obstet. Gynaec. Brit. Emp.* **64**, 373

MURRAY J.F. and SHILLINGFORD J.P. (1958) A comparison of the direct and extraction methods for the determination of T–1824 (Evans blue) in plasma and serum. *J. clin. Path.* **11**, 170

MURRAY M.B. (1924) *Child life investigations. The effect of maternal, social conditions and nutrition upon birth-weight and birth-length.* M.R.C. Special Report. Ser. No. 81. H.M.S.O., London

MUSSEY R.D. (1949) Nutrition and human reproduction. An historical review. *Amer. J. Obstet. Gynec.* **57**, 1037

NAISH F.C. (1948) *Breast feeding.* Oxford University Press, London

NAMBOODIRI N.K. and BALAKRISHNAN V. (1958–59a) On the effect of maternal age and parity on the birth weight of the offspring (Indian infants). *Ann. hum. Genet.* **23**, 189

NAMBOODIRI N.K. and BALAKRISHNAN V. (1958–59b) A contribution to the study of birth weight and survival of twins based on an Indian sample. *Ann. hum. Genet.* **23**, 334

NARANJO VARGAS P., CORNEJO F. and BERMEO J. (1953) El metabolismo basal en la embarazada y el feto. [Basal metabolism in pregnancy and in the foetus]. *Rev. esp. Fisiol.* **9**, 221

NATIONAL ACADEMY OF SCIENCES—NATIONAL RESEARCH COUNCIL (1958) *Recommended Dietary Allowances.* National Academy of Sciences—National Research Council. Publ. 589. Washington, D.C.

NAUNYN B. (1906) *Der Diabetes mellitus.* [Diabetes mellitus]. Afred Hölder, Vienna

NEEDHAM C.D., ROGAN M.C. and McDONALD I. (1955) Prediction of maximum breathing capacity from timed vital capacity. *Brit. J. Tuberc.* **49**, 30

NESER M.L. (1963) Weight gain during pregnancy of urban Bantu women. *S. Afr. med. J.* **37**, 900

NEWMAN R.L. (1957) Serum electrolytes in pregnancy, parturition and puerperium. *Obstet. and Gynec.* **10**, 51

NEWTON W.H. (1952) in *Marshall's Physiology of Reproduction.* Ed. A. S. Parkes. Vol. 2. 3rd Edition. Longmans, Green and Co, London

NICE M. (1935) Kidney function during normal pregnancy. I. The increased urea clearance of normal pregnancy. *J. clin. Invest.* **14**, 575

NICOL B.M. (1949) Nutrition of Nigerian peasant farmers, with special reference to the effects of vitamin A and riboflavin deficiency. *Brit. J. Nutr.* **3**, 25

NICOLAYSEN R. (1961) Kostholdsnormer. [Dietary standards]. *T. norske Laegeforen.* **81**, 1292

NILSSON A. (1920) Über sog. Kriegsamenörrhoe. [War amenorrhoea]. *Zbl. Gynäk.* **44**, 876

NOALL M.W., RIGGS T.R., WALKER L.M. and CHRISTENSEN H.N. (1957) Endocrine control of amino acid transfer. Distribution of an unmetabolizable amino acid. *Science* **124**, 1002

NOMOF N., HOPPER J. Jr., BROWN E., SCOTT K. and WENNESLAND R. (1954) Simultaneous determinations of the total volume of red blood cells by use of carbon monoxide and chromium^{51} in healthy and diseased human subjects. *J. clin. Invest.* **33**, 1382

NOVITSKI E. and KIMBALL A.W. (1958) Birth order, parental ages and sex of offspring. *Amer. J. hum. Genet.* **10**, 268

NUTRITION SOCIETY (1944a) The influence of diet on pregnancy and lactation in the mother, the growth and variability of the foetus, and post-natal development. Part 1. Pregnancy (a symposium). *Proc. Nutr. Soc.* **1**, 226–248

NUTRITION SOCIETY (1944b) Nutrition in pregnancy (a symposium). *Proc. Nutr. Soc.* **2**, 1–68

O'DONNELL V.J. and PREEDY J.R.K. (1961) The Oestrogens, in *Hormones in Blood.* Eds. Gray and Bacharach. Academic Press, New York

OLIVER M.F. and BOYD G.S. (1955) Plasma lipid and serum lipo protein patterns during pregnancy and puerperium. *Clin. Sci.* **14**, 15

OMATSU Y. (1957) Basal metabolism in pregnancy. *Kôbe J. med. Sci.* **27**, 21

ORAM S. and HOLT M. (1961) Innocent depression of the S-T segment and flattening of the T-wave during pregnancy. *J. Obstet. Gynaec. Brit. Commonw.* **68**, 765

ORR J.B. and GILKS J.L. (1931) Medical Research Council Special Report Series No. 155. H.M.S.O., London

OSLER M. and PEDERSEN J. (1960) The body composition of newborn infants of diabetic mothers. *Paediatrics* **26**, 985

OSORIO C. and MYANT N.B. (1960) The passage of thyroid hormone from mother to foetus and its relation to foetal development. *Brit. med. Bull.* **16**, 159

OTIS A.B. and PROCTOR D.F. (1948) Measurement of alveolar pressure in human subjects. *Amer. J. Physiol.* **152**, 106

OVERALL J.E. and WILLIAMS C.M. (1959) A note concerning sources of variance in determinations of human plasma volume. *J. Lab. clin. Med.* **54**, 186

PAABY P. (1959) Changes in the water content of serum and plasma during pregnancy. *Acta. Obstet. gynec. scand.* **38**, 297

PAABY P. (1960) Changes in serum proteins during pregnancy. *J. Obstet. Gynaec. Brit. Emp.* **67**, 43

PAGE E.W., GLENDENING M.B., DIGNAM W. and HARPER H.A. (1954) The causes of histidinuria in normal pregnancy. *Amer. J. Obstet. Gynec.* **68**, 110

PAINTIN D.B. (1962) The size of the total red cell volume in pregnancy. *J. Obstet. Gynaec. Brit. Commonw.* **69**, 719

PAINTIN D.B. (1963) The haematocrit ratio in pregnancy. *J. Obstet. Gynaec. Brit. Commonw.* **70**, 807

PALMER A. (1957) Chorionic gonadotropin. Its place in the treatment of infertility. *Fertil. and Steril.* **8**, 220

PALMER A.J. and WALKER A.H.C. (1949) The maternal circulation in normal pregnancy. *J. Obstet. Gynaec. Brit. Emp.* **56**, 537

PALMER R. and DEVILLIERS J. (1939) Action thermique des hormones sexuelles chez la femme. [Effect on temperature of sex hormones in women]. *C. R. Soc. Biol. (Paris)* **130**, 895

PANIGEL M. (1962) Placental perfusion experiments. *Amer. J. Obstet. Gynec.* **84**, 1664

PANUNZIO C. (1943) Are more males born in wartime? *Milbank mem. Fd. Quart.* **21**, 281

PARKES A.S. (1925–26) The physiological factors governing the proportions of the sexes in man. *Eugen. Rev.* **17**, 275

PASRICHA S. (1958) A survey of dietary intake in a group of poor, pregnant and lactating women. *Indian J. med. Res.* **46**, 605

PATTON W.E., ABELMANN W.H., FRANK N.R., BADGER T.L. and GAENSLER E.A. (1953) Pulmonary function in pregnancy. II. Comparison of the effects of pneumoperitoneum and pregnancy in young women with functionally normal lungs and serial observations during pregnancy and post-partum pneumoperitoneum. *Amer. Rev. Tuberc.* **67**, 755

PEARLMAN W.H. (1957a) [16-³H] progesterone metabolism in advanced pregnancy and in oophorectomized-hysterectomized women. *Biochem. J.* **67**, 1.

PEARLMAN W.H. (1957b) Circulating steroid hormone levels in relation to steroid hormone production. *Ciba Foundation Colloquia on Endocrinology*, **11**, 233

PEARSE A.G.E. (1953) Cytological and cytochemical investigations on the foetal and adult hypophysis in various physiological and pathological states. *J. Path. Bact.* **65**, 355

PEARSON K. (1899–1900) Data for the problem of evolution in man. III. On the magnitude of certain coefficients of correlation in man etc. *Proc. roy. Soc.* **66**, 23

PEOPLE'S LEAGUE OF HEALTH (1946) The nutrition of expectant and nursing mothers in relation to maternal and infant mortality and morbidity. *J. Obstet. Gynaec. Brit. Emp.* **53**, 498

PETERS J.P., HEINEMANN M. and MAN E.B. (1951) The lipids of serum in pregnancy. *J. clin. Invest.* **30**, 388

PETERS J.P. and VAN SLYKE D.D. (1946) *Quantitative Clinical Chemistry.* Interpretations Vol. 1, Second edition. Williams and Wilkins, Baltimore

PETERSEN H. and FRANK H. (1958) Untersuchungen über die Rückresorption des Histidins bei Schwangeren, bei der renalen Glycosurie und bei Kranken mit eingeschränkter Nierenfunktion. [Studies of reabsorption of histidine in pregnancy, in renal glycosuria and in patients with impaired renal function]. *Dtsch. Arch. klin. Med.* **205**, 70

PETERSON R.E., NOKES G., CHEN P.S. and BLACK R.L. (1960) Estrogens and adrenocortical function in man. *J. clin. Endocr.* **20**, 495

PHILLIPS L.L. and SKRODELIS V. (1958) The fibrinolytic enzyme system in normal, haemorrhagic and disease states. *J. clin. Invest.* **37**, 965

PINSON E.A. (1952) Water exchanges and barriers as studied by use of hydrogen isotopes. *Physiol. Rev.* **32**, 123

PINTO R.M., VOTTA R.A., MONTUORI E. and BALEIRON H. (1963) Oestrogens and the myometrium. *Brit. med. J.* ii, 934

PLASS E.D. and OBERST F.W. (1938) Respiration and pulmonary ventilation in normal non-pregnant, pregnant and puerperal women. *Amer. J. Obstet. Gynec.* **35**, 441

PLASS E.D. and YOAKAM W.A. (1929) Basal metabolism studies in normal pregnant women with normal and pathologic thyroid glands. *Trans. Amer. gynec. Soc.* **54**, 165

POCHIN E.E. (1952) The iodine uptake of the human thyroid throughout the menstrual cycle and in pregnancy. *Clin. Sci.* **11**, 441

POIDEVIN L.O.S. (1959) Striae gravidarum. Their relation to adrenal cortical hyperfunction. *Lancet* ii, 436

POO L.J., LEW W. and ADDIS T. (1939) Protein anabolism of organs and tissues during pregnancy and lactation. *J. biol. Chem.* **128**, 69

POTTER M.G. (1936) Observations of the gall-bladder and bile during pregnancy at term. *J. Amer. med. Ass.* **106**, 1070

POWELL J.F. (1944) Serum iron in health and disease. *Quart. J. Med.* **13**, 19

POZNANSKI R., BRZEZINSKI A. and GUGGENHEIM K. (1962) Value of flour enrichment to pregnant Israeli women. Calcium and riboflavin intake. *J. Amer. diet. Ass.* **40**, 120

PRADER A., TANNER J.M. and HARNACK G.A.V. (1963) Catch-up growth following illness or starvation. An example of developmental canalization in man. *J. Pediat.* **62**, 646

PRATT J.P., KAUCHER M., RICHARDS A.J., WILLIAMS H.H. and MACY I.G. (1946a) Composition of the human placenta. I. Proximate composition. *Amer. J. Obstet. Gynec.* **52**, 402

PRATT J.P., KAUCHER M., MOYER E., RICHARDS A.J. and WILLIAMS H.H. (1946b) Composition of the human placenta. II. Lipid content. *Amer. J. Obstet. Gynec.* **52**, 665

PREEDY J.R.K. and AITKEN E.H. (1956) The effect of estrogen on water and electrolyte metabolism. I. The normal. *J. clin. Invest.* **35**, 423

PRILL H.J. and GÖTZ F. (1961) Blood flow in the myometrium and endometrium of the uterus. *Amer. J. Obstet. Gynec.* **82**, 102

PRITCHARD J.A. and ADAMS R.H. (1960) Erythrocyte production and destruction during pregnancy. *Amer. J. Obstet. Gynec.* **79**, 750

PRITCHARD J.A., BARNES A.C. and BRIGHT R.H. (1955) The effect of the supine position on renal function in the near term pregnant woman. *J. clin. Invest.* **34**, 777

PRITCHARD J.A., WIGGINS K.M. and DICKEY J.C. (1960) Blood volume changes in pregnancy and the puerperium. I. Does sequestration of red blood cells accompany parturition? *Amer. J. Obstet. Gynec.* **80**, 956

PROCHOWNICK L. (1889) Ein Versuch zum Ersatz der künstlichen Frühgeburt. [An attempt towards the replacement of induced premature birth]. *Zbl. Gynäk.* **30**, 577

PROCHOWNICK L. (1901) Ueber Ernährungscuren in der Schwangerschaft. [Dietetics in pregnancy]. *Ther. Mh.* **15**, 387, 446

PROCHOWNICK L. (1917) Über Ernährungskuren in der Schwangerschaft. [Dietetics in pregnancy]. *Zbl. Gynäk.* **41**, 785

PRYSTOWSKY H. (1958) Fetal blood studies. VIII. Some observations on the transient fetal bradycardia accompanying uterine contractions in the human. *Bull. Johns. Hopk. Hosp.* **102**, 1

PRYSTOWSKY H. (1959) in *Oxygen supply to the human foetus*. Eds. J. Walker and A. C. Turnbull. Blackwell Scientific Publications, Oxford

PRYSTOWSKY H. (1960) in *The placenta and fetal membranes*. Ed. C. A. Villee. The Williams and Wilkins Co, Baltimore

PRYSTOWSKY H., HELLEGERS A. and BRUNS P. (1960) Fetal blood studies. 18. Supplementary observations on the oxygen pressure gradient between the maternal and fetal blood of humans. *Surg. Gynec. Obstet.* **110**, 495

PRYSTOWSKY H., HELLEGERS A.E. and BRUNS P. (1961) Fetal blood studies. 15. The carbon dioxide concentration gradient between the fetal and maternal blood of humans. *Amer. J. Obstet. Gynec.* **81**, 372

PSCHYREMBEL W. (1948) Zur Diagnose der Anenzephalus. [Diagnosis of Anencephalus]. *Zbl. Gynäk.* **70**, 408 (Proc.)

PUGLIATTI V. (1937) Le variazioni del peso corporeo durante la gravidanza normale e patologica. [Change of body weight during pregnancy, normal and pathological]. *Arte Ostet.* **51**, 33

PYKE D.A. (1956) Parity and the incidence of diabetes. *Lancet* **i**, 818

QUENOUILLE M.H., BOYNE A.W., FISHER W.B. and LEITCH I. (1951) *Statistical studies of recorded energy expenditure of man. Part 1. Basal metabolism related to sex, stature, age, climate and race*. Technical Communication No. 17. Commonwealth Bureau of Animal Nutrition, Rowett Institute, Bucksburn, Aberdeenshire, Scotland

QUILLIGAN E.J. and TYLER C. (1959) Postural effects on the cardiovascular status in pregnancy: A comparison of the lateral and supine postures. *Amer. J. Obstet. Gynec.* **78**, 465

RABINOWITCH I.M. (1936) Clinical and other observations on Canadian eskimos in the Eastern Arctic. *Canad. med. Ass. J.* **34**, 487

RÄIHÄ C.-E. (1959) Prematurity, its social consequences and our possibilities of decreasing the number of premature babies. *Étud. néo-natal.* **1**, 113

RÄIHÄ C.-E., JOHANSSON C.-E., LIND J. and VARA P. (1957) Heart volume during pregnancy with special consideration of its reduction. *Ann. Paediat. Fenn.* **3**, 65

RAINS A.J.H. (1961) Gallstones, an introduction to research into causes and remarks on some problems in treatment. *Ann. roy. Coll. Surg. Engl.* **29**, 85

RAJOO T.D. and NAIDU P.M. (1944) A study of 10,000 deliveries. *Indian. med. Gaz.* **79**, 373

RAMSEY E.M. (1959) Vascular anatomy of the utero-placental and foetal circulation, in *Oxygen supply to the human foetus*. Eds. J. Walker and A. C. Turnbull. Blackwell Scientific Publications, Oxford

RAMSEY E.M., CORNER G.W. Jr., LONG W.N. and STRAN H.M. (1959) Studies of amniotic fluid and intervillous space pressures in the rhesus monkey. *Amer. J. Obstet. Gynec.* **77**, 1016

RANDALL L.M. (1925) The weight factor in pregnancy. *Amer. J. Obstet. Gynec.* **9**, 529

RATH C.E., CATON W., REID D.E., FINCH C.A. and CONROY L. (1950) Hematological changes and iron metabolism of normal pregnancy. *Surg. Gynec. Obstet.* **90**, 320

RAYNAUD M. (1862) *On local asphyxia and symmetrical gangrene of the extremities*. Translated by Thomas Barlow, New Sydenham Society, 1888

RECHENBERGER J. and HEVELKE G. (1955) Tagesrhythmik des Serumeisens und Leber funktion. [Diurnal rhythm in serum iron and liver function]. *Dtsch. Z. Verdau.-u. Stoffwechselkr.* **15**, 12

REEVE E.B. (1947–48) Methods of estimating plasma and total red cell volume. *Nutr. Abstr. Rev.* **17**, 811

REGISTRAR GENERAL (1951) Classification of Occupations 1950. H.M.S.O., London

REGISTRAR GENERAL (1952) Statistical review of England and Wales for the year 1950. Tables Part II Civil. H.M.S.O., London

REGISTRAR GENERAL (1953, 1953a) Statistical review of England and Wales for the years 1951, 1952. Tables Part II Civil. H.M.S.O., London

REGISTRAR GENERAL (1955) Statistical review of England and Wales for the year 1953. Tables Part II Civil. H.M.S.O., London

REGISTRAR GENERAL (1956) Statistical review of England and Wales for the year 1954. Tables Part II Civil. H.M.S.O., London

REGISTRAR GENERAL (1956a) Census 1951. England and Wales. H.M.S.O., London

REGISTRAR GENERAL (1957) Statistical review of England and Wales for the year 1955. Tables Part II Civil. H.M.S.O., London

REGISTRAR GENERAL (1957a) Statistical review of England and Wales for the year 1956. Tables Part II Civil. H.M.S.O., London

REGISTRAR GENERAL (1958) Statistical review of England and Wales for the year 1956. Part III Commentary. H.M.S.O., London

REGISTRAR GENERAL (1959) Statistical review of England and Wales for the year 1957. Tables Part II Civil. H.M.S.O., London

REGISTRAR GENERAL (1960) Statistical review of England and Wales for the year 1958. Tables Part II Civil. H.M.S.O., London

REGISTRAR GENERAL (1960a) Statistical review of England and Wales for the year 1959. Tables Part II Civil. H.M.S.O., London

RENKONEN K.O., MÄKELÄ O. and LEHTOVAARA R. (1961) Factors affecting the human sex ratio. *Ann. Med. exp. Fenn.* **39**, 173

RENKONEN K.O. and LEHTOVAARA R. (1962) Further discussion of the incompatibility between the mother and her male offspring. *Ann. Med. exp. Fenn.* **40**, 352

ROBBINS J. and NELSON J.H. (1958) Thyroxine-binding by serum protein in pregnancy and in the newborn. *J. clin. Invest.* **37**, 153

ROBERTSON T.B. (1915) A comparison of the weights at birth of British infants born in the British Isles, the United States and Australia. (Preliminary Communication). Univ. California Publications in Physiology. Vol. 4, No. 20

ROBERTSON W.F. (1962) Thalidomide (Distaval) and vitamin-B deficiency. *Brit. med. J.* **i**, 792

ROBINSON H.R., GUTTMACHER A.F., HARRISON E.P.H. Jr. and SPENCE J.M. Jr (1943) Gain in weight during pregnancy. *Child Develpm.* **14**, 131

ROBLES R.H., PRATT J.H. and STARR G.F. (1961) Weight loss in ovaries and uteri after formaldehyde fixation. *Obstet. and Gynec.* **17**, 378

ROBSON E.B. (1953) The genetics of human birth weight. *Heredity* **7**, 149

ROBSON E.B. (1954–55) Birth weight in cousins. *Ann. hum. Genet.* **19**, 262

ROMNEY S.L., REID D.E., METCALFE J. and BURWELL C.S. (1955) Oxygen utilization by the human fetus in utero. *Amer. J. Obstet. Gynec.* **70**, 791

ROOT H.F. and ROOT H.K. (1923) The basal metabolism during pregnancy and the puerperium. *Arch. intern. Med.* **32**, 411

ROSCOE M.H. and DONALDSON G.M.M. (1946) The blood in pregnancy. Part II. The blood volume, cell volume and haemoglobin mass. *J. Obstet. Gynaec. Brit. Emp.* **53**, 527

ROSCOE M.H. and McKAY H.S. (1946) A dietary survey of pregnant women and schoolchildren in Edinburgh. *Edinb. med. J.* **53**, 565

ROSENTHAL S.L., ROWEN R. and VAZAKAS A.J. (1959) Comparative analysis of saliva in pregnant and non-pregnant women. 1. Calcium and pH. *J. dent. Res.* **38**, 883

RÖTTGER H. (1950) Kupfer bei Mutter und Kind. [Copper in mother and child]. *Arch. Gynäk.* **177**, 650

RÖTTGER H. (1953–54) Über den Wasserhaushalt in der physiologischen und toxischen Schwangerschaft. 1. Der Wasserhaushalt in der physiologischen Schwangerschaft. [Water metabolism in normal and toxaemic pregnancy. 1. Water metabolism in normal pregnancy]. *Arch. Gynäk.* **184**, 59

RÖTTGER H. and HECKENBACH E.M. (1957) Der Einfluss der sexual Hormone auf den Wasserhaushalt der Frau. [Effect of sex hormones on water metabolism in women]. *Arch. f. Gynäkol.* **190**, 95

ROY E.J. (1962) The concentration of oestrogens in maternal and foetal blood obtained at caesarean section, and the effect of hospitalization on maternal blood oestrogen levels. *J. Obstet. Gynaec. Brit. Commonw.* **69**, 196

RUBIN A., RUSSO N. and GOUCHER D. (1956) The effect of pregnancy upon pulmonary function in normal women. *Amer. J. Obstet. Gynec.* **72**, 963

RUSS E.M., EDER H.A. and BARR D.P. (1954) Protein-lipid relationships in human plasma. III. In pregnancy and the newborn. *J. clin. Invest.* **33**, 1662

SADOVSKY A., BERCOVICI B., RACHMILEWITZ M., GROSSOWICZ N. and ARONOVITCH J. (1959) Vitamin B$_{12}$ concentration in maternal and fetal blood. *Obstet. and Gynec.* **13**, 346

SAGARA T. (1961) Studies on weight at birth after world war II. *J. Nara. med. Ass.* **12**, 335

SALBER E.J. and BRADSHAW E.S. (1957) Birth weights of South African babies. *Brit. J. soc. Med.* **5**, 113

SALHANICK H.A. (1960) in *The Placenta and Fetal Membranes.* Ed. C. A. Villee. Williams and Wilkins, Baltimore

SANDIFORD I., WHEELER T. and BOOTHBY W.M. (1931) Metabolic studies during pregnancy and menstruation. *Amer. J. Physiol.* **96**, 191

SAVEL L.E. and ROTH E. (1962) Effects of smoking in pregnancy: a continuing retrospective study. *Obstet. and Gynec.* **20**, 313

SAXEN L. (1962) Virusinfektioners verkan pá fostret. [Effect of virus infections on the foetus]. *Nord. Med.* **67**, 536

SCAMMON R.E. and CALKINS L.A. (1929) *The development and growth of the external dimensions of the human body in the fetal period.* University of Minnesota Press, Minneapolis

SCHEINBERG I.H. and KOWALSKI H.J. (1950) The binding of thiocyanate to albumin in normal human serum and defibrinated blood with reference to the determination of 'thiocyanate space'. *J. clin. Invest.* **29**, 475

SCHLOERB P.R., FRIIS-HANSEN B.J., EDELMAN I.S., SOLOMON A.K. and MOORE F.D. (1950) Measurement of total body water in human subjects by deuterium oxide dilution: with consideration of dynamics of deuterium distribution. *J. clin. Invest.* **29**, 1296

SCHULL W.J. and NEEL J.V. (1958) Radiation and the sex ratio in man. *Science* **128**, 343

SCOTT J.A. and BENJAMIN B. (1948) Weight changes in pregnancy. *Lancet* **i**, 550

SCOTT J.H. (1954) Heat regulating function of the nasal mucous membrane. *J. Laryng.* **68**, 308

SEARLE A.G. (1958–59) The incidence of anencephaly in a polytypic population. *Ann. hum. Genet.* **23**, 279

SEGALOFF A., STERNBERG W.H. and GASKILL C.J. (1951) Effects of luteotropic doses of chorionic gonadotropin in women. *J. clin. Endocr.* **11**, 936

SEITCHIK J. and ALPER C. (1954) The body compartments of normal pregnant, edematous pregnant and pre-eclamptic women. *Amer. J. Obstet. Gynec.* **68**, 1540

SEITCHIK J. and ALPER C. (1956) The estimation of changes in body composition in normal pregnancy by measurement of body water. *Amer. J. Obstet. Gynec.* **71**, 1165

SEMPLE R.E., THOMSEN A.E.T. and BALL A.J. (1958) Description and evaluation of a dextran-dilution technique for the determination of plasma volume in the dog and man. *Clin. Sci.* **17**, 511

SENN L.Y. and KARLSON K.E. (1958) Methodologic and actual error of plasma volume determination. *Surgery* **44**, 1095

SHAN-YAH GIN (1948) Physical growth of Chinese infants. *J. Pediat.* **32**, 275

SHAW M.M. (1933) The birth weight of Africans. *E. Afr. med. J.* **10**, 32

SHEARMAN R.P. (1959) Some aspects of the urinary excretion of pregnanediol in pregnancy. *J. Obstet. Gynaec. Brit. Emp.* **66**, 1

SHEEHAN H.L. and FALKINER N.M. (1948) Splenic aneurysm and splenic enlargement in pregnancy. *Brit. med. J.* **2**, 1105

SHELDON J.H. (1949) Maternal obesity. *Lancet* **ii**, 869

SHELLEY H.J. (1961) Glycogen reserves and their changes at birth and in anoxia. *Brit. med. Bull.* **17**, 137

SHETTLES L.B. (1961) Conception and birth sex ratios. A review. *Obstet. and Gynec.* **18**, 122

SHIZUME K. and LERNER A.B. (1954) Determination of melanocyte-stimulating hormone in urine and blood. *J. clin. Endocr.* **14**, 1491

SHORT R.V. and ETON B. (1959) Progesterone in blood. III. Progesterone in the peripheral blood of pregnant women. *J. Endocr.* **18**, 418

SILVERSTEIN A.M. and LUKES R.J. (1962) Fetal response to antigenic stimulus. I. Plasmacellular and lymphoid reactions in the human fetus to intrauterine infection. *Lab. Invest.* **11**, 918

SILVERSTEIN A.M., UHR J.W., KRAMER K.L. and LUKES R.J. (1963) Fetal response to antigenic stimulus. II. Antibody production by the fetal lamb. *J. exp. Med.* **117**, 799

SIMPSON W.J. (1957) A preliminary report on cigarette smoking and the incidence of prematurity. *Amer. J. Obstet. Gynec.* **73**, 808

SIMS E.A.H. and KRANTZ K.E. (1958) Serial studies of renal function during pregnancy and the puerperium in normal women. *J. clin. Invest.* **37**, 1764

SIRI W.E. (1955) An apparatus for measuring human body volume. Donner Laboratory of Biophysics and Medical Physics, University of California. UCRL-3228

SIRI W.E. (1956) Body composition from fluid spaces and density: analysis of methods. Donner Laboratory, Univ. California. Pub. UCRL-3349

SJÖSTRAND T. (1953) Volume and distribution of blood and their significance in regulating the circulation. *Physiol. Rev.* **33**, 202

SJÖSTEDT S., ROOTH G. and CALIGARA F. (1960) The oxygen tension in the cord blood after normal delivery. *Acta obstet. gynec. scand.* **39**, 34

SLEMONS J.M. (1914) The involution of the uterus and its effect upon the nitrogen output of the urine. *Bull. Johns Hopk. Hosp.* **25**, 195

SLEMONS J.M. and FAGAN R.H. (1927) A study of the infants birth-weight and the mother's gain during pregnancy. *Amer. J. Obstet. Gynec.* **14**, 159

SMITH C.A. (1947) Effects of maternal undernutrition upon the newborn infant in Holland (1944–45). *J. Pediat.* **30**, 229

SMITH C.A. (1959) *The physiology of the newborn infant.* 3rd Ed. Charles, C. Thomas, Springfield

SMITH H.W. (1951) *The kidney. Structure and function in health and disease.* Oxford University Press, London

SMITH J.D. and MONTALVO J.M. (1961) Maternal-fetal relationships in normal and abnormal thyroid development of the newborn. *Amer. J. Med. Sci.* **241**, 769

SMITH M.D. (1952) The value of estimation of the serum iron in the investigation of anaemia. *Glasg. med. J.* **33**, 309

SNYDER R.G. (1961) The sex ratio of offspring of pilots of high performance military aircraft. *Hum. Biol.* **33**, 1

SOBERMAN R., BRODIE B.B., LEVY B.B., AXELROD J., HOLLANDER V. and STEELE J.M. (1949) Use of antipyrine in measurement of total body water in man. *J. biol. Chem.* **179**, 31

SOHAR E., SCADRON E. and LEVITT M.F. (1956) Changes in renal hemodynamics during normal pregnancy. *Clin. Res. Proc.* **4**, 142

SOLTH K. (1950) Die Veränderungen des Geburtsgewichtes im Laufe der letzten Jahrzehnte. [Changes in birth weight in the course of recent decades]. *Arch. Gynäk.* **177**, 678

SOMMERS S.C. (1959) Pituitary cell relations to body states. *Lab. Invest.* **8**, 588

SONTAG L.W., REYNOLDS E.L. and TORBET V. (1944) The relation of basal metabolic gain during pregnancy to non-pregnant basal metabolism. *Amer. J. Obstet. Gynec.* **48**, 315

SONTAG L.W. and WINES J. (1947) Relation of mothers' diets to status of their infants at birth and in infancy. *Amer. J. Obstet. Gynec.* **54**, 994

SOUPART P. (1960) Aminoacidémie and aminoacidurie au cours du cycle menstruel chez la femme normale. [Amino acids in blood and urine during the menstrual cycle in normal women]. *Clin. chim. Acta.* **5**, 235

SPARKMAN R.S. (1958) Rupture of the spleen in pregnancy. *Amer. J. Obstet. Gynec.* **76**, 587

SPEERT H., GRAFF S. and GRAFF A.M. (1951) Nutrition and premature labor. *Amer. J. Obstet. Gynec.* **62**, 1009

SPIGA-CLERICI A. (1937) Il metabolismo di base in gravidanza, travaglio, puerperio, allattamento. [Basal metabolism during pregnancy, labour, puerperium and suckling]. *Quad. Nutr.* **4**, 142

SPITZER W. (1933) Die Blutströmungsgeschwindigkeit in normaler und gestörter Schwangerschaft. Beitrag zur Funktionsprüfung des Herzens in der Schwangerschaft und vor der Geburt. [The rate of blood flow in normal and disturbed pregnancy. An examination of cardiac function during pregnancy and before birth]. *Arch. Gynäk.* **154**, 449

STAHLIE T.D. (1959) *Thai children under four.* Scheltema and Holkema, Amsterdam

STANDER H.J. and CADDEN J.F. (1932) The cardiac output in pregnant women. *Amer. J. Obstet. Gynec.* **24**, 13

STANDER H.J. and PASTORE J.B. (1940) Weight changes during pregnancy and puerperium. *Amer. J. Obstet. Gynec.* **39**, 928

STARKE J.S., SMITH J.B. and JOUBERT D.M. (1958) *The birth weight of lambs.* Union of South Africa, Dept. of Agriculture, Science Bull. No. 382

STARLING E.H. (1919) *Report on Food Conditions in Germany.* Cmd. 280. (State Papers 1919, liii). H.M.S.O., London

STATISTICAL BULLETIN OF THE METROPOLITAN LIFE INSURANCE CO. (1960) Chances of having a plural birth. **41**, Jan. 9

STEINBECK A.W. and THEILE H. (1962) Urinary steroids during pregnancy. *Acta endocr. (Kbh.)* **40**, 123

STENGLE J.M. and SCHADE A.L. (1957) Diurnal-nocturnal variations of certain blood constituents in normal human subjects: plasma iron, siderophilin, bilirubin, copper, total serum protein and albumin, haemoglobin and haematocrit. *Brit. J. Haemat.* **3**, 117

STERNBERG J. (1962) Placental transfers: modern methods of study. *Amer. J. Obstet. Gynec.* **84**, 1731

STEWART H.L. (1952) Duration of pregnancy and postmaturity. *J. Amer. med. Ass.* **148**, 1079

STIEVE H. (1932) Über die Neubildung von Muskelzellen in der Wand der schwangeren menschlichen Gebärmutter. [New formation of muscle cells in the wall of the pregnant human uterus]. *Zbl. Gynäk.* **56**, 1442

STOFFER R.P., KOENEKE I.A., CHESKY V.E. and HELLWIG C.A. (1957) The thyroid in pregnancy. *Amer. J. Obstet. Gynec.* **74**, 300

STONE M.L., PILIERO S.J., HAMMER H. and PORTNOY A. (1960) Epinephrine and norepinephrine in pregnancy. *Obstet. and Gynec.* **16**, 674

STREETER G.L. (1920) Weight, sitting height, head size, foot length and menstrual age of the human embryo. Contributions to Embryology, Vol. 11, No. 55. Carnegie Institution of Washington, Publication No. 274, Washington

STRUMIA M.M., COLWELL L.S. and DUGAN A. (1958) The measurement of erythropoesis in anaemias. I. The mixing time and the immediate post-transfusion disappearance of T-1824 dye and of Cr^{51}-tagged erythrocytes in relation to blood volume determination. *Blood.* **8**, 128

STURGEON P. (1959) Studies of iron requirements of infants. III. Influence of supplemental iron during normal pregnancy on mother and infant. *Brit. J. Haemat.* **5**, 31

SZENDI B. (1934) Über Menge, Verteilung und Bedeutung des Placenta-Glykogens in den verschiedenen Phasen der Schwangerschaft. [Amount, distribution and significance of placental glycogen in the several phases of pregnancy]. *Arch. Gynäk.* **158**, 409

TAGGART N. (1961a) Food habits in pregnancy. *Proc. Nutr. Soc.* **20**, 35

TAGGART N. (1961b) Skinfold measurements during human pregnancy. *Proc. Nutr. Soc.* **20**, xxx

TAIT L. (1875) Enlargement of the thyroid body in pregnancy. *Edinb. med. J.* **20**, 993

TAKAHASHI E. (1954) The effects of the age of the mother on the sex ratio at birth in Japan. *Ann. N.Y. Acad. Sci.* **57**, 531

TAYLOR H.L., ERICKSON L., HENSCHEL A. and KEYS A. (1945) The effect of bed rest on the blood volume of normal young men. *Amer. J. Physiol.* **144**, 227

THEOBALD G.W. and VERNEY E.B. (1935) Mechanical factors which affect the secretion of urine in mammals and their operation during pregnancy. *Quart. J. exp. Physiol.* **25**, 341

THOMPSON R.B. (1957) Seasonal incidence of megaloblastic anaemia of pregnancy and the puerperium. *Lancet* ii, 1171

THOMSON A.M. (1951) Human foetal growth. *Brit. J. Nutr.* **5**, 158

THOMSON A.M. (1958) Diet in pregnancy. 1. Dietary survey technique and the nutritive value of diets taken by primigravidae. *Brit. J. Nutr.* **12**, 446

THOMSON A.M. (1959a) Diet in pregnancy. 2. Assessment of the nutritive value of diets, especially in relation to differences between social classes. *Brit. J. Nutr.* **13**, 190

THOMSON A.M. (1959b) Diet in pregnancy. 3. Diet in relation to the course and outcome of pregnancy. *Brit. J. Nutr.* **13**, 509

THOMSON A.M. (1959c) Maternal stature and reproductive efficiency. *Eugen. Rev.* **51**, 3

THOMSON A.M. and BILLEWICZ W.Z. (1957) Clinical significance of weight trends during pregnancy. *Brit. med. J.* i, 243

440 THE PHYSIOLOGY OF HUMAN PREGNANCY

THOMSON A.M. and BILLEWICZ W.Z. (1961) Height, weight and food intake in man. *Brit. J. Nutr.* **15**, 241

THOMSON A.M. and BILLEWICZ W.Z. (1963) Nutritional status, maternal physique and reproductive efficiency. *Proc. Nutr. Soc.* **22**, 55

THOMSON A.M., CHUN D. and BAIRD D. (1963) Perinatal mortality in Hong Kong and Aberdeen, Scotland. *J. Obstet. Gynaec. Brit. Commonw.* **70**, 871

THOMSON A.M. and THOMSON W. (1949) Lambing in relation to the diet of the pregnant ewe. *Brit. J. Nutr.* **2**, 290

THOMSON K.J. and COHEN M.E. (1938) Studies on the circulation in pregnancy. II. Vital capacity observations in normal pregnant women. *Surg. Gynec. Obstet.* **66**, 591

THOMSON K.J., HIRSHEIMER A., GIBSON J.G. 2nd and EVANS W.A. Jr. (1938) Studies on the circulation in pregnancy. III. Blood volume changes in normal pregnant women. *Amer. J. Obstet. Gynec.* **36**, 48

THONNARD-NEUMANN E. (1961) The influence of hormones on the basophilic leukocytes. *Acta haemat. (Basel)* **25**, 261

TOMPKINS W.T. and WIEHL D.G. (1951) Nutritional deficiencies as a causal factor in toxemia and premature labor. *Amer. J. Obstet. Gynec.* **62**, 898

TOMPKINS W.T., WIEHL D.G. and MITCHELL R.M. (1955) The underweight patient as an increased obstetric hazard. *Amer. J. Obstet. Gynec.* **69**, 114

TOVEY J.E. (1959) The significance of electrophoretic serum protein changes in pregnancy. *J. Obstet. Gynaec. Brit. Emp.* **66**, 981

TRICOMI V., SERR D. and SOLISH G. (1960) The ratio of male to female embryos as determined by the sex chromatin. *Amer. J. Obstet. Gynec.* **79**, 504

TRILLAT P. (1928) Des variations de poids chez la femme enceinte. [Changes in weight in pregnant women]. *Progr. méd. (Paris)* **49**, 2029

TROEN P. (1961a) Perfusion studies of the human placenta. II. Metabolism of C-14 17β-estradiol with and without added human chorionic gonadotropin. *J. clin. Endocr.* **21**, 895

TROEN P. (1961b) Perfusion studies of the human placenta. III. Production of free and conjugated Porter-Silber chromogens. *J. clin. Endocr.* **21**, 1511

TROEN P. and GORDON E.E. (1958) Perfusion studies of the human placenta. I. Effect of estradiol and human chorionic gonadotropin on citric acid metabolism. *J. clin. Invest.* **37**, 1516

TROLLE D. (1955) Experimental and clinical investigations on the pregnanediol excretion in human urine. *Acta endocr. (Kbh.)* **19**, 217

TULSKY A.S. and KOFF A.K. (1957) Some observations on the role of the corpus luteum in early human pregnancy. *Fertil. and Steril.* **8**, 118

TURNBULL E.P.N. and BAIRD D. (1957) Maternal age and foetal oxygenation. *Brit. med. J.* **ii**, 1021

TURNER A.H., NEWTON M.I. and HAYNES F.W. (1930) The circulatory reaction to gravity in healthy young women. Evidence regarding its precision and its instability. *Amer. J. Physiol.* **94**, 507

TUTTLE S.G., RUFIN F. and BETTARELLO A. (1961) The physiology of heartburn. *Ann. intern. Med.* **55**, 292

TYLER J.M. (1960) The effect of progesterone on the respiration of patients with emphysema and hypercapnia. *J. clin. Invest.* **39**, 34

Tysoe F.W. and Lowenstein L. (1950) Blood volume and hematologic studies in pregnancy and the puerperium. *Amer. J. Obstet. Gynec.* **60**, 1187

Uhr J.W., Dancis J., Franklin E.C., Finkelstein M.S. and Lewis E.W. (1962) The antibody response to bacteriophage QX174 in newborn premature infants. *J. clin. Invest.* **41**, 1509

Umland K. (1948) Beitrag zur Frage des Einflusses der mütterlichen Ernährung auf Gewicht, Grösse und Tragezeit der Neugeborenen. [Contribution to the question of the effect of maternal diet on weight, length and time carried of the newborn]. *Zbl. Gynak.* **70**, 465

U.S. Department of Health, Education and Welfare (1962) *Vital Statistics of the United States* 1960. Vol. 1, Section 2. U.S. Government Printing Office, Washington

Uttley K.H. (1940) The birth weight of full term Cantonese babies. *Chin. med. J.* **58**, 582

Valiente S. and Muñoz M. (1962) Valor nutritivo de la dieta de 800 embarazadas chilenas y su relación can el peso y la talla de los ninos. [Nutritive value of the diet of 800 pregnant Chilean women and its relation to the weight and length of the infants]. *Nutrición, Bromatol. Toxicol.* **1**, 63

Vallance-Owen J. and Lilley M.D. (1961) Insulin antagonism in the plasma of obese diabetics and prediabetics. *Lancet* **1**, 806

Van der Rijst M.P.J. (rapporteur) (1962) Onderzoek naar de voeding van zwangere vrouwen en de gezondheidstoestand van moeders en kinderen te Amsterdam in de jaren 1950 en 1951, verricht in opdracht van de Gemeentelijke Geneeskundige en Gezondheidsdienst. [Study of the diet of pregnant women and the health of mothers and infants in Amsterdam in the years 1950 and 1951, made on request of the city medical and health service]. *Voeding* **23**, 695

Van de Wiele R.L., Gurpide E., Kelly W.G., Laragh H.J. and Lieberman S. (1960) The secretory rate of progesterone and aldosterone in normal and abnormal pregnancy. *Acta endocr. (Kbh.)* Suppl. 51, 159

van Rood J.J., van Leeuwen A. and Eernisse J.G. (1959) Leucocyte antibodies in sera of pregnant women. *Vox. Sang. (Basel)* **4**, 427

Van Slyke D.D. (1959) in *Oxygen supply to the human foetus.* Eds. J. Walker and A. C. Turnbull. Blackwell Scientific Publications, Oxford

Vasicka A., Quilligan E.J., Aznar R., Lipsitz P.J. and Bloor B.M. (1960) Oxygen tension in maternal and fetal blood, amniotic fluid, and cerebrospinal fluid of the mother and the baby. *Amer. J. Obstet. Gynec.* **79**, 1041

Veal J.R. and Hussey H.H. (1941) The venous circulation in the lower extremities during pregnancy. *Surg. Gynec. Obstet.* **72**, 841

Velardo J.T. (1960) Pacemaker action of the ovarian hormones in reproductive processes: II. The estrogens and progesterones during pregnancy. *Fertil. and Steril.* **11**, 343

Venkatachalam P.S. (1962a) Maternal nutritional status and its effect on the newborn. *Bull. Wld. Hlth. Org.* **26**, 193

Venkatachalam P.S. (1962b) A study of the diet, nutrition and health of the people of the Chimbu area (New Guinea highlands). Territory of Papua and New Guinea, Dept. Publ. Hlth. Monograph No. 4

Venkatachalam P.S., Shankar K. and Gopalan C. (1960) Changes in body weight and body composition during pregnancy. *Indian J. med. Res.* **48**, 511

VENNING E.H., SYBULSKI S., POLLAK V.E. and RYAN R.J. (1959) Aldosterone excretion in two adrenalectomized pregnant women. *J. clin. Endocr.* **19**, 1486

VENTURA S. and KLOPPER A. (1951a) Iron metabolism in pregnancy: the behaviour of haemoglobin, serum iron, the iron-binding capacity of serum proteins, serum copper and free erythrocyte protoporphyrin in normal pregnancy. *J. Obstet. Gynec. Brit. Emp.* **58**, 173

VENTURA S. and KLOPPER A. (1951b) Iron metabolism in pregnancy. 2. The behaviour of serum iron in pregnancy after the administration of iron compounds by mouth and intravenously. *S. Afr. med. J.* **25**, 969

VEREL D., BURY J.D. and HOPE A. (1956) Blood volume changes in pregnancy and the puerperium. *Clin. Sci.* **15**, 1

VERLOOP M.C., BLOKHUIS E.W.M. and BOS C.C. (1959a) Causes of the difference in haemoglobin and serum-iron between men and women. *Acta Haematol. (Basel)* **21**, 199

VERLOOP M.C., BLOKHUIS E.W.M. and BOS C.C. (1959b) Cause of the 'physiological' anaemia of pregnancy. *Acta haemat. (Basel)* **22**, 158

VILLEE C.A. (1953) The metabolism of human placenta in vitro. *J. biol. Chem.* **205**, 113

VON STUDNITZ W. (1955) Studies on serum lipids and lipoproteins in pregnancy. *Scand. J. clin. Lab. Invest.* **7**, 329

VORYS N., ULLERY J.C. and HANUSEK G.E. (1961) The cardiac output changes in various positions in pregnancy. *Amer. J. Obstet. Gynec.* **82**, 1312

WAGNER G. and FUCHS F. (1962) The volume of amniotic fluid in the first half of human pregnancy. *J. Obstet. Gynaec. Brit. Commonw.* **69**, 131

WALKER J. (1954a) Foetal anoxia. *J. Obstet. Gynaec. Brit. Emp.* **61**, 162

WALKER J. (1954b) in *Cold Spring Harbor Symposia on Quantitative Biology Vol. XIX. The Mammalian Foetus: Physiological Aspects of Development.* The Biological Laboratory, Cold Spring Harbor, L.I., New York

WALKER J. and TURNBULL E.P.N. (1953) Haemoglobin and red cells in the human foetus. *Lancet* **2**, 312

WALLER H. (1939) *Clinical Studies in Lactation.* William Heinemann Ltd., London

WALLER H. (1946) The early failure of breast feeding. A clinical study of its causes and their prevention. *Arch. Dis. Childh.* **21**, 1

WALLRAFF E.B., BRODIE E.C. and BORDEN A.L. (1950) Urinary excretion of amino-acids in pregnancy. *J. clin. Invest.* **29**, 1542

WALSH R.J., ARNOLD B.J., LANCASTER H.O., COOTE M.A. and COTTER H. (1953) *A study of haemoglobin values in New South Wales, with observations on haematocrit and sedimentation rate values.* National Health and Medical Research Council Special Report Series No. 5. Australasian Med. Pub. Co. Sydney

WALTON A. and HAMMOND J. (1938) The maternal effects on growth and conformation in Shire horse—Shetland pony crosses. *Proc. roy. Soc. B* **125**, 311

WASSERMAN L.R., RASHKOFF I.A., LEAVITT D., MAYER J. and PORT S. (1952)

The rate of removal of radioactive iron from the plasma—an index of erythropoiesis. *J. clin. Invest.* **31**, 32

WATERFIELD R.L. (1931) The effects of posture on the circulating blood volume. *J. Physiol.* **72**, 110

WATERHOUSE J.A.H. and HOGBEN L. (1947) Incompatability of mother and foetus with respect to iso-agglutinogen A and its antibody. *Brit. J. soc. Med.* **1**, 1

WATERS E.G. (1942) Weight studies in pregnancy. *Amer. J. Obstet. Gynec.* **43**, 826

WATSON W.C. (1957) Serum lipids in pregnancy and the puerperium. *Clin. Sci.* **16**, 475

WEINBERG W. (1909) Die Anlage zur Mehrlingsgeburt bein Menschen und ihre Vererbung. [The anlage for multiple births in man and its inheritance]. *Arch. Rassen-u. Gesellschaftsbiol.* **6**, 322

WELSH C.A., WELLEN I. and TAYLOR H.C. (1942) The filtration rate, effective renal blood flow, tubular excretory mass and phenol red clearance in normal pregnancy. *J. clin. Invest.* **21**, 57

WERKÖ L., BUCHT H., LAGERLÖF H. and HOLMGREN A. (1948) Cirkulationen vid graviditet. [The circulation in pregnancy]. *Nord. Med.* **40**, 1868

WERKÖ L., LAGERLÖF H., BUCHT H., WEHLE B. and HOLMGREN A. (1949) Comparison of Fick and Hamilton methods for determinations of cardiac output in man. *Scand. J. clin. Lab. Invest.* **1**, 109

WHITBY L.E.H. and BRITTON C.J.C. (1957) *Disorders of the Blood.* 8th Edition. J. and A. Churchill, London

WHITE R. (1950) Blood volume in pregnancy. *Edinb. med. J.* 57, Trans 14

WIDDAS W.F. (1961) Transport mechanisms in the foetus. *Brit. med. Bull.* **17**, 107

WIDDOWSON E.M. and McCANCE R.A. (1936) Iron in human nutrition. *J. Hyg. (London)* **36**, 13

WIDDOWSON E.M. and SPRAY C.M. (1951) Chemical development *in utero*. *Arch. Dis. Childh.* **26**, 205

WIDE L. (1962) An immunological method for the assay of human chorionic gonadotrophin. *Acta endocr. (Kbh.)* **41**, Suppl. 70

WIDLUND G. (1945) The cardio-pulmonal function during pregnancy. *Acta obstet. gynec. scand.* **25**, Suppl. 1

WILKIN P. (1957) Étude des factures physiques conditionnant la perméabilité placentaire. [Study of the physical factors that determine permeability of the placenta]. *Bull. Féd. Gynéc. Obstét. franç.* **9**, 33

WILLIAMS P.F. and FRALIN F.G. (1942) Nutrition study in pregnancy. Dietary analyses of seven-day food intake records of 514 pregnant women, comparison of actual food intakes with variously stated requirements, and relationship of food intake to various obstetric factors. *Amer. J. Obstet. Gynec.* **43**, 1

WILLS L., HILL G., BINGHAM K., MIALL M. and WRIGLEY J. (1947) Haemoglobin levels in pregnancy. The effect of the rationing scheme and routine administration of iron. *Brit. J. Nutr.* **1**, 126

WILSON K.M. (1916) Nitrogen metabolism during pregnancy. *Bull. Johns Hopk. Hosp.* **27**, 121

WOKES F., BADENOCH J. and SINCLAIR H.M. (1955) Human dietary deficiency of vitamin B_{12}. *Amer. J. clin. Nutr.* **3**, 375

WOLF S. (1943) The relation of gastric function to nausea in man. *J. clin. Invest.* **22**, 877

WOODBURY R.A., AHLQUIST R.D., ABREV B., TORPIN R. and WATSON W.G. (1946) The inactivation of pitocin and pitressin by human pregnancy blood. *J. Pharmacol. exp. Ther.* **86**, 359

WOODHILL J.M., VAN DEN BERG A.S., BURKE B.S. and STARE F.J. (1955) Nutrition studies of pregnant Australian women. *Amer. J. Obstet. Gynec.* **70**, 987

WOODRUFF M.F.A. (1957) Transplantation immunity and the immunological problem of pregnancy. *Proc. roy. Soc.* B **148**, 68

WRIGHT H.P., OSBORN S.B. and EDMONDS D.G. (1950) Changes in the rate of flow of venous blood in the leg during pregnancy, measured with radioactive sodium. *Surg. Gynec. Obstet.* **90**, 481

WYERS P.J.H. and VAN MUNSTER P.J.J. (1961) The disappearance of Evans blue dye from the blood in normal and nephrotic subjects. *J. Lab. clin. Med.* **58**, 375

YAMAZAKI E., NOGUCHI A. and SLINGERLAND D.W. (1961) Thyrotropin in the serum of mother and fetus. *J. clin. Endocr.* **21**, 1013

YANAGI K., HAYAMI H., SUZUKI S. and NAGAMINE S. (1951) Studies on dietary allowances for Japanese. I. Allowances of calories and protein for various ages, sexes, activities, pregnancy and lactation. *Ann. Rept. Nat. Inst. Nutrition 1949-50.* Nat. Inst. Nutrition, Toyamacho, Tokyo

YOSHIMURA H. (1958) Seasonal changes in human body fluids. *Jap. J. Physiol.* **8**, 165

ZABRISKIE J.R. (1963) Effect of cigarette smoking during pregnancy. *Obstet. and Gynec.* **21**, 405

ZACHARIAE F. (1959) *Acid mucopolysaccharides in the female genital system and their rôle in the mechanism of ovulation.* Periodica, Copenhagen

ZANDER J. (1959) Gestagens in human pregnancy. *Recent Progress in Hormone Research.* Ed. G. Pincus. Academic Press, New York

ZANGEMEISTER W. (1911) Die Altersbestimmung des Fötus nach graphischer Methode. [Estimation of the age of the foetus by a graphic method]. *Z. Geburtsh. Gynäk.* **69**, 127

ZANGEMEISTER W. (1916) Ueber das Körpergewicht Schwangerer, nebst Bemerkungen über den Hydrops gravidarum. [Body weight of pregnant women, with remarks on hydrops gravidarum]. *Z. Geburtsh. Gynäk.* **78**, 325

ZARROW M.X., HOLSTROM E.G. and SALHANICK H.A. (1955) The concentration of relaxin in the blood serum and other tissues of women during pregnancy. *J. clin. Endocr.* **15**, 22

ZARROW M.X. and YOCHIM J. (1961) Dilation of the uterine cervix of the rat and accompanying changes during the estrous cycle, pregnancy and following treatment with estradiol, progesterone and relaxin. *Endocrinology* **69**, 292

ZATUCHNI J. (1951) The electrocardiogram in pregnancy and the puerperium. *Amer. Heart J.* **42**, 11

ZILLIACUS H., WIDHOLM O. and PESONEN S. (1954) The concentration of chorionic gonadotrophin in the urine and in the placenta of Rh negative immunized mothers. *Acta endocr. (Kbh.)* **16**, 343

ZIMMERMAN H.A. (1950) A preliminary report on intracardiac catheterization studies during pregnancy. *J. Lab. clin. Med.* **36**, 1007

ZIPF R.E., WEBBER J.M. and GROVE G.R. (1955) A comparison of routine plasma volume determination methods using radioiodinated human serum albumin and Evans blue dye (T–1824). *J. Lab. clin. Med.* **45**, 800

ZUCKERMAN S., VAN WAGENEN G. and GARDINER R.H. (1938) The sexual skin of the rhesus monkey. *Proc. zool. Soc. Lond.* A. **108**, 385

Index